Atypical Language Development in Romance Languages

Atypical Language Development in Romance Languages

Edited by

Eva Aguilar-Mediavilla
Lucía Buil-Legaz
Raúl López-Penadés
Victor A. Sanchez-Azanza
Daniel Adrover-Roig
University of Balearic Islands

John Benjamins Publishing Company
Amsterdam / Philadelphia

The paper used in this publication meets the minimum requirements of the American National Standard for Information Sciences – Permanence of Paper for Printed Library Materials, ANSI z39.48-1984.

DOI 10.1075/z.223

Cataloging-in-Publication Data available from Library of Congress:
LCCN 2019005526 (PRINT) / 2019015426 (E-BOOK)

ISBN 978 90 272 0321 2 (HB)
ISBN 978 90 272 6249 3 (E-BOOK)

John Benjamins Publishing Company · https://benjamins.com

Table of contents

Introduction to atypical language development in romance languages

Eva Aguilar-Mediavilla, Lucía Buil-Legaz, Raúl López-Penadés, Victor A. Sanchez-Azanza and Daniel Adrover-Roig
University of Balearic Islands

This chapter presents a state of the art in atypical language development in Romance languages and introduces, as well, the chapters in this book. The first part describes the aim of the book. The second part describes typical language acquisition in Romance language and their main differences with English. Finally, the third section focuses on four clinical conditions that show atypical language development: prematurity, Specific Language Impairment, hearing loss, and genetic syndromes.

Keywords: atypical language development, Romance languages, prematurity, Specific Language Impairment, hearing loss, genetic syndromes

Introduction

Most of the research on child language development in the last century has been conducted in English (Berman, 2014). However, in the eighties of the last century, the need for cross-linguistic studies in language acquisition was revealed (Bavin, 1995; Berman & Slobin, 1994; Lieven, 1994). Thus, during the last forty decades, languages' acquisition studies in languages different from English have grown vastly (Berman, 2014; Guo et al., 2009). Romance language acquisition studies have also bloomed, especially with the constitution of the *Asociación para el estudio de la adquisición del lenguaje* (AEAL; Association for the study of language acquisition) driven by their congresses (*I Encuentro sobre la adquisición de las lenguas del estado* in 1995) and publications (Aguilar-Mediavilla, Adrover-Roig, Buil-Legaz, & López-Penadés, 2016; Diez-itza, 2007; Mayor-Cinca, Zubiauz de de Pedro, & Díez, 2005; Pérez-Pereira, 1996). Studies of language acquisition in other languages and cross-linguistic studies have shown that some results about language development in English may not be transferred into other languages (Bates,

https://doi.org/10.1075/z.223.01agu

Devescovi, & Wulfeck, 2001; Berman, 2014; Lieven, 2010). Despite the increase in the number of studies, there is still little research about atypical language development in other languages, especially in Romance languages. Some previous research can be found in cross-linguistic studies of Leonard (2015) regarding children with Specific Language Impairment. However, less is known with respect to other clinical populations that also show atypical language development. Therefore, this book aims to fill the current void in these studies, give them visibility and show the last research in atypical language development in Romance languages.

Typical language acquisition in Romance languages

One of the most important differences between English and Romance languages is that Romance languages are characterized for having a very extensive morphology. Languages with rich morphology are called fusion languages, and other language families form part of these types of languages, such as Baltic languages (e.g., Russian). Romance languages mark two genders and two numbers for nominal morphology; and have categories of person, number, time and grammatical mode – generally varying the inflectional form according to verb conjugation – for verbal morphology. Besides, there must be concordances of gender and number between the noun and the adjective, and between the number of the subject and the number expressed in the verb. Although the basic order is Subject-Verb-Object (SVO), most times the subject is omitted contrary to English where the subject is obligatory. In addition, nouns use to be preceded by a determiner, except in Rumanian. Considering the phonological form of these languages, most times morphological marks in Romance languages are new syllables added at the end of the word, even sometimes these are heavy syllables – for example, compra (he buy)-compra*rán* (they buy) –, therefore these marks are very salient. Contrary to this, most morphological marks in English are non-syllabic consonants (which do not form a new syllable) that are added to a final unstressed syllable with a very short duration (e.g. play-*ed*; play-*s*); and grammatical words are usually unstressed syllables or contractions (e.g., *the* cat; *it's* funny).

Results of early cross-linguistic studies of typical language acquisition in Romance languages contrasted with the implicit idea that assumed that morphological acquisitions were slower than those in English due to their complex morphology (Serra-Raventós, Serrat Sellabona, Solé Planas, Bel Leal, & Aparici Aznar, 2000). These early comparative studies showed that children acquiring Romance languages were faster using some morphological forms (e.g. using the past, Mueller Gathercole, Sebastián, & Soto, 1999) than English children, and even used longer utterances (Devescovi et al., 2003).

Following a usage-based approach (constructivist point of view of language acquisition), this early appearing of morphological forms in children speaking Romance languages does not mean that children have acquired completely this morphological forms (Tomasello, 2003). It only reflects the fact that the morphological marks are more phonologically salient and more frequent in the input that children listen, that is to say, an interaction between input (language form) and use by the children. This makes more probable that children learning Romance languages use them earlier than those learning English. Nevertheless, these early appearances are not true acquisitions, but crystalized forms or semi-learned forms, that only later will form part of a productive system (Tomasello, 2003).

López-Ornat (1998) proposed four phases to explain typical morphological development in Romance languages. At phase 1, the child uses amalgams and unanalysed units only; these can include non-inflected verb forms, such as infinitive and imperative, but also some other crystalized forms can appear. At Phase 2, called "defective rule/prerule" phase, "grammaticalization" begins, and the child begins to contrast impersonal/non-finite forms (infinitives, imperatives) with personal/finite forms (mostly, first and third person singular forms). In phase 3, the child applies "rigid rules" in which over-regularizations occur; and finally, in phase 4, "flexible rules" are present, in which the child makes no errors of any kind.

This interpretation of language development could be framed into a more general point of view on cognitive development, the neuroconstructivist approach (Karmiloff-Smith, 1992). Neuroconstructivism proposes that language modularity arises from the ontogenetic development and it is the brain that sculpts their form from their function, that is to say, brain specialization is a result of cognitive development through the use. Therefore, in this theory, genes interact with the ambient, with usage as a key factor, to explain language development. Hence, this book adheres to this theoretical framework of language development: neuroconstructivism and based-usage approach that could be considered inside a cognitive-functional paradigm of language development.

Atypical language development

Preterm children

The first part of the present book explores the linguistic and communicative characteristics of preterm children learning Romance languages. The World Health Organization defines preterm birth by gestational age, with extremely preterm <28 weeks of gestation, very preterm 28–32 weeks, and moderate to late preterm 32–37 weeks of gestation. Prematurity is a major global health problem, being the leading cause of death in children under five years of age worldwide (Liu et al., 2016). Preterm children are not a homogeneous group, and to date, there is not a consistent profile of their linguistic and cognitive capacities, particularly in the moderate and late preterm categories. The variety of profiles is dependent on the high heterogeneity of variables that can modulate individual differences in language delay, executive functioning, and language comprehension. Such variables include gestational age, birth weight, the presence of brain lesion, perinatal difficulties, low socioeconomic status, male gender, and the lack of breast feeding (Spittle, Orton, Anderson, Boyd, & Doyle, 2015). Impairments in cognitive function are often difficult to detect because some premature children without signs of neurodevelopmental difficulties in early childhood could manifest school problems, which might persist even during adulthood (Serenius et al., 2016). Thus, this section aims at providing a clearer picture of the variety of profiles in preterm children learning Romance languages, which might be of great help to establish adequate prevention and intervention programs that will redound in a better quality of life.

Chapter 1 (Guarini, & Sansavini) provides a neuroconstructivist framework that allows understanding the heterogeneity of profiles and the bulk of developmental trajectories and individual differences found in language and literacy in preterm children, most of them learning Romance languages, such as Italian. It is worth mentioning that by 36 months, gestational age at birth has less impact on cognition and receptive language than chronological age; however, expressive language is still a function of the degree of prematurity, indicating that prematurity differentially affects various aspects of language development (Ionio et al., 2016). Thus, this chapter emphasizes the importance of considering a multiplicity of interrelated factors, such as gestational age, neonatal maturity as well as social and relational variables when assessing premature children. In particular, the neuroconstructivist approach can help to better understand the difficulties in the development of language production, for which the contingent and symmetric interaction are very relevant. Since both the interpretation of facial expressions and body language are impaired in preterm children (Williamson & Jakobson, 2014), dyadic interactions might be of lower quality. It is also important to consider that parental education, fine motor skills, and object exploration are crucial for the development of the preterm child. Understanding that preterm children are not a homogeneous group is particularly relevant because their trajectory of language delay tends to worsen with age and continues until adolescence, or even longer, in contrast to full-term children. Among other linguistic domains, literacy is affected at the beginning of primary school, and very preterm children appear to be particularly vulnerable to spelling deficits. Therefore, it is of key importance to monitor developmental trajectories in these infants and to encourage effective early intervention programmes with a special interest in positive body experiences, early exposure to language and maternal voice (Webb, Heller, Benson, & Lahav, 2015), together with adequate environmental stimuli and contingent social relations, especially when prematurity is severe. Language delays in children are often related to speed processing deficits and a selective damage to executive control (EC). For instance, preterm children with low gestational age and low birth weight are at risk of having reduced volume in brain regions dedicated to EC, and EC deficits are proportional to the degree of prematurity (Aarnoudse-Moens, Weisglas-Kuperus, van Goudoever, & Oosterlaan, 2009).

In a similar vein, Chapter 2 (Pérez-Pereira, Peralbo & Veleiro) aims at establishing a relationship between the development of EC, language, general cognition and other environmental factors in a sample of healthy late preterm and full-term children between 4 and 5 years of age learning Galician and/or Spanish. The authors stress the importance of measuring general cognitive abilities and underline the notion that preterm children are a heterogeneous group, as explained in Chapter 1. Their results seem to contrast other works conducted with extremely or very preterm children (see Taylor & Clark, 2016) showing that healthy late preterm children learning Galician do not experience difficulties in vocabulary and grammar comprehension, morphosyntactic production, verbal memory, non-verbal working memory or inhibition. This chapter reports that general cognitive abilities strongly determine vocabulary comprehension in healthy preterm children, while rule governed-grammar and understanding depend on non-verbal working memory component of EC. In fact, recent investigations show that EC at the beginning of schooling fully accounted for the lower academic achievement at age 9 in preterm children (Clark & Woodward, 2015), and even EC tests but not IQ measures are predictors of the propensity to behaviour problems in extremely preterm children (Scott et al., 2012).

Thus, several dimensions of language development in preterm children are influenced by a wide array of cognitive factors. In this sense, Chapter 3 (Resches, Pérez Pereira, Cruz Guerrero, & Fernández Prieto) provides a temporal perspective on this mutual influence over time, and highlights the importance of cognitive development, maternal education, and early expressive vocabulary as the most important factors to predict receptive language development (RLD) in preterm children learning Galician and/or Spanish. Although the pattern of results is not always consistent in the field of language and prematurity (van Noort-van der Spek, Franken, & Weisglas-Kuperus, 2012), findings on grammar, lexicon and semantics yield a robust pattern of results (Sansavini, Guarini, & Caselli, 2011). This chapter explores the risk of language delay in healthy preterm and full-term children with a longitudinal study that included small children learning Galician ranging from 10 to 60 months of age. Results of this work show that at early ages

(22–30 months) the prevalence of RLD between preterm and full-term children is equivalent. However, at age five, a receptive grammar delay is more frequently observed in preterm children, a result that stresses the high instability in the prevalence of RLD throughout time.

Finally, Chapter 4 (Bosch, Teixidó & Agut) explores receptive language acquisition in nine-month-old full-term and moderately preterm infants learning Catalan and/or Spanish. Early capacities for receptive language are affected by prematurity, such as the lack of perceptual narrowing for non-native phonemes, which is linked to the appearance of linguistic problems at two years of age (Jansson-Verkasalo et al., 2010). Also, premature children experience difficulties when segmenting words, even when results are corrected by age (Bosch, 2011). This chapter explores word segmentation and word mapping in preterm children while recording their gaze during an audio-visual dual task. The analysis of fixation times suggests that full-term infants can learn novel words by segmenting them from fluent speech and mapping these word-forms to possible referents. However, it seems that this ability is not yet mature for preterm infants, probably due to the high demands of the task. The authors discuss the potential consequences of these results on the low speed at which novel words are gradually incorporated in moderately preterm infants, which is not attributable to cognitive deficits. Intervention in preterm children is effective (Koldewijn et al., 2010) and thus, difficulties can be compensated. The authors suggest that intervention can benefit from reducing the demands of speech segmentation, especially in controlled contexts that allow the enhancement of the word learning processes.

Specific Language Impairment

The second part of this book is centred in children with Specific Language Impairment (SLI). SLI is a disorder that affects between 5 and 7% of the population and limits comprehension and/or production involving difficulties in one, several or all language components, especially morphosyntax in the absence of cognitive, motor or sensory deficits (Leonard, 2014a). The factors that are normally associated with language problems, such as hearing or neurological damage, or low non-verbal IQ, are not affected (American Psychiatric Association (APA), 2013; Bishop, 2004; Leonard, 2015; Schwartz, 2009).

One aspect that is often related as a warning sign of the appearance of language difficulties in children, which can later lead to a diagnosis of SLI, is not receiving enough stimulation in early developmental stages, especially when children are in a sensitive period of language acquisition. In this sense, the role of the family in the development of the posterior language must be considered. Cross-linguistic studies on SLI have shown differences in the type of errors among children with SLI speaking different languages, emphasizing the importance of studies in different languages and not only in English (Leonard, 2014b, 2015).

The first chapter of this second part of the book, (Chapter 5, Auza-Benavides, Peñaloza, & Murata) explores whether the level of maternal education (ME) can influence the later development of the language. It has been observed that the socioeconomic level of the family is a relevant factor in the development of children (Conger & Conger, 2002; Repetti, Taylor, & Seeman, 2002) and that a low socioeconomic level can cause greater probability of suffering from cognitive problems, including language difficulties (Ackerman, Brown, & Izard, 2004; Dearing, McCartney, & Taylor, 2002). Previous studies showed that mothers with higher education were more sensitive to the need of their children to be cognitively stimulated (Bradley & Corwyn, 2005; Raviv, Kessenich, & Morrison, 2004; Tamis-LeMonda, Shannon, Cabrera, & Lamb, 2004). However, ME level represents family vulnerability and seems to be an adequate alert of child development signal, but it is not usually a variable studied since SLI excludes any socio-environmental remarks (Bishop, 2014). Therefore, authors consider relevant to know if the ME is a factor that influences the lexical and grammatical measures obtained from narratives samples and whether it influences the diagnosis of SLI in a Spanish monolingual sample. Results suggested that the relationship between ME and any linguistic phenomenon is modulated by the interaction with other environmental factors since the low performance in language skills in terms of morphosyntax and lexical diversity are related not only to the presence of the SLI diagnosis but also to a precarious educational background. However, the level of ME does not affect directly the lexical diversity or morphosyntax. Thus, authors suggested that there is a high heterogeneity and dynamic interaction with environmental factors that may or may not influence the development of children's language difficulties (Conger & Donellan, 2002; Parise & Maillart, 2009; Petersen & Gardner, 2011). A recent study assessing grammaticality in monolingual Spanish-speaking children with SLI have shown that it is important to differentiate the procedures to elicit the morphosyntax, since this can affect children utterances and, therefore, their diagnosis (Jackson-Maldonado & Maldonado, 2017).

Morphosyntax seems to be always altered in children with SLI, however, there is a group within the disorder that have significant difficulties with pragmatics, which can sometimes lead to confusion. In this vein, Chapter 6 (Andrés-Roqueta & Clemente) explored the existence of deficits in the understanding of idioms in children with Language Impairment (LI) and the role of receptive and expressive language skills (grammar, vocabulary, and pragmatics) in this pragmatic ability to determine whether the lack of ability to understand idioms could be extended to SLI in general, or whether it is more related to children with SLI that have greater levels of pragmatic impairment (PLI). Results suggested the existence of a diminished understanding of idioms in both children with PLI and children with SLI as compared to children with typical language development (TD). Thus, PLI children were prone to incorrectly assign literal meanings to idioms irrespective of pragmatic demands (i.e., they failed to reach adequate figurative meanings to both verbally and visually presented idioms). Furthermore, PLI children showed diminished understanding of idioms, even as compared to SLI children, under high pragmatic demands (verbal presentation of idioms). Children with SLI also showed more literality than TD children but only under low pragmatic demands (visual presentation of idioms). Regarding the role of language skills, correlational analyses showed that receptive structural language skills (especially grammar) and pragmatic receptive skills are crucial for the understanding of idioms in children with LI.

One of the skills that often entail difficulty for children with language deficits is the narrative, due to its great complexity as it involves several language and communication abilities that are usually affected in children with language disorders. Thus, in order to explore this dimension of language, Chapter 7 (Balčiūnienė & Kornev) aims to analyse the narrative skills of children with language impairment in Russian, from a dynamic approach. Although the focus of the book is placed in the Romance languages, we decided to include this chapter since it is a not so studied language, but it is also a fusion language with a very rich morphology. In this chapter, authors examine data of storytelling and retelling according to a wordless picture sequences in a group of children with SLI, children with dyslexia and a group of TD. Narrative studies have shown that younger children or children with disorders have more difficulties (Duinmeijer, De Jong, & Scheper, 2012; Fey, Catts, Proctor-Williams, Tomblin, & Zhang, 2004; Fiestas, Bedore, Peña, & Nagy, 2005; Thorne, Coggins, Carmichael Olson, & Astley, 2007) due to limitations related to language competence, a deficit of cognitive resources and an influence of the communicative context and communication intention (Gonzalez, Cáceres, Bento-Gaz, & Befi-Lopes, 2012; Holm, Crosbie, & Dodd, 2007; Kapa, Plante, & Doubleday, 2017). Taking this into account, it could be expected that children in the SLI group showed greater difficulty when performing the task. Results revealed that children produced shorter and less complete utterances and structures, especially in the first session. The ratio of verbs produced is related to the total number of words, in the sense that the higher the number of verbs, the rarer they were. Considering the central role of the verb phrase in the description of events (Berman & Slobin, 1987), this skill might prevent children with SLI from creating productive but still lexically rich narratives.

In this vein, Chapter 8 (Andreu, Ahufinger, Ferinu, Pacheco, Colomé & Sanz Torrent) explores how do children with SLI process the verb information. This chapter analysed a more specific aspect of the morphosyntax comprehension, specifically the real-time comprehension. This task involves the rapid activation of conceptual and linguistic information, including verbs knowledge and the ability to anticipate sentence information (Andreu, Sanz-Torrent, & Trueswell, 2012). The aim of this work is to analyse how verb information is used during real-time comprehension of sentences in Spanish children with SLI. The results, shown through the study of eye movements using visual world paradigm, suggested that children with SLI showed ability to use verb-specific semantic information during spoken sentence comprehension to anticipate referents similarly to the other groups without disorder. The authors discuss these results suggesting that children with SLI present less atypical comprehension than would be expected due to their language competence.

Deaf children

Another relevant factor leading to atypical language development is hearing loss (HL), which is known to balk the acquisition of language in children. In this vein, since linguistic inputs are crucial in the formation of language, reduced audibility is related to a poorer productive and receptive language development (Stevenson, McCann, Watkin, Worsfold, & Kennedy, 2010). As a brief introduction, HL is mainly characterized as sensorineural, conductive or mixed. The sensorineural hearing loss is the most frequent form, and it is commonly produced by the deterioration of hair cells in the tonotopically-arranged cochlea. On the other hand, conductive HL involves the block or interference of the mechanical reception of sound in the outer or middle ear, producing inadequate transduction of aural information. While sensorineural HL usually impairs the correct hearing of high frequencies, conductive HL affects mainly low frequencies. In those cases in which sensorineural and conductive HL co-occur, the condition is identified as mixed. Moreover, there are also cases of central auditory dysfunction, a product of a damaged auditory cortex or the VIII cranial nerve. As a result, children with any of the previously depicted forms of HL have mild to severe problems understanding communicative interactions. In addition, HL might be caused by genetic or acquired factors. Regarding the genetic causes of HL, this condition is mainly inherited via an autosomal recessive (e.g., mutations in *GJB2*) or dominant (e.g., mutations in *WFS1*) trait (Kochhar, Hildebrand, & Smith, 2007). Among the acquired HL causes, a variety of factors may underlie the appearance of HL as a cause, such as a wide range of intrauterine (e.g., congenital cytomegalovirus) or postnatal infections, head injuries, or even impacted cerumen (Delgado Domínguez & Grupo PrevInfad/PAPPS Infancia y Adolescencia, 2011; Petersen, Jørgensen, & Ovesen, 2015).

Early studies performed on children with HL showed an association between several language-related difficulties and experiencing HL. For example, these children have been reported to have poor verbal skills, particularly in expressive vocabulary (Davis, Elfenbein, Schum, & Bentler, 1986), where the more severe the HL is, the less vocabulary they have (Kiese-Himmel, 2008). Moreover, these children, despite speaking with intelligibility, show deficits in articulation, morphology, and syntax, difficulties thought to be related to their altered aural input (Elfenbein, Hardin-Jones, & Davis, 1994). Fortunately, in the past three decades, a huge effort has been made to identify and start early interventions in the life of these children. Along with the universal hearing screening of newborns, the introduction of hearing devices seems to have positively impacted the development of language in children with HL, even though their social wellbeing remains affected (Sorkin, Gates-Ulanet, & Mellon, 2015). Note that there are differences between distinct hearing devices and technologies. In short, while hearing aids (HA) amplify environmental sound, cochlear implants (CI) transform sound into electronic stimulation through the auditory nerve. Children with HA do apparently benefit from their use, showing better speech and language development (Tomblin, Oleson, Ambrose, Walker, & Moeller, 2014). Regarding children with CI, it seems that these devices promote speech perception of language and communication (May-Mederake, 2012; Niparko et al., 2010), being this effect more robust in early implantation (Ruben, 2018). Still, when children using HA and CI are compared, the former benefit more than the latter from the hearing technologies in almost every language domain (Fitzpatrick et al., 2012). However, it has to be noted that, in general, children using HA tend to experience milder HL than their CI peers. Moreover, children with CI show morphological, pragmatic and syntactic difficulties (Boons et al., 2013), as well as divergent phonological processes (Asad, Purdy, Ballard, Fairgray, & Bowen, 2018), when compared to normal hearing matched samples.

However, as with almost every other linguistic-related phenomenon or condition, studies in HL are eminently conducted in children speaking West Germanic languages, English mostly. Hence, given the differences between the latter and Romance language families depicted at the beginning of this chapter, more research is needed in order to set clear HL clinical profiles in Romance language-speaking children. Furthermore, the World Health Organization (World Health Organisation, 2018) estimates that the prevalence of disabling HL in children in the regions in which Romance languages are spoken as the first language is below the World's mean (1.7%), including Latin America and the Caribbean (1.6%), North America and Western Europe (0.5%), and Central and East Europe (1.5%). Nevertheless, that same institution predicts that the incidence of HL will very likely increase in the future. Altogether, these factors make HL an important concern that should be profoundly investigated in order to palliate its present and upcoming effects.

In this book, two investigations that shed light on interesting aspects regarding HL in children speaking Romance languages can be found. On the one hand, Chapter 9 (Sidera, Serrat, Amadó & Morgan) presents a study clarifying the associations between several language abilities and emotion recognition of children at different ages. Moreover, due to psychosocial difficulties experienced by children with HL (Netten et al., 2015; Sorkin et al., 2015), the authors of this chapter did also investigate whether linguistic and emotion recognition developmental patterns between children of different ages with and without HL were distinct, how they differed, and to what extent. On the other hand, Chapter 10 (Lara Díaz, Rivera & Rodríguez) aims at determining the relation between HL and executive functions in children who use CI, and to provide clinicians with a profile of processes in which these children are more likely to show deficits. Furthermore, this study explores the visual fixation of children who use CI given that children with HL are not able to locate spatial auditory information (Hoffman, Tiddens, & Quittner, 2018), hence altering their attentional visual strategies.

Genetic syndromes

Finally, this book focuses in Genetic syndromes that course with cognitive impairment. Throughout the last decades, it has been proposed that the definition and research of intellectual disability should be focused on exploring syndrome-specific neurodevelopmental profiles rather than general impairments or delays (Schalock & Luckasson, 2004). In this vein, the study of language deficits associated with intellectual disability is currently focused on the comparison of profiles of different syndromes such as Down, Williams, and fragile X syndromes. These syndromes are genetic in nature, and cause, along with other genetic disorders, approximately 40% of cases of intellectual disability (Toth, de Lacy, & King, 2016).

Down syndrome (DS) is the most common genetic syndrome causing intellectual disability (occurring approximately 1 per 1000 live births; Orphanet, 2018). It is characterised by moderate to severe intellectual disability and it is caused, in most of the cases, by an extra 21st chromosome (Trisomy 21). DS is accompanied by deficits in several language domains. Although lexical comprehension of children with DS seems to be somewhat preserved, they often show impoverished lexical production and deficient grammar processing (Arias-Trejo & Barrón-Martínez, 2017; Næss, Lyster, Hulme, & Melby-Lervåg, 2011) as compared to non-verbal mental age-matched controls. Beyond, several models have shown a strong lexicon-grammar relationship for the emergence of grammar on DS and TD children. Notwithstanding, some authors have proposed the existence of a dissociation between lexical and grammatical systems only in DS (Bates, Dale, & Thal, 1995), thus advocating for a modular model of language acquisition. Recent research suggests the existence of associations between grammar and lexicon in Romance language-speaking children with DS (Galeote, Soto, Sebastián, Checa, & Sánchez-Palacios, 2014), yet simultaneously highlights the idea that this relation is perhaps more complex in those children. This complexity encourages refined research by exploring vocabulary composition for a better understanding of this linkage. This is the case of Chapter 11 (Jackson-Maldonado, Galeote, & Flores), where the relation of vocabulary and grammar was explored in a group of Spanish-speaking Mexican pre-school children with DS. Children were assessed employing a parental report, paying special attention to vocabulary categories (nouns, predicates, social words, and closed-class words) as well as the length and complexity of utterances. Results evidenced a general association between the lexicon and grammar in children with DS. In turn, the exploration of individual cases yielded diverse outcomes suggesting that vocabulary size does not consistently predict grammatical maturity in children with DS. This study emphasizes the considerable variability of language development profiles among DS individuals.

Williams syndrome (WS) is also a relevant cause of intellectual disability but its prevalence is lower than in DS (WS prevalence is estimated in 1 in 10,000 live births; Orphanet, 2018). It is characterized by mild to moderate intellectual disability and it is caused by a deletion of about 17 genes in the 7q11.23 region of chromosome 7 (Donnai & Karmiloff-Smith, 2000). Despite the fact that it has been claimed that individuals with WS show preserved language abilities, there is limited evidence about TD in several language domains such as morphosyntax, phonology, and pragmatics (See Brock, 2007, for a review). Indeed, research in Romance languages has usually reported atypical morphosyntactic errors (Diez-Itza, Martínez, Fernández-Urquiza, & Antón, 2017), thus contrasting the language preservation hypothesis. These findings intensify the debate about typical or atypical nature of the morphosyntactic profile of WS and challenge the idea of modularity of language in respect to other cognitive functions. A better understanding of WS linguistic characterization could be gained by comparative studies exploring language profiles of individuals with different syndromes associated with intellectual disability. Following this rationale, Chapter 12 (Diez-Itza, Miranda, Pérez, & Martínez) reports a comparative study examining morphological profiles of Spanish-speaking adolescents with WS or DS, and TD children paired by sex and verbal age. Speech samples were obtained from spontaneous conversations in natural settings. Distribution of the part-of-speech categories and frequency and type of morphological errors were analysed. Results evidenced a specific impairment of grammatical morphology in DS adolescents who showed atypical characteristics in the distribution of the part-of-speech categories and the frequency of omission of free morphemes. The morphological profile of the adolescents with WS also presented certain atypical features that were similar to those observed in the DS group, such as the high relative proportion of errors in free morphemes. Moreover, WS-specific atypical features were also found, such as the high relative proportion of addition errors. Furthermore, the morphological profiles of the WS and DS groups would not correspond to a developmental delay since they presented differential characteristics compared to those of TD children. Authors interpret these distinct morphological profiles as the consequences of atypical trajectories of development.

Atypical development of language in WS seems to affect not only morphological outcomes but also other domains of language. WS individuals are usually described as being extremely friendly (Jones et al., 2000) and seem to easily engage in social interactions. However, their conversations tend to be inappropriate and superficial (Diez-Itza, Martínez, Pérez, & Fernández-Urquiza, 2018), suggesting the existence of problems regarding the pragmatic component of language. Congruently, some disturbances have been found when studying language production either during conversations or during narrative tasks (see Brock, 2007, for a review). During narration tasks, children with WS usually show a lack of integration and a lack of use of cognitive inference mechanisms while showing a greater use of social engagement devices and emotional inferences (Reilly, Losh, Bellugi, & Wulfeck, 2004). Findings in Romance languages seem to be language-dependent, hence the investigation of narrative and social language in WS are in need of new studies in order to clarify possible pragmatic difficulties in this population. Chapter 13 (Shiro, Diez-Itza, & Fernández-Urquiza) aimed to explore the pragmatic profile of Spanish-speaking WS population as compared to that of TD children matched for verbal abilities. The narrative organisation and evaluative devices were explored revealing no differences between WS and TD in terms of macro-structural narrative skills but in microelements that contribute to the overall coherence. Moreover, children with WS tended to increase the use of evaluative devices only when referring to emotional states, not differing from TD in other kinds of evaluative expressions. Authors conclude that the use of evaluative devices in narratives constitutes a relative strength in WS of which therapeutic interventions could benefit.

Conclusions

This book depicted recent research in language development in a wide range of difficulties that course with language problems (preterm children, SLI, hearing impairment, and genetic syndromes) in populations learning different Romance languages: Italian, Spanish, Catalan, and Galician, besides a Slavic language (Russian). Therefore, this book adds a new step that covers the lack of studies in atypical language development of Romance languages.

Acknowledgements

This chapter and this books has been supported by the Spanish government (MINECO/AEI) and the ERDF, UE (European Regional Development Fund) [SEJ2006-12616], [EDU2013-45174-P] and [EDU2017-85909-P], and also by the University of Balearic Islands, the department of Pedagogy and Applied Psychology, and the Institute of Research and Innovation in Education (IRIE).

References

Aarnoudse-Moens, C. S. H., Weisglas-Kuperus, N., van Goudoever, J. B., & Oosterlaan, J. 2009. Meta-analysis of neurobehavioral outcomes in very preterm and/or very low birth weight children. *Pediatrics* 124(2), 717–728. https://doi.org/10.1542/peds.2008-2816

Ackerman, B. P., Brown, E. D., & Izard, C. E. 2004. The relations between contextual risk, earned income, and the school adjustment of children from economically disadvantaged families. *Developmental Psychology* 40(2), 204–216. https://doi.org/10.1037/0012-1649.40.2.204

Aguilar-Mediavilla, E., Adrover-Roig, D., Buil-Legaz, L., & López-Penadés, R. 2016. *Proceedings of the VIII International Conference of Language Acquisiction, Palma, UIB*. Palma: UIB.

American Psychiatric Association (APA). 2013. DSM-5. <http://www.psychiatry.org/dsm5> (8 October, 2018).

Andreu, L., Sanz-Torrent, M., & Trueswell, J. C. 2012. Anticipatory sentence processing in children with specific language impairment: Evidence from eye movements during listening. *Applied Psycholinguistics* 34(1), 5–44. https://doi.org/10.1017/S0142716411000592

Arias-Trejo, N., & Barrón-Martínez, J. B. 2017. Language skills in Down Syndrome. En A. Auza Benavides & R. G. Schwartz (Ed.), *Language development and disorders in Spanish-speaking children* (pp. 329–341). New York, NY: Springer. https://doi.org/10.1007/978-3-319-53646-0

Asad, A. N., Purdy, S. C., Ballard, E., Fairgray, L., & Bowen, C. 2018. Phonological processes in the speech of school-age children with hearing loss: Comparisons with children with normal hearing. *Journal of Communication Disorders*. https://doi.org/10.1016/j.jcomdis.2018.04.004

Bates, E., Dale, P. S., & Thal, D. J. 1995. Individual differences and their implications for theories of language development. En P. Fletcher & B. MacWhinney (Ed.), *The handbook of child language* (pp. 96–151). Oxford: Blackwell.

Bates, E., Devescovi, A., & Wulfeck, B. 2001. Psycholinguistics: A cross-language perspective. *Annual Review of Psychology* 52, 369–398. https://doi.org/10.1146/annurev.psych.52.1.369

Bavin, E. L. 1995. Language acquisition in crosslinguistic perspective. *Annual Review of Anthropology* 24(1): 373–396. https://doi.org/10.1146/annurev.an.24.100195.002105

Berman, R. A. 2014. Cross-linguistic comparisons in child language research. *Journal of Child Language* 41(S1), 26–37. https://doi.org/10.1017/S0305000914000208

Berman, R. A., & Slobin, D. I. 1987. *Five ways of learning to talk about events: A crosslinguistic study of children's narratives* (Cognitive Science Report, Vol. 46). Berkeley, CA: Institute of Cognitive Studies.

Berman, R. A., & Slobin, D. I. 1994. *Relating events in narrative: A cross-linguistic developmental study*. Hillsdale, NJ: Lawrence Erlbaum Associates.

Bishop, D. V. M. 2004. Specific language impairments: Diagnotic dilemmas. En *Classification of developmental language disorders: Theoretical issues and clinical implications* (pp. 309–326). Mahwah, NJ: Lawrence Erlbaum Associates.

Bishop, D. V. M. 2014. Ten questions about terminology for children with unexplained language problems. *International Journal of Language & Communication Disorders* 49(4), 381–415. https://doi.org/10.1111/1460-6984.12101

Boons, T., De Raeve, L., Langereis, M., Peeraer, L., Wouters, J., & van Wieringen, A. 2013. Expressive vocabulary, morphology, syntax and narrative skills in profoundly deaf children after early cochlear implantation. *Research in Developmental Disabilities* 34(6), 2008–2022. https://doi.org/10.1016/j.ridd.2013.03.003

Bosch, L. 2011. Precursors to language in preterm infants. En *Progress in brain research* (Vol. 189, pp. 239–257). Burlington, VT: Academic Press. https://doi.org/10.1016/B978-0-444-53884-0.00028-2

Bradley, R. H., & Corwyn, R. F. 2005. Productive activity and the prevention of behavior problems. *Developmental Psychology* 41(1), 89–98. https://doi.org/10.1037/0012-1649.41.1.89

Brock, J. 2007. Language abilities in Williams syndrome: A critical review. *Development and Psychopathology* 19(01), 97–127. https://doi.org/10.1017/S095457940707006X

Clark, C. A. C., & Woodward, L. J. 2015. Relation of perinatal risk and early parenting to executive control at the transition to school. *Developmental Science* 18(4), 525–542. https://doi.org/10.1111/desc.12232

Conger, R. D., & Conger, K. J. 2002. Resilience in midwestern families: Selected findings from the first decade of a prospective, longitudinal study. *Journal of Marriage and Family* 64(2), 361–373. https://doi.org/10.1111/j.1741-3737.2002.00361.x

Davis, J. M., Elfenbein, J. L., Schum, R., & Bentler, R. A. 1986. Effects of mild and moderate hearing impairments on language, educational, and psychosocial behavior of children. *Journal of Speech and Hearing Disorders* 51(1), 53. https://doi.org/10.1044/jshd.5101.53

Dearing, E., McCartney, K., & Taylor, B. A. 2002. Change in family income-to-needs matters more for children with less. *Child Development* 72(6), 1779–1793. <http://www.ncbi.nlm.nih.gov/pubmed/11768145> https://doi.org/10.1111/1467-8624.00378

Delgado Domínguez, J., & Grupo PrevInfad/PAPPS Infancia y Adolescencia. 2011. Detección precoz de la hipoacusia infantil. *Revista Pediatría de Atención Primaria* 13(50), 279–297.

Devescovi, A., Caselli, M. C., Marchione, D., Pasqualetti, P., Reilly, J., & Bates, E. 2003. A cross-linguistic study of the relaitonship between grammar and lexical development. *Manuscript, Center for Reseach in Language*, University of California, San Diego.

Diez-itza, E. 2007. *Estudios de desarrollo del lenguaje y educación*. Oviedo: Universidad de Oviedo ICE.

Díez-Itza, E., Martínez, V., Fernández-Urquiza, M., & Antón, A. 2017. Morphological profile of Williams syndrome: Typical or atypical? In A. Auza-Benavides & R. G. Schwartz (Ed.), *Language development and disorders in Spanish- speaking children* (pp. 311–327). New York, NY: Springer. https://doi.org/10.1007/978-3-319-53646-0_15

Díez-Itza, E., Martínez, V., Pérez, V., & Fernández-Urquiza, M. 2018. Explicit oral narrative intervention for students with Williams syndrome. *Frontiers in Psychology* 8(JAN), 1–18. https://doi.org/10.3389/fpsyg.2017.02337

Donnai, D., & Karmiloff-Smith, A. 2000. Williams syndrome: From gentotype through to the cognitive phenotype. *American Journal of Medical Genetics* 97(2), 164–171. https://doi.org/10.1002/1096-8628(200022)97:2<164::AID-AJMG8>3.0.CO;2-F

Duinmeijer, I., de Jong, J., & Scheper, A. 2012. Narrative abilities, memory and attention in children with a specific language impairment. *International Journal of Language and Communication Disorders* 47(5), 542–555. https://doi.org/10.1111/j.1460-6984.2012.00164.x

Elfenbein, J. L., Hardin-Jones, M. A., & Davis, J. M. 1994. Oral communication skills of children who are hard of hearing. *Journal of Speech Language and Hearing Research* 37(1), 216. https://doi.org/10.1044/jshr.3701.216

Fey, M. E., Catts, H. W., Proctor-Williams, K., Tomblin, J. B., & Zhang, X. 2004. Oral and written story composition skills of children with language impairment. *Journal of Speech, Language, and Hearing Research : JSLHR* 47(6), 1301–1318. <http://www.ncbi.nlm.nih.gov/pubmed/15842012> https://doi.org/10.1044/1092-4388(2004/098)

Fiestas, C. E., Bedore, L. M., Peña, E. D., & Nagy, V. J. 2005. Use of mazes in the narrative language samples of bilingual and monolingual 4- to 7-year old children. In J. Cohen, K. T. McAlister, K. Rolstad, & J. MacSwan (Eds.), *Proceedings of the 4th International Symposium on Bilingualism* (pp. 730–740). Somerville, MA: Cascadilla.

Fitzpatrick, E. M., Olds, J., Gaboury, I., McCrae, R., Schramm, D., & Durieux-Smith, A. 2012. Comparison of outcomes in children with hearing aids and cochlear implants. *Cochlear Implants International* 13(1), 5–15. https://doi.org/10.1179/146701011X12950038111611

Galeote, M., Soto, P., Sebastián, E., Checa, E., & Sánchez-Palacios, C. 2014. Early grammatical development in Spanish children with Down syndrome. *Journal of Child Language* 41(01), 111–131. https://doi.org/10.1017/S0305000912000591

Gonzalez, D. O., Cáceres, A. M., Bento-Gaz, A. C. P., & Befi-Lopes, D. M. 2012. The complexity of narrative interferes in the use of conjunctions in children with specific language impairment. *Jornal da Sociedade Brasileira de Fonoaudiologia* 24(2), 152–156. <http://www.ncbi.nlm.nih.gov/pubmed/22832683> https://doi.org/10.1590/S2179-64912012000200011

Guo, J., Lieven, E. V. M., Budwig, N., Ervin-Tripp, S., Nakamura, K., & Ozcaliskan, S. 2009. *Crosslinguistic approaches to the psychology of language: Research in the tradition of Dan Isaac Slobin*. New York, NY: Psychology Press. <https://books.google.cz/books?id=W-B4AgAAQBAJ&pg=PA119-IA2&lpg=PA119-IA2&dq=slovin+frog+crosslinguistic&source=bl&ots=7T9afSFY8B&sig=i27-LgApsO8CLAIRUm8iQe5fgJ8&hl=es&sa=X&ved=2ahUKEwjz7cPh2-XdAhVDnRoKHfVYAkEQ6AEwA3oECAYQAQ#v=onepage&q=slovinfrogcro>

Hoffman, M., Tiddens, E., & Quittner, A. L. 2018. Comparisons of visual attention in school-age children with cochlear implants versus hearing peers and normative data. *Hearing Research* 359, 91–100. https://doi.org/10.1016/j.heares.2018.01.002

Holm, A., Crosbie, S., & Dodd, B. 2007. Differentiating normal variability from inconsistency in children's speech: Normative data. *International Journal of Language & Communication Disorders* 42(4), 467–486. https://doi.org/10.1080/13682820600988967

Ionio, C., Riboni, E., Confalonieri, E., Dallatomasina, C., Mascheroni, E., Bonanomi, A., … Comi, G. 2016. Paths of cognitive and language development in healthy preterm infants. *Infant Behavior and Development* 44, 199–207. https://doi.org/10.1016/j.infbeh.2016.07.004

Jackson-Maldonado, D., & Maldonado, R. 2017. Grammaticality differences between Spanish-speaking children with specific language impairment and their typically developing peers. *International Journal of Language and Communication Disorders* 52(6), 750–765. https://doi.org/10.1111/1460-6984.12312

Jansson-Verkasalo, E., Ruusuvirta, T., Huotilainen, M., Alku, P., Kushnerenko, E., Suominen, K., … Hallman, M. 2010. Atypical perceptual narrowing in prematurely born infants is associated with compromised language acquisition at 2 years of age. *BMC Neuroscience* 11(1), 88. https://doi.org/10.1186/1471-2202-11-88

Jones, W., Bellugi, U., Lai, Z., Chiles, M., Reilly, J., Lincoln, A., & Adolphs, R. 2000. II. Hypersociability in Williams Syndrome. *Journal of Cognitive Neuroscience* 12(supplement 1), 30–46. https://doi.org/10.1162/089892900561968

Kapa, L. L., Plante, E., & Doubleday, K. 2017. Applying an integrative framework of executive function to preschoolers with Specific Language Impairment. *Journal of Speech Language and Hearing Research* 60(8), 2170. https://doi.org/10.1044/2017_JSLHR-L-16-0027

Karmiloff-Smith, A. 1992. *Beyond modularity: A developmental perspective on cognitive science.* Cambridge, MA: The MIT Press; Bradford Books.

Kiese-Himmel, C. 2008. Receptive (aural) vocabulary development in children with permanent bilateral sensorineural hearing impairment. *The Journal of Laryngology & Otology* 122(5). https://doi.org/10.1017/S0022215107000321

Kochhar, A., Hildebrand, M. S., & Smith, R. J. H. 2007. Clinical aspects of hereditary hearing loss. *Genetics in Medicine* 9(7), 393–408. https://doi.org/10.1097/GIM.0b013e318098 0bd0

Koldewijn, K., van Wassenaer, A., Wolf, M.-J., Meijssen, D., Houtzager, B., Beelen, A., … Nollet, F. 2010. A Neurobehavioral intervention and assessment program in very low birth weight infants: Outcome at 24 months. *The Journal of Pediatrics* 156(3), 359–365. https://doi.org/10.1016/j.jpeds.2009.09.009

Leonard, L. B. 2014a. Children with Specific Language Impairment and their contribution to the study of language development. *Journal of Child Language* 41(S1), 38–47. https://doi.org/10.1017/S0305000914000130

Leonard, L. B. 2014b. Specific Language Impairment across languages. *Child Development Perspectives* 8(1), 1–5. https://doi.org/10.1111/cdep.12053

Leonard, L. B. 2015. *Specific Language Impairment* (2nd ed.). Cambridge, MA: The MIT Press.

Lieven, E. V. M. 1994. Crosslinguistic and crosscultural aspects of language addressed to children. En C. Gallaway & B. J. Richards (Ed.), *Input and interaction in language acquisition* (pp. 56–73). Cambridge: Cambridge University Press. https://doi.org/10.1017/CBO9780511620690.005

Lieven, E. V. M. 2010. Language development in a cross-linguistic context. In M. Kail & M. Hickmann (Eds.), *Language acquisition across linguistic and cognitive systems* (pp. 91–108). Amsterdam: John Benjamins. https://doi.org/10.1075/lald.52.08lie

Liu, L., Oza, S., Hogan, D., Chu, Y., Perin, J., Zhu, J., … Black, R. E. 2016. Global, regional, and national causes of under-5 mortality in 2000–15: An updated systematic analysis with implications for the Sustainable Development Goals. *The Lancet* 388(10063), 3027–3035. https://doi.org/10.1016/S0140-6736(16)31593-8

López-Ornat, S. 1998. La adquisición del lenguaje. Nuevas perspectivas. En F. Cuetos-Vega & M. de Vega (Ed.), *Avances en la psicolingüística del español.* Madrid: Siglo XXI.

May-Mederake, B. 2012. Early intervention and assessment of speech and language development in young children with cochlear implants. *International Journal of Pediatric Otorhinolaryngology* 76(7), 939–946. https://doi.org/10.1016/j.ijporl.2012.02.051

Mayor-Cinca, M. A., Zubiauz de de Pedro, B., & Díez, E. 2005. *Estudios sobre la adquisición del lenguaje.* Salamanca: Universidad de Salamanca.

Mueller Gathercole, V. C., Sebastián, E., & Soto, P. 1999. The early acquisition of Spanish verbal morphology: Across-the-board or piecemeal knowledge? *International Journal of Bilingualism* 3(2–3), 133–182. https://doi.org/10.1177/13670069990030020401

Næss, K. A. B., Lyster, S. A. H., Hulme, C., & Melby-Lervåg, M. 2011. Language and verbal short-term memory skills in children with Down syndrome: A meta-analytic review. *Research in Developmental Disabilities* 32(6), 2225–2234. https://doi.org/10.1016/j.ridd.2011.05.014

Netten, A. P., Rieffe, C., Theunissen, S. C. P. M., Soede, W., Dirks, E., Korver, A. M. H., … Frijns, J. H. M. 2015. Early identification: Language skills and social functioning in deaf and hard of hearing preschool children. *International Journal of Pediatric Otorhinolaryngology* 79(12), 2221–2226. https://doi.org/10.1016/j.ijporl.2015.10.008

Niparko, J. K., Tobey, E. A., Thal, D. J., Eisenberg, L. S., Wang, N.-Y., Quittner, A. L., & Fink, N. E. 2010. Spoken language development in children following Cochlear implantation. *JAMA* 303(15), 1498–1506. <http://www.jama.com> https://doi.org/10.1001/jama.2010.451

Orphanet. 2018. *Prevalence and incidence of rare diseases: Bibliographic data* (Orphanet Report Series 2). <www.orpha.net>

Parisse, C. & Maillart, C. (2009). Specific language impairment as systemic developmental disorders. *Journal of Neurolinguistics* 22(2), 109-122. https://doi.org/10.1016/j.jneuroling.2008.07.004

Pérez-Pereira, M. 1996. *Estudios sobre la adquisición del castellano, catalán, esquera y gallego. Actas del I Encuentro Internacional sobre Adquisición de las lenguas del Estado*. Santiago de Compostela: Universidad de Santiago de Compostela.

Petersen, N. K., Jørgensen, A. W., & Ovesen, T. 2015. Prevalence of various etiologies of hearing loss among cochlear implant recipients: Systematic review and meta-analysis. *International Journal of Audiology* 54(12), 924–932. https://doi.org/10.3109/14992027.2015.1091094

Peterson, D. B. & Gardner, C. M. (2011). Trastornos específicos del lenguaje: una revisión. *Revista Chilena de Fonoaudiología* 10, 19-32. https://doi.org/10.5354/0719-4692.2011.17348

Raviv, T., Kessenich, M., & Morrison, F. J. 2004. A mediational model of the association between socioeconomic status and three-year-old language abilities: The role of parenting factors. *Early Childhood Research Quarterly* 19(4), 528–547. https://doi.org/10.1016/j.ecresq.2004.10.007

Reilly, J., Losh, M., Bellugi, U., & Wulfeck, B. 2004. 'Frog, where are you?' Narratives in children with specific language impairment, early focal brain injury, and Williams syndrome. *Brain and Language* 88(2), 229–247. https://doi.org/10.1016/S0093-934X(03)00101-9

Repetti, R. L., Taylor, S. E., & Seeman, T. E. 2002. Risky families: Family social environments and the mental and physical health of offspring. *Psychological Bulletin* 128(2), 330–366. https://doi.org/10.1037//0033-2909.128.2.330

Ruben, R. J. 2018. Language development in the pediatric cochlear implant patient. *Laryngoscope Investigative Otolaryngology* 3(3), 209–213. https://doi.org/10.1002/lio2.156

Sansavini, A., Guarini, A., & Caselli, M. C. 2011. Preterm birth: Neuropsychological profiles and atypical developmental pathways. *Developmental Disabilities Research Reviews* 17(2), 102–113. https://doi.org/10.1002/ddrr.1105

Schalock, R. L., & Luckasson, R. 2004. American Association on Mental Retardation's Definition, Classification, and System of Supports and its relation to international trends and issues in the field of intellectual disabilities. *Journal of Policy and Practice in Intellectual Disabilities* 1(3), 136–146. https://doi.org/10.1111/j.1741-1130.2004.04028.x

Schwartz, R. G. 2009. *Handbook on child language disorders*. New York NY: Psychology Press.

Scott, M. N., Taylor, H. G., Fristad, M. A., Klein, N., Espy, K. A., Minich, N., & Hack, M. 2012. Behavior disorders in extremely preterm/extremely low birth weight children in kindergarten. *Journal of Developmental & Behavioral Pediatrics* 33(3), 202–213. https://doi.org/10.1097/DBP.0b013e3182475287

Serenius, F., Ewald, U., Farooqi, A., Fellman, V., Hafström, M., Hellgren, K., … 2016. Extremely preterm infants in Sweden study group. Neurodevelopmental outcomes among extremely preterm infants 6.5 years after active perinatal care in Sweden. *JAMA Pediatrics* 170(10), 954. https://doi.org/10.1001/jamapediatrics.2016.1210

Serra-Raventós, M., Serrat Sellabona, E., Solé Planas, R., Bel Leal, A., & Aparici Aznar, M. 2000. *La adquisición del lenguaje*. Barcelona: Ariel.

Sorkin, D. L., Gates-Ulanet, P., & Mellon, N. K. 2015. Psychosocial aspects of hearing loss in Children. *Otolaryngologic Clinics of North America* 48(6), 1073–1080. https://doi.org/10.1016/j.otc.2015.07.008

Spittle, A., Orton, J., Anderson, P. J., Boyd, R., & Doyle, L. W. 2015. Early developmental intervention programmes provided post hospital discharge to prevent motor and cognitive impairment in preterm infants. *Cochrane Database of Systematic Reviews* 776(11), CD005495. https://doi.org/10.1002/14651858.CD005495.pub4

Stevenson, J., McCann, D., Watkin, P., Worsfold, S., & Kennedy, C. 2010. The relationship between language development and behaviour problems in children with hearing loss. *Journal of Child Psychology and Psychiatry* 51(1), 77–83. https://doi.org/10.1111/j.1469-7610.2009.02124.x

Tamis-LeMonda, C. S., Shannon, J. D., Cabrera, N. J., & Lamb, M. E. 2004. Fathers and mothers at play with their 2- and 3-year-olds: contributions to language and cognitive development. *Child Development* 75(6), 1806–1820. https://doi.org/10.1111/j.1467-8624.2004.00818.x

Taylor, H. G., & Clark, C. A. C. 2016. Executive function in children born preterm: Risk factors and implications for outcome. *Seminars in Perinatology* 40(8), 520–529. https://doi.org/10.1053/j.semperi.2016.09.004

Thorne, J. C., Coggins, T. E., Carmichael Olson, H., & Astley, S. J. 2007. Exploring the utility of narrative analysis in diagnostic decision making: Picture-bound reference, elaboration, and fetal alcohol spectrum disorders. *Journal of Speech Language and Hearing Research* 50(2), 459. https://doi.org/10.1044/1092-4388(2007/032)

Tomasello, M. 2003. *Constructing a language : A usage-based theory of language acquisition*. Cambridge, MA: Harvard University Press. <http://www.hup.harvard.edu/catalog.php?isbn=9780674017641>

Tomblin, J. B., Oleson, J. J., Ambrose, S. E., Walker, E., & Moeller, M. P. 2014. The influence of hearing aids on the speech and language development of children with hearing loss. *JAMA Otolaryngology–Head & Neck Surgery* 140(5), 403. https://doi.org/10.1001/jamaoto.2014.267

Toth, K., de Lacy, N., & King, B. H. 2016. Intelectual disability. In M. K. Dulcan (Ed.), *Dulcan's textbook of child and adolescent psychiatry* (pp. 105–133). Arlington VA: American Psychiatric Publishing. https://doi.org/10.1176/appi.books.9781615370306.md07

van Noort-van der Spek, I. L., Franken, M.-C. J. P., & Weisglas-Kuperus, N. 2012. Language functions in preterm-born children: A systematic review and meta-analysis. *Pediatrics* 129(4), 745–754. https://doi.org/10.1542/peds.2011-1728

Webb, A. R., Heller, H. T., Benson, C. B., & Lahav, A. 2015. Mother's voice and heartbeat sounds elicit auditory plasticity in the human brain before full gestation. *Proceedings of the National Academy of Sciences of the United States of America* 112(10), 3152–3157. https://doi.org/10.1073/pnas.1414924112

Williamson, K. E., & Jakobson, L. S. 2014. Social perception in children born at very low birthweight and its relationship with social/behavioral outcomes. *Journal of Child Psychology and Psychiatry* 55(9), 990–998. https://doi.org/10.1111/jcpp.12210

World Health Organisation. 2018. *Addressing the rising prevalence of hearing loss*. <http://www.who.int/iris/handle/10665/260336>

PART I

Preterm children

Neuroconstructivism to understand the effect of very preterm birth on language and literacy

Annalisa Guarini, Mariagrazia Zuccarini and Alessandra Sansavini
Department of Psychology, University of Bologna, Italy

The preterm population is not characterised by an initial delay that recovers during development, but by atypical developmental trajectories, that can be understood through the neuroconstructivist approach. The neuropsychological profiles of very preterm infants show a great heterogeneity, depending on neonatal immaturity, medical complications, environmental, relational and social factors. The developmental trajectory of very preterm children is described in relation to the acquisition and consolidation of language and literacy from early infancy to adolescence. Indexes for early individuation of language and literacy delays, as well as for planning focused interventions, are discussed.

Keywords: demands, moderately preterm, word learning mechanism

Rethinking preterm birth with the neuroconstructivist approach

Preterm birth is defined by the World Health Organization when babies are born alive before 37 weeks of gestational age (GA); the rate of preterm birth ranges from 5% to 18% across 184 countries (March of Dimes, 2012). Different subcategories of preterm birth were defined in function of GA (extremely preterm, <28 weeks; very preterm, from 28 to <32 weeks; moderate to late preterm from 32 to <37 weeks, March of Dimes, 2012).

Preterm birth constitutes a risk condition for cerebral, physical and neuropsychological development (March of Dimes, 2012) that can be understood through the neuroconstructivist framework (Sansavini, Guarini & Caselli, 2011). Neuroconstructivism argued that development is determined by the interplay of multiple biological and environmental constraints interacting at different levels (genes, brain, body, and environment, Karmiloff-Smith, 1998; Westermann et al., 2007). In preterm infants atypical constraints occur in a critical period of rapid

https://doi.org/10.1075/z.223.02gua

development of the neural system (Volpe, 2009) determining an atypical developmental trajectory (Sansavini, Guarini, & Caselli, 2011) resulting from the adaptation to multiple altered constraints (Karmiloff-Smith, 1998). In other words, preterm birth forces brain and body to adapt to an artificial environment characterised by hypo-stimulation (e.g., absence of rhythmic and kinaesthetic stimulations) and over-stimulation (e.g., light, noise, painful and invasive medical interventions, Sansavini, Guarini, & Caselli, 2011) affecting cerebral, physical and neuropsychological development. Neuroconstructivism can also explain the wide heterogeneity observed in the neuropsychological profiles of preterm infants (Guarini & Sansavini, 2010; Sansavini, Guarini, & Caselli, 2011) in function of different levels of neonatal immaturity, medical complications and the environmental and social characteristics to which the child is exposed, such as the level of parental education and their responsiveness to the child's communicative signals (Bozzette, 2007).

This risk condition associated to preterm birth can affect the development of communication and language, since the auditory system and the neural circuits involved in the development of language are particularly vulnerable in the last trimester of gestation, when preterm newborns live in an extra-uterine artificial environment (Vohr, 2014). The early exposure to an artificial environment of a biologically immature system increases the risk of atypical development pathways (Sansavini, Guarini, & Caselli, 2011). This vulnerability can be amplified by environmental characteristics (e.g., exposure to a noisy environment and lack of rhythmic stimulation, such as maternal heart rate) and fewer communication opportunities with parents and people who take care of the newborn (Sansavini et al., 2017; Vohr, 2014).

The atypical developmental trajectory of very preterm children in communication, language and literacy is described in the following paragraphs of the present chapter. In the last paragraph, focused interventions proposed to preterm children and their parents are described in order to indicate good practices for creating an enriched environment and ehancing protective factors.

Effects of preterm birth on communication and language development

As shown by many studies conducted in several countries and by recent meta-analyses and reviews, preterm birth has an impact on the development of communication and language since early childhood and persists until adolescence (Barre et al., 2011; Sansavini, Guarini, & Caselli, 2011; Sansavini & Faldella, 2013; Sansavini et al., 2017; van Noort van der Spek et al., 2012). Most effects have been found on extremely preterm and very preterm infants, but some also on moderate (32–33 weeks GA) and late preterm (34–36 weeks GA) infants. Language difficulties of very preterm children are often associated with early perceptual, cognitive, communicative, and motor problems that may have cascading effects on later more complex abilities (Sansavini, Guarini & Caselli, 2011).

Speech perception skills, such as discrimination, recognition and tuning on the phonetic units and the prosodic characteristics of the mother tongue, as well as word segmentation, develop in the first year of life (Bosch, 2011). When corrected age has been used (i.e., referring to the expected date of birth of 40 weeks GA), only slight delays have been found in very preterm infants, showing that the development of speech perception skills is much affected by neurobiological maturation (Bosch, 2011; Peña et al., 2010).

By contrast, early gestural and vocal production is less developed between the first and second year of life in extremely preterm and very preterm children with respect to full-term children, even when using corrected age (Benassi et al., 2016; Sansavini et al., 2011, Sansavini, Bello et al., 2015). Gesture and word production at 12 and 18 months is predictive of word production at 24 months indicating the importance of monitoring and supporting these skills from early stages of development (Sansavini et al., 2011; Stolt et al., 2014).

The ability to share attention with the caregiver on a common focus is fragile in extremely preterm and very preterm children and strongly affected by mother-infant interaction modalities. Synchrony, symmetric co-regulation and cooperation in mother-infant interaction, constitute important protective factors for communication development (Forcada-Guex et al., 2006; Landry et al., 1996; Sansavini, Zavagli et al., 2015). In particular, maternal contingent and highly relevant responses (i.e., those with a repeated label) following infants' spontaneous communicative behaviors support communication development in extremely preterm infants, being related with their receptive and expressive communication skills at 12 months and expressive communication skills at 24 months (Benassi et al., 2018).

Fine and gross motor skills are also often compromised in very preterm and extremely preterm children since the early years of life, affecting the ability to explore objects that is crucial to the construction of cognitive and linguistic categories (Ruff et al., 1984; Sansavini et al., 2014; Zuccarini et al., 2016). Recently, studies on extremely preterm infants have found concurrent and longitudinal relationships between fine motor skills and communication development: global fine motor skills were positively associated with communication skills, specifically with pointing and representational gestures, at 12 months (Benassi et al., 2016), whereas active object exploration behaviors at 6 months were associated with gesture and language abilities at 12 months (Zuccarini et al., 2018) and with linguistic and cognitive skills at 24 months (Zuccarini et al., 2017).

Studies conducted in different countries with extremely preterm and very preterm children between the second and third year of life, have shown a less advanced development with respect to full-term children in phonology, lexicon and grammar, both in comprehension and production (D'Odorico et al., 2011; Foster-Cohen et al., 2007; Sansavini et al., 2010, 2011, Sansavini, Bello et al. 2015; Stolt et al., 2009, 2017). The risk of language delay in very preterm children increases from 20–25% at two and a half years to 30–35% at three and a half years, whereas in the same period it decreases from 13% to 7% in full-term children (Sansavini et al., 2010), highlighting the importance of monitoring language development of preterm children during this period. Language delay in very preterm children is often associated with delays in basic information processing skills, such as lexical processing speed (Marchman et al., 2016) and in cognitive skills, such as executive functions (Aarnoudse-Moens et al., 2009; Dall'Oglio et al., 2010), with a higher severity in case of neurological damage (Woodward et al., 2009). These findings suggest the importance of assessing basic general abilities alongside specific language skills to outline the neuropsychological profile of these children and schedule early interventions in multiple developmental domains.

Lexicon, grammar and phonological skills continue to be affected by a very preterm birth during preschool and school age (Guarini et al., 2009, 2010, 2016) with scores ranging from 0.38 to 0.77 standard deviations (SD) lower than those of full-term children (Barre et al., 2011; van Noort-van der Spek et al., 2012). Towards the end of preschool age, difficulties also arise in phonological awareness (Guarini et al., 2009) and pragmatic skills, for example in the narrative of figurative stories (Guarini et al., 2016). These difficulties are often associated with cognitive difficulties, particularly with working memory skills (Guarini et al., 2016; Sansavini et al., 2007; Wolke & Meyer, 1999).

The differences between very preterm and full-term children in the above mentioned language skills often remain up to adolescence even in the absence of severe neurological impairment or disability and regardless of parental socio-economic level. However, as far as lexical comprehension is concerned, a study showed a recovery in adolescence, associated with high level of maternal education, presence of both parents in the family, and absence of neurosensory damage, suggesting that protective environmental factors may have compensatory effects on some aspects of linguistic development (Luu et al., 2011; van Noort-van der Spek et al., 2012).

Some delays have also been found in moderate and late preterm children: their language skills, even if better than those of very preterm children, were lower than those of full-term children (Putnick et al., 2016). Since individual differences in language development in the preterm population become gradually stable between 2 and 4 years of age and remain stable up to 8 years, it is important to detect early language delays and plan targeted interventions starting from preschool age (Putnick et al., 2016).

Acquisition and consolidation of literacy

Several reviews revealed that preterm birth affects not only language but also literacy skills. Delays were found in the acquisition and consolidation of reading and spelling processes with different developmental trajectories in function of gestational age (Guarini & Sansavini, 2010; Sansavini, Guarini & Caselli, 2011). In extremely preterm children delays emerge in primary school and up tp secondary school, with a mean of 15 points lower than that of their full-term peers (Johnson et al., 2009). A different picture emerges in very preterm children who have greater difficulties in the spelling process (–0.76 SD), than in the reading process (–0.48 SD; Aarnoudse-Moens et al., 2009; Guarini et al., 2010). Delays in spelling are already present in the acquisition phase, with lower performances in handwriting due to difficulties in fine-motor coordination and visual-motor integration (Feder et al., 2005), and they persist up to secondary school (Chaudhari et al., 2004). Some difficulties were also described in moderate preterm children (de Jong et al., 2012), even if a partial recovery in reading decoding (Rose et al., 2011) and spelling (Tideman, 2000) has been observed in secondary school.

However, most studies have been conducted with native English-speaking children, exposed to an opaque orthography. Very few studies have been carried out in preterm children exposed to a language with a transparent orthography, such as Italian, highlighting the importance of interpreting the results obtained according to the specificity of the mother tongue. Italian very preterm children showed delays in spelling, with errors in word, non-word and sentence tasks at 8 years of age. In reading, speed was affected whereas decoding was accurate as that of full-term peers (Guarini et al., 2010). These results suggest that the effect of preterm birth on reading in a language with transparent orthography is particularly evident in speed, as already found in dyslexic children native speakers of orthographically regular languages (Zoccolotti et al., 1999).

As revealed by a recent meta-analysis, delays in very preterm children involved not only decoding, but also comprehension of written texts (Kovachy et al., 2015), revealing that difficulties in reading comprehension were not recovered, but they increased with increasing age-related difficulties (Kovachy et al., 2015).

Starting from these considerations, the process of reading and spelling of preterm infants required to be monitored both in the acquisition phase and in the consolidation phase, since a higher rate of impairments across multiple curriculum areas are frequent among preterm children (Litt et al., 2005; Pritchard et al., 2009). In addition, the role of cognitive variables, such as processing speed and executive functions, should be taken into account, since they mediate the role of preterm birth in learning difficulties (Loe et al., 2012; Rose et al., 2011). In addition, extremely preterm children are at high risk for comorbidity between learning disabilities and intellectual disabilities (Johnson et al., 2016). The role of preterm birth on literacy was also mediated by language acquisition, since phonological awareness and grammar comprehension showed significant correlations with literacy processes at 8 years of age (Guarini et al., 2010). In addition, phonological awareness and lexicon, before entering primary school, are predictive of literacy skills two years later(Guarini & Sansavini, 2012). Eventually, additional variables may influence learning, such as motivation, and self-efficacy, since preterm children appear to benefit less from learning opportunities and show more motivational problems (Taylor et al., 2000).

Interventions

The studies described in the previous paragraphs outline the importance of monitoring the development of oral and written language of preterm infants and, in particular, of very preterm and extremely preterm infants, from early infancy to adolescence. Follow-up programs should be implemented in order to detect developmental delays and to propose customized interventions from the first years of life onwards (Sansavini & Faldella, 2013).

As shown by a recent review (Spittle et al., 2015), early intervention programs begin within the first 12 months of life and are focused on infant development and/or parent-infant relationship. Notwithstanding the great heterogeneity of these interventions, their positive impact on later cognitive outcomes until at least preschool age has been shown (Spittle et al., 2015). Indeed, preterm infants involved in these programs reported higher cognitive scores than infants who received a standard follow-up program (0.32 SD in infancy and 0.43 SD at preschool age). However, these differences were no longer evident at school age and adulthood (Spittle et al., 2015). Interestingly, interventions focused on both infant development and parent-infant relationship show a higher positive impact on later outcomes (Spittle et al., 2015).

NIDCAP (Newborn Individualized Developmental Care Assessment Programme) is an early intervention programme widely used in Neonatal Intensive Care Units (NICU). This is a family-centered and personalised intervention aiming at enhancing parental care and preterm infant well-being and reducing stress conditions of the NICU (Als, 2009; Als et al., 2012). Significant positive effects of NIDCAP on neurodevelopmental outcomes of preterm infants were found between 9 and 12 months (Jacobs et al., 2002), whereas evidence at later ages is still scarce (Ohlsson & Jacobs, 2013).

Benefits on infants' self-regulation, improving sleep-wake cycle, arousal modulation and sustained exploration of the environment at 6 months, have also been shown through the implementation of Kangaroo Mother Care, which aims at promoting skin-to-skin contact between preterm infants and their caregivers (Feldman et al., 2002). A significant positive effect of this early intervention has been found both in increasing maternal attachment behaviour and child autonomic functioning in the first year of life and on cognition, executive functions and mother–child reciprocity up to 10 years (Feldman et al., 2014). The Kangaroo Mother Care was endorsed by the World Health Organization in 2003 as an intervention highly recommended and as an effective solution to reduce deaths among preterm infants (March of Dimes, 2012).

Early intervention programs focused on enhancing parent-infant relationship and parent coping have shown positive effects on infants' neurodevelopmental outcomes at least up to 36 months of age (Vanderveen et al., 2009). A study by Brooks-Gunn et al. (1992) showed that an intervention programme on parent–child relationship improved cognitive (visual-motor and spatial skills) and language skills of low-birth weight preterm infants at 24 and 36 months, with some differences in treatment efficacy in function of birth-weight and ethnic group. Parent-infant interventions have shown positive effects also on parental outcomes, reducing maternal anxiety and depressive symptoms and increasing their self-efficacy (Benzies et al., 2013).

In recent years, interventions to improve specific competences of very preterm children have been designed.

For istance, infant massage, proposed in the NICU following a specific protocol, accelerates brain activity and visual function, such as visual acuity, in preterm infants (Guzzetta et al., 2009, 2011).

Recent research suggests that encouraging parents to talk and sing to their newborn during hospitalization in the NICU is very promising for language development (Filippa et al., 2013). Very preterm infants increase vocal production between 32 and 36 weeks when parents talk to them and the amount of parental language in NICU is associated with child language and cognitive development at 7 and 18 months (Caskey et al., 2014) suggesting that a positive early auditory experience contributes to cerebral maturation and neuropsychological development.

Some interventions were also conducted to improve specific cognitive functions that are particularly vulnerable in pre-school preterm infants, such as working memory. Very preterm children, who followed a computerized cognitive training at pre-school age, improved several skills that had an impact on later achievement, such as auditory attention, phonological awareness, visual and verbal memory and sentences repetition (Grunewaldt et al., 2013).

Further research is needed to replicate these studies and examine the long-term effects of interventions on developmental trajectories of preterm children.

Conclusions

The present chapter describes preterm birth and its effects on language and literacy development within the neuroconstructivist framework. Since preterm birth exposes the newborn to atypical constraints, an atypical developmental trajectory is shaped with possible delays in language and literacy from the first years of life to adolescence. Some abilities may be particularly affected with a high variability in function of neonatal immaturity, medical complications and social risk factors. An important role of speed processing and executive functions is also described, revealing strict relationships among domains, as already described in other populations with atypical development (Karmiloff-Smith, 1998). As suggested by the neuroconstructivist framework, positive body experiences, adequate environmental stimuli, and positive social interactions can improve the outcomes of preterm infants, indicating the importance to design and promote effective early intervention.

Authors contributions

Conceived and designed the content of the manuscript, wrote and revised the paper: AG AS. Wrote the paragraph on interventions: MZ AG AS.

References

Aarnoudse-Moens, C. S. H., Weisglas-Kuperus, N., van Goudoever, J. B., & Oosterlann, J. 2009. Meta-analysis of neurobehavioral outcomes in very preterm and/or very low birth weight children. *Pediatrics* 124, 717–728. https://doi.org/10.1542/peds.2008-2816

Als, H. 2009. *Program Guide- Newborn Individualized Developmental Care and Assessment Program (NIDCAP): An education and training program for health care professionals.* Boston, MA: Copyright, NIDCAP Federation International.

Als, H., Duffy, F. H., McAnulty, G., Butler, S. C., Lightbody, L., Kosta, S., Weisenfeld, N. I., Robertson, R., Parad, R. B., Ringer, S. A., Blickman, J. G., Zurakowski, D., & Warfield, S. K. 2012. NIDCAP improves brain function and structure in preterm infants with severe intrautherine growth restriction. *Journal of Perinatology* 32, 797–803. https://doi.org/10.1038/jp.2011.201

Barre, N., Morgan, A., Doyle, L. W., & Anderson, P. J. 2011. Language abilities in children who were very preterm and/or very low birth weight: A meta-analysis. *Journal of Pediatrics* 158, 766–774. https://doi.org/10.1016/j.jpeds.2010.10.032

Benassi, E., Guarini, A., Savini, S., Iverson, J. M., Caselli, M. C., Alessandroni, R., Faldella, G., & Sansavini, A. 2018. Maternal responses and development of communication skills in extremely preterm infants. *First Language* 38(2), 175–197 (First Published November 9, 2017). https://doi.org/10.1177/0142723717736449

Benassi, E., Savini, S., Iverson, J. M., Guarini, A., Caselli, M. C., Alessandroni, R., Faldella, G., & Sansavini, A. 2016. Early communicative behaviors and their relationship to motor skills in extremely preterm infants. *Research in Developmental Disabilities* 48, 132–144. https://doi.org/10.1016/j.ridd.2015.10.017

Benzies, K. M., Magill-Evans, J. E., Hayden, K. A., & Ballantyne, M. 2013. Key components of early intervention programs for preterm and their parents: a systematic review and meta-analysis. *BMD Pregnancy & Childbirth* 13, 1–15. https://doi.org/10.1186/1471-2393-13-S1-S10

Bosch, L. 2011. Precursors to language in preterm infants: Speech perception abilities in the first year of life. *Progress in Brain Research* 189, 239–257. https://doi.org/10.1016/B978-0-444-53884-0.00028-2

Bozzette, M. 2007. A review of research on premature infant-mother interaction. *Newborn and Infant Nursing Reviews* 7, 49–55. https://doi.org/10.1053/j.nainr.2006.12.002

Brooks-Gunn, J., Liaw, F., & Klebanov, P. K. 1992. Effects of early intervention on cognitive function of low birth weight preterm infants. *Journal of Pediatrics* 120, 350–359. https://doi.org/10.1016/S0022-3476(05)80896-0

Caskey, M., Stephens, B., Tucker, R., & Vohr, B. 2014. Adult talk in the NICU with preterm infants and developmental outcomes. *Pediatrics* 133, 578–584. https://doi.org/10.1542/peds.2013-0104

Chaudhari, S., Otiv, M., Chitale, A., Pandit, A., & Hoge, M. 2004. Pune low birth weight study-cognitive abilities and educational performance at twelve years. *Indian Pediatrics* 41, 121–128.

D'Odorico, L., Majorano, M., Fasolo, M., Salerni, N., & Suttora, C. 2011. Characteristics of phonological development as a risk factor for language development in Italian-speaking pre-term children: A longitudinal study. *Clinical Linguistics & Phonetics* 25, 53–65. https://doi.org/10.3109/02699206.2010.511759

Dall'Oglio, A. M., Rossiello, B., Coletti, M. F., Bultrini, M., De Marchis, C., Ravà, L., Caselli, C., Paris, S., & Cuttini, M. 2010. Do healthy preterm children need neuropsychological follow-up? Preschool outcomes compared with term peers. *Developmental Medicine & Child Neurology* 52, 955–961. https://doi.org/10.1111/j.1469-8749.2010.03730.x

de Jong, M., Verhoeven, M., & van Baar, A. L. 2012. School outcome, cognitive functioning, and behaviour problems in moderate and late preterm children and adults: A review. *Seminars in Fetal & Neonatal Medicine* 17, 163–169. https://doi.org/10.1016/j.siny.2012.02.003

Feder, K. P., Majnemer, A., Bourbonnais, D., Platt, R., Blayney, M., & Synnes, A. 2005. Handwriting performance in preterm children compared with term peers at age 6 to 7 years. *Developmental Medicine and Child Neurology* 47, 163–170. https://doi.org/10.1017/S0012162205000307

Feldman, R., Rosenthal, Z., & Eidelman, A. I. 2014. Maternal-preterm skin-to-skin contact enhances child physiologic organization and cognitive control across the first 10 years of life. *Biological Psychiatry* 75, 56–64. https://doi.org/10.1016/j.biopsych.2013.08.012

Feldman, R., Weller, A., Sirota, L., & Eidelman, A. I. 2002. Skin-to-skin contact (kangaroo care) promotes self-regulation in premature infants: sleep-wake cyclicity, arousal modulation, and sustained exploration. *Developmental Psychology* 38, 194–207. https://doi.org/10.1037/0012-1649.38.2.194

Filippa, M., Devouche, E., Arioni, C., Imberty, M., & Gratier M. 2013. Live maternal speech and singing have beneficial effects on hospitalized preterm infants. *Acta Pediatrica, International Journal of Pediatrics* 102, 1017–1020. https://doi.org/10.1111/apa.12356.

Forcada-Guex, M., Pierrehumbert, B., Borghini, A., Moessinger, A., & Muller-Nix C. 2006. Early dyadic patterns of mother-infant interactions and outcomes of prematurity at 18 months. *Pediatrics* 118, 107–114. https://doi.org/10.1542/peds.2005-1145

Foster-Cohen, S., Edgin, J. O., Champion, P. R., & Woodward, L. J. 2007. Early delayed language development in very preterm infants: Evidence from the MacArthur-Bates CDI. *Journal of Child Language* 34, 655–675. https://doi.org/10.1017/S0305000907008070

Grunewaldt, K. H., Løhaugen, G. C. C., Austeng, D., Brubakk, A. M., & Skranes, J. 2013. Working memory training improves cognitive function in VLBW preschoolers. *Pediatrics* 131, e747–e754. https://doi.org/10.1542/peds.2012-1965

Guarini, A., Marini, A., Savini, S., Alessandroni, R., Faldella, G., & Sansavini, A. 2016. Linguistic features in children born very preterm at preschool age. *Developmental Medicine & Child Neurology* 58, 949–956. https://doi.org/10.1111/dmcn.13118

Guarini, A., & Sansavini, A. 2010. Sviluppo cognitivo e competenze linguistiche orali e scritte nei nati pretermine: Traiettorie evolutive a rischio o atipiche? *Psicologia Clinica dello Sviluppo* 14, 3–32. https://doi.org/10.1449/32002

Guarini, A., & Sansavini, A. 2012. Language, executive functions and short-term memory on literacy among very preterm infants: A longitudinal study. *Journal of Applied Psycholinguistics* 3, 67–81.

Guarini, A., Sansavini, A., Fabbri, C., Alessandroni, R., Faldella, G., & Karmiloff-Smith, A. 2009. Reconsidering the impact of preterm birth on language outcome. *Early Human Development* 85, 639–645. https://doi.org/10.1016/j.earlhumdev.2009.08.061

Guarini, A., Sansavini, A., Fabbri, C., Savini, S., Alessandroni, R., Faldella G., & Karmiloff-Smith, A. 2010. Long-term effects of preterm birth on language and literacy at eight years. *Journal of Child Language* 37, 865–885. https://doi.org/10.1017/S0305000909990109

Guzzetta, A., Baldini, S., Bancale, A., Baroncelli, L., Ciucci, F., Ghirri, P., Putignano, E., Sale, A., Viegi, A., Berardi, N., Boldrini, A., Cioni, G., & Maffei, L. 2009. Massage accelerates brain development and the maturation of visual function. *The Journal of Neuroscience* 29, 6042–6051. https://doi.org/10.1523/JNEUROSCI.5548-08.2009

Guzzetta, A., D'Acunto, M., Carotenuto, M., Berardi, N., Bancale, A., Biagioni, E., Boldrini, A., Ghirri, P., Maffei, L., & Cioni, G. 2011. The effects of preterm infant massage on brain electrical activity. *Developmental Medicine & Child Neurology* 53, 46–51. https://doi.org/10.1111/j.1469-8749.2011.04065.x

Jacobs, S. E., Sokol, J., & Ohlsson, A. 2002. The Newborn Individualized Developmental Care and Assessment Program is not supported by meta-analysis of the data. *Journal of Pediatrics* 140, 699–706. https://doi.org/10.1067/mpd.2002.123667

Johnson, S., Strauss, V., Gilmore, C., Jaekel, J., Marlow, N., & Wolke, D. 2016. Learning disabilities among extremely preterm children without neurosensory impairment: Comorbidity, neuropsychological profiles and scholastic outcomes. *Early Human Development* 103, 69–75. https://doi.org/10.1016/j.earlhumdev.2016.07.009

Johnson, S., Hennessy, E., Smith, R., Trikic, R., Wolke, D., & Marlow, N. 2009. Academic attainment and special educational needs in extremely preterm children at 11 years. The EPICure study. *Archives of Disease in Childhood-Fetal and Neonatal Edition* 94, 283–289. https://doi.org/10.1136/adc.2008.152793

Karmiloff-Smith, A. 1998. Development itself is the key to understanding developmental disorders. *Trends in Cognitive Science* 10, 389–398. https://doi.org/10.1016/S1364-6613(98)01230-3

Kovachy, V. N., Adams, J. N., Tamaresis, J. S., & Feldman, H. M. 2015. Reading abilities in school-aged preterm children: A review and meta-analysis. *Developmental Medicine & Child Neurology* 57, 410–419. https://doi.org/10.1111/dmcn.12652

Landry, S. H., Garner, P. W., Swank, P. R., & Baldwin, C. D. 1996. Effects of maternal scaffolding during joint toy play with preterm and full-term infants. *Merrill-Palmer Quarterly* 42, 177–199.

Litt, J. H., Taylor, N., & Hack, K. M. 2005. Learning disabilities in children with very low birthweight: Prevalence, neuropsychological correlates, and educational interventions. *Journal of Learning Disabilities* 38, 130–141. https://doi.org/10.1177/00222194050380020301

Loe, I. M., Lee, E. S., Luna, B., & Feldman, H. M. 2012. Executive function skills are associated with reading and parent-rated child function in children born prematurely. *Early Human Development* 88, 111–118. https://doi.org/10.1016/j.earlhumdev.2011.07.018

Luu, T. M., Vohr, B. R., Allan, W., Schneider, K. C., & Ment, L. R. 2011. Evidence for catch-up in cognition and receptive vocabulary among adolescents born very preterm. *Pediatrics* 128, 313–322. https://doi.org/10.1542/peds.2010-2655

March of Dimes, PMNCH, Save the Children, WHO. 2012. *Born too soon: The global action report on preterm birth*, edited by C. P. Howson, M. V. Kinney, & J. E. Lawn. Geneva: World Health Organization.

Marchman, V. A., Adams, K. A., Loi, E. C., Fernald, A., & Feldman, H. M. 2016. Early language processing efficiency predicts later receptive vocabulary outcomes in children born preterm. *Child Neuropsychology* 22, 649–665. https://doi.org/10.1080/09297049.2015.1038987

Ohlsson, A., & Jacobs, S. E. 2013. NIDCAP: A systematic review and meta-analyses of randomized controlled trials. *Pediatrics* 131, 881–893. https://doi.org/10.1542/peds.2012-2121

Peña, M., Pittaluga, E., & Mehler, J. 2010. Language acquisition in premature and full-term infants. *Proceedings of the National Academy of Sciences* 107, 3823–3828. https://doi.org/10.1073/pnas.0914326107

Pritchard, V. E., Clark, C. A. C., Liberty, K., Champion, P. R., Wilson, K., & Woodward, L. J. 2009. Early school based learning difficulties in children born very preterm. *Early Human Development* 85, 215–224. https://doi.org/10.1016/j.earlhumdev.2008.10.004

Putnick, D. L., Bornstein, M. H., Eryigit-Madzwamuse, S., & Wolke, D. 2016. Long-term stability of language performance in very preterm, moderate-late preterm, and term children. *The Journal of Pediatrics* 181, 74–79. https://doi.org/10.1016/j.jpeds.2016.09.006

Rose, S. A., Feldman, J. F., & Jankowski, J. J. 2011. Modelling a cascade of effects: The role of speed and executive functioning in preterm/ full-term differences in academic achievement. *Developmental Science* 14, 1161–1175. https://doi.org/10.1111/j.1467-7687.2011.01068.x

Ruff, H. A., McCarton, C., Kurtzberg, D., & Vaughan, H. G. 1984. Preterm infants' manipulative exploration of objects. *Child Development* 55, 1166–1173. https://doi.org/10.2307/1129985

Sansavini, A., Bello, A., Guarini, A., Savini, S., Alessandroni, R., Faldella, G., & Caselli, M. C. 2015. Noun and predicate comprehension/production and gestures in extremely preterm children at two years of age: Are they delayed? *Journal of Communication Disorders* 58, 126–142. https://doi.org/10.1016/j.jcomdis.2015.06.010

Sansavini, A., & Faldella, G. 2013. (a cura di), *Lo sviluppo dei bambini nati pretermine. Aspetti neuropsicologici, metodi di valutazione e interventi*. Milano: Franco Angeli.

Sansavini, A., Guarini, A., Alessandroni, R., Faldella, G., Giovanelli, G., & Salvioli. G. P. 2007. Are early grammatical and phonological working memory abilities affected by preterm birth? *Journal of Communication Disorders* 40, 239–256. https://doi.org/10.1016/j.jcomdis.2006.06.009

Sansavini, A., Guarini, A., & Caselli, M. C. 2011. Preterm birth: Neuropsychological profiles and atypical developmental pathways. *Developmental Disabilities Research Reviews* 17, 102–113. https://doi.org/10.1002/ddrr.1105

Sansavini, A., Guarini, A., Justice, L. M., Savini, S., Broccoli, S., Alessandroni, R., & Faldella, G. 2010. Does preterm birth increase a child's risk for language impairment? *Early Human Development* 86, 765–772. https://doi.org/10.1016/j.earlhumdev.2010.08.014

Sansavini, A., Guarini, A., Savini, S., Broccoli, S., Justice, L. M., Alessandroni, R., & Faldella, G. 2011. Longitudinal trajectories of gestural and linguistic abilities in very preterm infants in the second year of life. *Neuropsychologia* 49, 3677–3688. https://doi.org/10.1016/j.neuropsychologia.2011.09.023

Sansavini A., Guarini, A., Savini, S., Alessandroni, R., & Faldella, G. 2017. Sviluppo e ritardi della comunicazione, del linguaggio e della letto-scrittura nei bambini nati pretermine. In F. Ferrari (a cura di), *Il neonato pretermine: Disordini dello sviluppo e interventi precoci*. Milano: Franco Angeli.

Sansavini, A., Pentimonti, J., Justice, L. M., Guarini, A., Savini, S., Alessandroni, R., & Faldella, G. 2014. Language, motor and cognitive development of extremely preterm children: Modeling individual growth trajectories over the first three years of life. *Journal of Communication Disorders* 49, 55–68. https://doi.org/10.1016/j.jcomdis.2014.02.005

Sansavini, A., Savini, S., Guarini, A., Broccoli, S., Justice, L., Alessandroni, R., & Faldella, G. 2011. The effect of gestational age on developmental outcomes: A longitudinal study in the first two years of life. *Child Care Health Development* 37, 26–36. https://doi.org/10.1111/j.1365-2214.2010.01143.x

Sansavini, A., Zavagli, V., Guarini, A., Savini, S., Alessandroni, R., & Faldella G. 2015. Dyadic co-regulation, affective intensity and infant's development at 12 months: A comparison among extremely preterm and full-term dyads. *Infant Behavior and Development* 40, 29–40. https://doi.org/10.1016/j.infbeh.2015.03.005

Spittle, A., Orton, J., Anderson, P. J., Boyd, R., & Doyle, L. W. 2015. Early developmental intervention programs provided post hospital discharge to prevent motor and cognitive impairment in preterm infants (Review). *Cochrane Database of Systematic Reviews* 11, 1–72. https://doi.org/10.1002/14651858.CD005495.pub4.

Stolt, S., Haataja, L., Lapinleimu, H., & Lehtonen, L. 2009. The early lexical development and its predictive value to language skills at two years in very-low-birth-weight children. *Journal of Communication Disorders* 42, 107–123. https://doi.org/10.1016/j.jcomdis.2008.10.002

Stolt, S., Makila, A. M., Matomaki, J., Lehtonen, L., Lapinleimu, H., & Haataja, L. 2014. The development and predictive value of gestures in very-low-birth- weight children: A longitudinal study. *International Journal of Speech and Language Pathology* 16, 121–131. https://doi.org/10.3109/17549507.2013.794861

Stolt, S., Savini, S., Guarini, A., Caselli, M. C., Matomaki, J., Lapinleimu, H., Haataja, L., Lehtonen, L., Alessandroni, R., Faldella, G., & Sansavini, A. 2017. Does the native language influence lexical composition in very preterm children at the age of two years? A cross-linguistic comparison study of Italian and Finnish children. *First Language* 37, 368–390. https://doi.org/10.1177/0142723717698006

Taylor, H. G., Klein, N., Minich, N. M., & Hack, M. 2000. Middle school age outcomes in children with very low birthweight. *Child Development* 71, 1495–1511. https://doi.org/10.1111/1467-8624.00242

Tideman, E. 2000. Longitudinal follow-up of children born preterm: Cognitive development at age 19. *Early Human Development* 58, 81–90. https://doi.org/10.1016/S0378-3782(00)00055-4

van Noort-van der Spek, I. L., Franken, M. C., & Weisglas-Kuperus, N. 2012. Language functions in preterm-born children: A systematic review and meta-analysis. *Pediatrics* 129, 745–754. https://doi.org/10.1542/peds.2011-1728

Vanderveen, J. A., Bassler, D., Robertson, C. M., & Kirpalani, H. 2009. Early intervention involving parents to improve neurodevelopmental outcomes of premature infants: A meta-analysis. *Journal of Perinatology* 29, 343–351. https://doi.org/10.1038/jp.2008.229

Vohr, B. 2014. Speech and language outcomes of very preterm infants. *Seminars in Fetal and Neonatal Medicine* 19, 78–83. https://doi.org/10.1016/j.siny.2013.10.007

Volpe, J. J. 2009. Brain injury in premature infants: A complex amalgam of destructive and developmental disturbances. *Lancet Neurology* 8, 110–124. https://doi.org/10.1016/S1474-4422(08)70294-1

Westermann, G., Mareschal, D., Johnson, M. H., Sirois, S., Spratling, M. W., & Thomas, M. S. C. 2007. Neurocostructivism. *Developmental Science* 10, 75–83. https://doi.org/10.1111/j.1467-7687.2007.00567.x

Wolke, D., & Meyer, R. 1999. Cognitive status, language attainment, and prereading skills of 6-year-old very preterm children and their peers: The Bavarian Longitudinal Study. *Developmental Medicine & Child Neurology* 41, 94–109. https://doi.org/10.1017/S0012162299000201

Woodward, L. J., Moor, S., Hood, K. M., Champion, P. R., Foster-Cohen, S., Inder, T., & Austin, N. C. 2009. Very preterm children show impairments across multiple neurodevelopmental domains by age 4 years. *Archives of Disease in Childhood. Fetal & Neonatal Edition* 94, 339–344. https://doi.org/10.1136/adc.2008.146282

Zoccolotti, P., De Luca, M., Di Pace, E., Judica, A., Orlandi, M., & Spinelli, D. 1999. Markers of developmental surface dyslexia in a language (Italian) with high grapheme–phoneme correspondence. *Applied Psycholinguistics* 20, 191–216. https://doi.org/10.1017/S0142716499002027

Zuccarini, M., Guarini, A., Savini, S., Iverson, J. M., Aureli, T., Alessandroni, R., Faldella, G., & Sansavini, A. 2017. Object exploration in extremely preterm infants between 6 and 9 months and relation to cognitive and language development at 24 months. *Research in Developmental Disabilities* 68, 140–152. https://doi.org/10.1016/j.ridd.2017.06.002

Zuccarini, M., Sansavini, A., Iverson, J. M., Savini, S., Guarini, A., Alessandroni, R., Faldella, G., & Aureli, T. 2016. Object engagement and manipulation in extremely preterm and full term infants at 6 months of age. *Research in Developmental Disabilities* 55, 173–184. https://doi.org/10.1016/j.ridd.2016.04.001

Zuccarini, M., Guarini, A., Iverson, J. M., Benassi, E., Savini, S., Alessandroni, R., Faldella, G., & Sansavini, A. 2018. Does early object exploration support gesture and language development in extremely preterm and full-term infants? *Journal of Communication Disorders*, 76, 91–100. https://doi.org/10.1016/j.jcomdis.2018.09.004

Prematurity, executive functions and language

A study with low risk preterm children

Miguel Pérez-Pereira,[1] Manuel Peralbo[2] and Alberto Veleiro[2]
[1]University of Santiago de Compostela / [2]University of A Coruña

This chapter aims to compare language development and executive functions (EFs) in healthy preterm (PT) and full-term (FT) children, and to explore the influence of EFs and other factors on language abilities. One group of 111 low-risk PT children and another group of 34 FT children were followed from 4 to 5 years of age, and predictors of language abilities were analysed. The PT children in our study did not obtain significantly lower results than the FT children in any EF task. Cognitive score was the main predictor of linguistic results. EFs, verbal memory and non-verbal working memory in particular, had a moderately significant effect on morphosyntactic production and on grammar understanding. The results seem to reinforce the declarative/procedural model.

Keywords: preterm children, executive functions, language development, predictive factors, dual models

Introduction

In this chapter, we will study the performance of low-risk preterm (PT) children with different gestational ages and a group of full-term children in different executive functions (EFs; working memory and inhibitory control) and language abilities. The effect of different predictive factors on language performance (with special attention to EFs) is also studied in relation to dual models of language processing (Ullman, 2001). Ullman (2001) proposes that different processing mechanisms (procedural memory versus declarative memory) are responsible for the learning of different language abilities (rule governed -syntax, regular morphology- versus more item based -vocabulary, irregular verbs-, respectively). Procedural memory and EFs are rooted in the same cerebral areas, and therefore syntax and regular morphology are supposed to be more affected by EFs than vocabulary learning.

https://doi.org/10.1075/z.223.03per

Executive functions (EFs) include a series of processes which underlie planned and conscious goal directed behaviour, responses to novel or difficult situations, and also the capacity of inhibition of behaviours which distract us from the goal. Thus, EFs are related to what is needed to get a purposeful control of thought, emotions and actions. EFs are self-regulated high order cognitive processes, which help in the supervision and control of thought and action. These abilities include inhibitory control, working memory (WM), attention control, cognitive flexibility and behaviour supervision (Miyake, Friedman, Emerson, Witzki, & Howerter, 2000).

The prefrontal cortex seems to be involved in executive control, although other non-frontal areas, such as the basal ganglia, also have an important role (Carlson, 2005). Different regions of the prefrontal cortex seem to be involved in the functioning of different EFs. For instance, the dorsolateral prefrontal cortex is involved in working memory, and the ventromedial region in inhibitory control (Nigg, 2006).

Research on EFs has also focused on atypical populations, such as preterm children. Although the studies carried out on the topic vary greatly in methods, PT children show deficits in EFs such as inhibitory control, working memory, verbal fluency, planning, switching and attention when compared to full term children (Anderson & Doyle, 2004; Bohm, Smedler, & Forssberg, 2004; Mulder, Pitchford, Hagger, & Marlow 2009), even after controlling for IQ and maternal education, or excluding those PT children with neurosensory impairments (Aarnoudse-Moens, Smidts, Oosterlaan, Duivenvoorden, & Weisglas-Kuperus, 2009).

According to the model of WM proposed by Gathercole and Baddeley (1990), the phonological loop predicts linguistic abilities such as vocabulary size and the sentence length (Adams & Gathercole, 1995, 1996; Archibald & Gathercole, 2007; Gathercole, Service, Hitch, Adams, & Martin, 1999). Although the relationship between the phonological loop and linguistic abilities decreases with age, the relationships between working memory, vocabulary acquisition and language processing still continues throughout time (Gathercole, 2007; Montgomery, 2003).

Working memory (WM) has been found to be worse in PT children than in FT children from early age to adolescence (Lowe, MacLean, Shaffer, & Watterberg, 2009; Luu, Ment, Allan, Schneider, & Vohr, 2011; Saavalainen et al., 2007; Woodward, Edgin, Thompson, & Inder, 2005). Sansavini and colleagues (Sansavini, Guarini, Alessandroni, Faldella, Giovanelli, & Salvioli, 2007) found that very preterm children (Gestational age (GA) ≤ 33 weeks) without severe deficits obtained lower results than the comparison group of FT children in phonological working memory, as well as in grammatical and cognitive abilities, at 3;6 years of age. Recently, Hodel, Senich, Jokinen, Sasson, Morris and Thomas (2017) found that moderately preterm babies of 9 months of age demonstrated poorer memory (but not complex attention and inhibition) than FT children.

The difficulties of PT children in working memory are higher when the complexity of the task increases (Baron Kerns, Müller, Ahronovich, & Litman, 2012), when the gestational age is lower, and when the risk of neonatal damage is high (Beauchamp et al., 2008, Luciana, Lindeke, Georgief, Mills, & Nelson, 1999; Woodward, Clark, Bora, & Inder, 2012). These deficits in working memory in PT children were found not only in studies using experimental tasks, but also in studies using rating scales (Ritter, Nelle, Perrig, Steinlin, & Everts, 2014; Scott et al., 2012).

In relation to inhibitory control, several studies indicate that differences between very preterm children and FT children are higher at preschool age than at school age, although these differences continue at this later age (Aarnoudse-Moens, Duivenvoorden, Weisglas-Kuperus, Van Goudoever, and Oosterlaan, 2012; Mulder, Pitchford, & Marlow, 2011). Other studies (Baron et al., 2012) found that extremely low birth weight children performed worse than term-born on working memory and inhibition tasks at 3 years of age. Additionally, late-preterm children (GA between 34–36 weeks) performed worse compared with FT on measures of complex working memory but this did not occur when considering inhibition measures (Baron et al., 2012).

Although a few exceptions exist (Hodel et al., 2017), most of these studies on EFs in PT children were carried out with very or extremely preterm children. It is still necessary, however, to see if these difficulties in language skills or in EFs exist at a preschool age when the PT children studied are not at risk, that is, if they do not have additional severe biomedical problems and are not extremely preterm children.

In relation to language development, most research carried out with extremely or very preterm children, who constitute 20% of all the PT children, has found that these children show lower results in receptive and expressive language in comparison to FT children (Barre, Morgan, Doyle, & Foster-Cohen, 2011; Friesen, Champion, & Woodward, 2010; Howard et al., 2011; Luoma, Herrgard, Martikainen, & Ahonen, 1998; Mikkola et al., 2005, van Noort-van der Spek, Franken, & Weisglas-Kuperus, 2012). The results of studies carried out with samples of PT children of a wider spectrum or with a GA above 31 weeks have found, however, different results, and in many cases no significant differences have been found between PT and FT children (Cattani et al., 2010; Menyuk, Liebergott, Schultz, Chesnick & Ferrier, 1991; Pérez-Pereira, Fernández, Gómez-Taibo, & Resches, 2014; Pérez-Pereira & Cruz, 2018; Sansavini, Guarini, Alessandroni, Faldella, Giovanelli, & Salvioli, 2006).

Evidence exists that there is a link between executive functions and language development in typically developing young children (Bohlmann, Maier, & Palacios, 2015; Fuhs & Day, 2011; Weiland, Barata, & Yoshikawa, 2014). The effects of EFs on language vary depending on the linguistic ability studied and the EF dimension studied as well as on the demands of the working memory (Adams, 1996) or the inhibitory control tasks (Fuhs & Day, 2011). For instance, syntactic abilities seem to be related to attention, memory, inhibition and flexibility (Taylor, 2002), and past formation and irregular verbs were found to be related to inhibitory control (Ibbotson & Kearvell-White, 2015). White, Alexander and Greenfield (2017), who studied a sample of children attending Head Start, found a clear relationship between EF, vocabulary and syntax, and language learning.

Different studies claimed that the combination of deficits in working memory and inhibition affect the capacity of processing language (Marton, Kelmenson, & Pinkhasova, 2007; Marton, Campanelli, Eichorn, Scheuer, & Yoon, 2014), particularly when working memory tasks involve simultaneous processing (Im-Bolter, Johnson, & Pascual-Leone, 2006). Additional evidence in favor of the relationship between EFs and language has to do with the fact that preschool children with specific language impairment show deficits in EFs (D'Odorico, Assanelli, Franco, & Jacob, 2007; Roello, Ferretti, Colonnello, & Levi, 2015; Vugs, Hendriks, Cuperus, & Verhoeven, 2014; Vissers, Koolen, Hermans, Schepper, & Knoors, 2015).

Very scarce studies have been carried out to study the relationships between EFs and language development in preterm children. Sansavini et al. (2007) found a close relationship between phonological working memory and grammar in both very preterm and FT children at 3;6 years of age. Guarini and Sansavini (2012) found that language (vocabulary, grammar, and phonological awareness) and short-term verbal memory had a predictive role on literacy for very preterm and FT children. Pérez-Pereira, Peralbo, and Veleiro (2017) found that verbal memory and inhibition have a moderate predictive effect on understanding grammar, while non-verbal working memory has an effect on morphosyntactic production for low risk PT and FT children.

There are a series of factors that were found to affect the performance in EFs and language. Several studies found an effect of maternal education level on EF abilities (Sansavini et al., 2007; Aarnoudse-Moens et al., 2009), with children who have mothers with higher education performing better in EF tests. Gestational age and birth weight (BW) were also found to have an effect on the performance of executive function tasks (Baron et al., 2012; Duvall, Erickson, MacLean, & Lowe, 2015; Mulder et al., 2009) and language development (Foster-Cohen, Edgin, Champion, & Woodward, 2007; Kern & Gayraud, 2007). Children with low GA or/and BW (very preterm or extremely preterm) tend to have lower performance than children with higher GA or/and BW or FT children. PT children with brain injury, which is highly associated with very low BW or/and GA, also have more difficulties in EF (Woodward et al., 2005, 2012). Gender has also been found to affect neurodevelopmental outcomes of PT children (Aylward, 2005), with boys presenting more difficulties than girls. The effect of these variables will also be taken into consideration in the present research.

In contrast to Gathercole and Baddeley's model (Gathercole & Baddeley, 1990), dual models of language, such as the declarative/procedural model (Ullman, 2001), state that the mental lexicon and the learning of irregular verbs depend on declarative memory, which is rooted in the temporal lobe, whereas the rule-governed combination of words by the mental grammar and the learning of regular pasts involves procedural memory, which is rooted in the frontal cortex and basal ganglia (Ullman, 2001). Therefore, performance differences in executive functions, linked to prefrontal cortex areas, should affect certain linguistic abilities, such as grammar processing, but not on others, such as vocabulary. It is possible, however, that with time alternative neural pathways have a compensatory effect on the functioning of EFs (Réveillon et al., 2015).

In the present study, the results will be discussed from the viewpoint of the declarative/procedural model.

The aims of the study are:

1. To study receptive and expressive language abilities of one group of low-risk PT children and another group of FT children at 5 years of age.
2. To relate their language skills to some executive functions assessed at 4 and 5 years of age.
3. At the same time, other variables (cognition and quality of home environment) have also been studied to control their possible effect.

According to the declarative/procedural model, we expect that receptive and expressive grammatical abilities will be more dependent on EFs than vocabulary comprehension.

Method

Participants

The participants form part of a longitudinal sample of children who have been followed since birth. The children were assessed when they were 4 years and 5 years old (± 1 month). At 4 years of age, there were 111 preterm children and 34 full-term children. At 5 years of age, there were 109 preterm and 33 full-term children.

The PT children had a mean GA of 32.6 weeks (*SD* = 2.5) and a mean BW of 1712 grams (*SD* = 428). The FT children had a mean GA of 39.8 weeks (*SD* = 1.5) and a mean BW of 3377 grams (*SD* = 443).

The PT and FT groups did not differ in terms of mother's education (X^2 (1) = 8.66, $p = .194$), gender (X^2 (1) = .000, $p = .997$) and Apgar score (t (197) = −.909, $p = .365$). The PT and FT groups lived in similar sociolinguistic conditions. For the comparison of mother's education, the children's mothers were put into three groups: (1) Basic education, (2) High school and professional training, and (3) University degree.

A series of exclusion/inclusion criteria were used to select the group of PT children. Those children with the following characteristics were not included: cerebral palsy, periventricular leukomalacia (PVL), intraventricular hemorrhage (IVH) greater than grade II, hydrocephalus, encephalopathy, genetic malformations, chromosomal syndromes and metabolic syndromes associated with mental retardation, important motor or sensory (vision or hearing) impairments, or Apgar scores below 6 at 5 minutes. This circumstance makes the group of PT children a low-risk group.

The full-term children could be considered as a typically developing group.

For the ANOVA analyses, the children were sorted into 4 GA groups (Blencowe et al., 2013):

1. PT children with GA equal or lower than 31 weeks (VPR and EPR children). There were 36 and 35 children in this group at 4 and 5 years of age, respectively.
2. PT children with GAs of 32 or 33 weeks. There were 33 and 32 children in this group at 4 and 5 years of age, respectively.
3. PT children with GAs between 34 and 36 weeks. There were 42 children at 4 and 5 years of age
4. FT children with GA equal to or higher than 37 weeks. This group was formed by 34 and 33 children at 4 and 5 years of age, respectively.

Instruments

The following instruments were used to assess language skills.

The Spanish version of the Peabody Picture Vocabulary Test (Dunn, Dunn, & Arribas, 2005) was used to assess vocabulary comprehension.

The test *Comprensión de Estructuras Gramaticales* (CEG; Mendoza, Carballo, Muñoz, & Fresneda, 2005), similar to the well known TROG (Test of Reception of Grammar; Bishop, 2003), was used to assess the comprehension of syntactic structures.

The production subscale of the *Test de Morfo-sintaxis* de Aguado (TSA; Aguado, 1999) was used to assess morphological and syntactic production skills.

The following instruments were used to assess the executive functions:

The verbal working memory task (*memoria secuencial auditiva*) which forms part of the EDAF (*Evaluación de la Discriminación Auditiva y Fonológica*; Brancal, Alcantud, Ferrer, & Quiroga, 2005). The child has to repeat a sequence of words, which progressively increases in number.

The CORSI ordering task (Kessels, van Zandvoort, Postma, Kappelle, & de Haan, 2000; Farrell-Pagulayan, Busch, Medina, Bartok, & Krikorian, 2006) assessed non-verbal working memory. Colored blocks are highlighted in a given sequence. The children must repeat the sequence. The total raw score and the memory span score were used for the analysis.

The go/no-go task (Rueda et al., 2004) explored sustained attention and inhibitory control. The child is told to respond by pressing a key every time that a certain stimulus is presented (go stimulus) and to withhold the response in those trials where an alternative stimulus (no-go) appears. The total number of correct responses as well as the reaction time (RT), and the number of errors committed (no-go trials in which a response was produced) were used.

Also, other tests were used to measure other possible predictive factors.

The Spanish version (Moreno, 1992) of the HOME scale (Observation for Measurement of the Environment-Revised edition: Caldwell & Bradley, 1984) explored the quality of home environment. The total score was used in the analyses.

The Spanish version of the Batelle Developmental Inventory (BDI) (Newborg, Stock, & Wnek, 1996) was applied to assess cognitive development.

Procedure

The children were assessed in their homes by a trained psychologist. The HOME scale and the verbal working memory task (EDAF) were administered when the children were 4 years of age (± 1 month). The remaining tests to assess language abilities, executive functions and cognitive abilities were administered when the children were 5 years old (± 1 month). Approval by the Galician Ethics Committee of Clinical Research and parents' consent were obtained before the beginning of the investigation.

Analyses performed

One factor ANOVA was performed to compare the results obtained by the different GA groups in the different tasks applied, and controlling for cognitive development (BDI score) when necessary.

Three linear regression analyses were performed to identify those factors which could act as predictors of language abilities. The dependent variables (DV) were, in turn, (1) The raw scores obtained in vocabulary comprehension (Peabody), (2) the scores obtained in grammar understanding (CEG), and (3) the scores obtained in morpho-syntactic production (TSA). The effect of several independent variables was tested in 3 models. In Model 1, gender, gestational age in weeks (numerical variable), the quality of the home environment (HOME score) and the cognitive score of the BDI were included. In Model 2 the score obtained in the verbal working memory task (EDAF), the total score in the CORSI (non-verbal working memory), and the memory span score obtained in the CORSI were added. Finally, in Model 3 the total number of correct responses as well as the reaction time (RT), and the number of errors committed in the Go/no-go task (sustained attention and inhibitory control) were added.

Birth weight was not included as independent variable because BW and GA measures were very highly correlated. Therefore, the use of BW for the analysis would be redundant.

Results

Table 1 shows the results obtained by the different GA groups (mean and standard deviation) in the tasks administered, as well as the results of the ANOVA. As can be observed, there were no significant differences in any measure, except at comprehension of syntactic structures (CEG). When we controlled for cognition and the Batelle's cognitive raw score was introduced as a co-variable, no significant difference was found in the ANOVA among the four GA groups, even in the results obtained in the CEG ($F = 2.35$, $p = .075$, $\eta^2 = .050$).

The results of the linear regression analysis for vocabulary comprehension as DV are shown in Table 2.

The results indicate that the variables introduced in Model 1 have a significant effect on vocabulary comprehension, and explain .172 of the variance. Cognitive development is the only variable which has a single significant effect on vocabulary comprehension. When memory variables (verbal memory, CORSI total score and CORSI memory span) are introduced in Model 2, the variance explained increases .035 (change in R^2), and the variance explained reaches .207. Obviously, Model 2 has a significant effect, although the change in F is not significant. Cognitive development is the only variable with a single significant effect. The variables added in Model 3 (go/no-go accuracy, the reaction time at correct responses, and go/no-go errors) hardly increment the variance explained on vocabulary comprehension (change in $R^2 = .001$) at all.

Table 1. Mean (standard deviation) and ANOVA comparisons for the different tasks

	GA Group Mean (SD)				*F*	df	Sig	Partial Eta Squared
	≤31	32–33	34–36	≥37				
N*	35	32	42	33				
Peabody	56.26 (13.07)	57.00 (12.11)	57.86 (11.42)	62.00 (12.59)	1.46	3, 138	.23	.03
CEG	48.65 (13.48)	47.13 (9.16)	44.40 (13.88)	52.06 (7.33)	2.80	3, 136	.04	.06
TSA production	39.71 (15.99)	41.55 (11.29)	38.41 (15.86)	43.59 (8.17)	.98	3, 134	.40	.02
Cognitive score BDI	84.48 (8.54)	85.58 (5.34)	82.40 (15.64)	85.91 (3.17)	.94	3,135	.41	.02
HOME scale	48.14 (3.35)	49.12 (3.87)	49.40 (3.48)	49.97 (2.46)	1.86	3,141	.13	.04
CORSI Total score	10.50 (7.42)	9.25 (8.30)	11.78 (8.48)	10.65 (7.61)	.54	3, 124	.66	.01
CORSI Memory Span	2.53 (.90)	2.39 (.94)	2.68 (.96)	2.65 (.80)	.62	3, 124	.60	.01
Verbal memory	5.41 (2.36)	5.28 (2.79)	5.98 (2.51)	5.79 (2.54)	.59	3, 138	.63	.01
Go/Nogo (Accuracy)	73.10 (11.34)	68.81 (12.17)	73.53 (10.55)	70.39 (18.17)	.87	3, 125	.46	.02
Go/Nogo (Errors)	26.90 (11.34)	35.04 (24.39)	26.48 (10.55)	26.58 (13.90)	2.10	3, 125	.10	.05
Go/Nogo RT (msecs)	730.84 (200.11)	730.15 (181.79)	788.43 (124.33)	754.82 (209.28)	.82	3, 125	.49	.02

* N is offered for the tasks administered at 5 years of age. The HOME scale and the verbal memory task were administered when the children were 4 years old and, at this age, there was one more child in each GA group, except in the GA group 34–36, in which there were 42 children as well.
CEG: Raw score obtained in the test Comprensión de Estructuras Gramaticales (grammar comprehension)
TSA production: Raw score obtained in the production section of the Test de Sintaxis de Aguado (morphosyntax production).
Cognitive score BDI: Raw score in the cognitive scale of the Batelle Developmental Inventories (BDI)
Go/Nogo RT: reaction time in milliseconds obtained in the Go/Nogo task.

Table 2. Linear regression analysis: Predictors of vocabulary comprehension

Predictors of vocabulary comprehension	Standardized β	Sig.	R^2	Change in R^2	Change in F	Signif. change in F	F	df	p
Model 1			.172	.172	5.346	.001	5.346	4,103	.001
Gender	–.107	.244							
GA	.141	.119							
BDI Cognitive score	.388	.000							
HOME score	.016	.864							
Model 2			.207	.035	1.471	.227	3.727	3,100	.001
Gender	–.100	.278							
GA	.150	.099							
BDI Cognitive score	.364	.000							
HOME score	–.001	.988							
Verbal memory	.181	.060							
CORSI total score	.185	.366							
CORSI memory span	–.191	.368							
Model 3			.208	.001	.029	.575	2.541	3,97	.009
Gender	–.101	.289							
GA	.148	.113							
BDI Cognitive score	.367	.000							
HOME score	.000	.996							
Verbal memory	.181	.066							
CORSI total score	.187	.374							
CORSI memory span	–.185	.395							
Go/no-go errors	.032	.838							
Go/no-go accuracy	.002	.990							
RT accuracy Go/no-go	.009	.930							

About grammar understanding, the results of the regression analysis show that the variables introduced in Model 1 explained .165 of the variance of grammar understanding (see Table 3). Again, cognitive development is the only variable which has a single significant effect. Model 1 has a significant effect on grammar understanding. When memory variables are added in Model 2, the variance explained reaches .261 (change in R^2 = .096), and change in F (.096) is significant (p = .006). The variables which have a single significant effect in Model 2 (standardised β)

Table 3. Linear regression analysis: Predictors of grammar understanding

Predictors of grammar understanding	Standardized β	Sig.	R^2	Change in R^2	Change in F	Signif. change in F	F	df	p
Model 1			.165	.165	5.079	.001	5.079	4,103	.001
Gender	.151	.104							
GA	.116	.204							
BDI Cognitive score	.345	.000							
HOME score	–.035	.703							
Model 2			.261	.096	4.332	.006	5.041	3,100	.000
Gender	.149	.098							
GA	.100	.251							
BDI Cognitive score	.273	.004							
HOME score	–.068	.442							
Verbal memory	.288	.002							
CORSI total score	–.236	.232							
CORSI memory span	.243	.237							
Model 3			.288	.027	1.221	.306	3.918	3,97	.000
Gender	.143	.238							
GA	.104	.238							
BDI Cognitive score	.255	.007							
HOME score	–.074	.404							
Verbal memory	.294	.002							
CORSI total score	–.233	.242							
CORSI memory span	.196	.343							
Go/no-go errors	–228	.124							
Go/no-go accuracy	–.071	.640							
RT accuracy Go/no-go	–.014	.884							

are cognitive development and verbal memory. The increment of the variance explained when the Go/no-go variables are added in Model 3 is very reduced (change in $R^2 = .027$), and change in F is not significant.

About morphosyntactic production, the regression analysis shows that the variables introduced in Model 1 have a significant effect on this dependent variable, and explain .244 of the variance in the TSA score (see Table 4). In addition to cognitive development, the quality of the home environment (HOME scale score)

Table 4. Linear regression analysis: Predictors of morphosyntactic production

Predictors of morphosyntactic production	Standardized β	Sig.	R^2	Change in R^2	Change in F	Signif. change in F	F	df	p
Model 1			.244	.244	8.232	.000	8.232	4,102	.000
Gender	.080	.365							
GA	.072	.404							
BDI Cognitive score	.432	.000							
HOME score	–.222	.013							
Model 2			.329	.085	4.204	.008	6.949	3,99	.000
Gender	.062	.467							
GA	.048	.567							
BDI Cognitive score	.344	.000							
HOME score	–.252	.004							
Verbal memory	.168	.059							
CORSI total score	–.395	.038							
CORSI memory span	.494	.013							
Model 3			.350	.021	1.034	.381	5.179	3,96	.000
Gender	.048	.575							
GA	.031	.717							
BDI Cognitive score	.347	.000							
HOME score	–.254	.004							
Verbal memory	.168	.060							
CORSI total score	–.356	.065							
CORSI memory span	.498	.013							
Go/no-go errors	.098	.488							
Go/no-go accuracy	–.052	.720							
RT accuracy Go/no-go	.137	.146							

also has a significant effect (standardized β $p = .013$)). When the memory variables are introduced in Model 2, the variance explained ascends up to .329 (change in $R^2 = .082$), and change in F reaches significance ($p = .008$). The variables which have a single significant effect on morphosyntactic production are cognitive development, the HOME score, CORSI total score and CORSI memory span. Verbal memory shows a trend ($p = .059$). The addition of the measures taken in the go/no-go task (sustained attention and inhibitory control) in Model 3 increments the variance explained only by .021 (change in R^2), and the total variance explained reaches .350. Change in F does not reach significance.

Discussion

There was no significant difference between the four GA groups in vocabulary comprehension (Peabody Vocabulary Test), comprehension of grammar (CEG) and in morphosyntactic production (TSA). Therefore, the results we found with low-risk PT children differ from those found in other studies with extremely preterm or very preterm children (Foster-Cohen et al., 2010; Howard et al., 2011; Luoma et al., 1998; Mikkola et al., 2005; Noort-van der Spek, Franken, & Weisglas-Kuperus, 2012; Sansavini et al., 2007).

No differences were found in verbal memory, non-verbal working memory or inhibition, which contrasts with the results obtained by other studies carried out with extremely preterm or very preterm children (Aarnoudse-Moens et al., 2009; Baron et al., 2012; Böhm, Smedler, & Forssberg, 2004; Marlow, Hennessy, Bracewell, & Wolke, 2007; Ni, Huang, & Guo, 2011; Lowe et al., 2009; Woodward et al., 2005, Sansavini et al., 2007). These results indicate that EF and language development of low-risk PT children are not so affected as is the case with extremely or very preterm children.

Differences in the sample characteristics may be responsible for the differences found in language, EFs and cognition. When additional handicaps are excluded, preterm birth does not seem to have such dramatic consequences on development. Also, the samples of the majority of previous studies were composed of very or extremely preterm children, who have a higher probability of suffering additional problems (which not always were excluded or under control).

The results of the linear regression analyses indicate that gestational age did not have any significant effect on the linguistic results obtained by the children. This is in contrast to the results obtained in other studies with very preterm or extremely preterm children (Foster Cohen et al., 2010).

Vocabulary comprehension seems to be mainly determined by general cognitive abilities, and the role of EF is minimal. In contrast, verbal memory ability has a strong predictive effect on the comprehension of grammar structures (Sansavini et al., 2007). To have a good score on the test of comprehension of grammar (CEG), the child needs to retain elements of the syntactic structure to understand its meaning.

Similarly, EFs also have a significant effect on morphosyntactic production. The memory processes, which play a more important role in the production of morphosyntax, are of a nonverbal type (CORSI), probably more linked to general working memory processes. These results give support to the potential importance of working memory processes for the active comprehension and production of language (Gathercole & Baddeley, 1990). In a more interesting way these results seem to give support to the declarative/procedural model (Ullman, 2001), which predicts that vocabulary abilities depend on declarative memory, which is rooted in the temporal lobe, whereas the rule-governed grammar understanding and production involves procedural memory, which is rooted in the frontal cortex and basal ganglia, the same areas which are involved in the functioning of executive functions. The fact that EFs play a role in the prediction of grammar understanding and morphosyntactic production, but not in the prediction of vocabulary comprehension, seems to give support to the declarative/procedural model.

On the other hand, the fact that cognitive ability has an important effect on the prediction of all the linguistic abilities explored (vocabulary comprehension, grammar understanding and production) points to the effect of general processing resources on language abilities (Im-Bolter, Johnson, & Pascual-Leone, 2006; Marton, Kelmenson, & Pinkhasova, 2007; Vugs et al., 2014).

Inhibitory control and sustained attention do not seem to have a significant effect on language performance.

The quality of the home environment has a significant effect only on morphosyntactic production. However, its effect is paradoxical, since the standardised β value is negative, which means that children from high-quality homes get low results in the TSA, and those children from low-quality homes get high results in the TSA. In any case, this result has to be taken with caution since the mean results in the HOME scale (see Table 1) were located in the 1st quartile, and the variance was low, which means that the quality of home environments was high in general terms and that the differences in the HOME scale were reduced.

Conclusions

The present paper indicates that low risk PT children do not have poorer scores than FT children in cognition, in any of the EFs analysed, or in language. These results are a good counterbalance to previous studies carried out with higher risk PT children, and highlight that the population of PT children cannot be considered as a homogeneous group.

The most interesting result, in our view, is that EFs play a relevant role in language development, although their effects vary depending on the dimension of language studied. The effect of certain EFs on grammar comprehension and production does not diminish the important role that general cognitive skills have in the prediction of language skills.

Our results seem to support the distinction between declarative and procedural processes. It would be necessary to study other EFs and other linguistic abilities to reinforce this model.

References

Aarnoudse-Moens, C. S. H., Smidts, D. P., Oosterlaan, J., Duivenvoorden, H. J., & Weisglas-Kuperus, N. 2009. Executive functions in very preterm children at early school age. *Journal of Abnormal. Child Psychology* 37, 981–999. https://doi.org/10.1007/s10802-009-9327-z

Aarnoudse-Moens, C. S., Duivenvoorden, H. J., Weisglas-Kuperus, N., Van Goudoever, J. B., & Oosterlaan, J. 2012. The profile of executive function in very preterm children at 4 to 12 years. *Developmental Medicine and Child Neurology* 54(3), 247–253. https://doi.org/10.1111/j.1469-8749.2011.04150.x

Adams, A.-M. 1996. Phonological working memory and spoken language development in young children. *Quarterly Journal of Experimental Psychology A* 49, 216–233.

Adams, A.-M., & Gathercole, S. E. 1995. Phonological working memory and speech production in young children. *Journal of Speech and Hearing Research* 38, 493–414.

Adams, A.-M., & Gathercole, S. E. 1996. Phonological working memory and spoken language development in children. *Quarterly Journal of Experimental Psychology* 49A, 216–233. https://doi.org/10.1080/713755610

Anderson, P. J., & Doyle, L. W. 2004. Executive functioning in school-aged children who were born very preterm or with extremely low birth weight in the 1990s. *Pediatrics* 114(1), 50–57. https://doi.org/10.1542/peds.114.1.50

Aguado, G. 1999. *Desarrollo de la morfosintaxis en el niño (TSA).* Madrid: CEPE.

Aylward, G. P. 2005. Neurodevelopmental outcomes of infants born prematurely. *Developmental and Behavioral Pediatrics* 26(6), 427–440. https://doi.org/10.1097/00004703-200512000-00008

Baron, I. S., Kerns, K. A., Müller, U., Ahronovich, M. D., & Litman, F. R. 2012. Executive functions in extremely low birth weight and late-preterm preschoolers: Effects on working memory and response inhibition. *Child Neuropsychology* 18, 586–599. https://doi.org/10.1080/09297049.2011.631906

Barre, N., Morgan, A., Doyle, L. W., & Anderson, P. J. 2011. Language abilities in children who were very preterm and/or very low birth weight: A meta-analysis. *Journal of Pediatrics* 158(5), 766-U100. https://doi.org/10.1016/j.jpeds.2010.10.032

Beauchamp, M. H., Thompson, D. K., Howard, K., Doyle, L. W., Egan, G. F., Inder, T. E., & Anderson, P. J. 2008. Preterm infant hippocampal volumes correlate with later working memory deficits. *Brain* 131, 2986–2994. https://doi.org/10.1093/brain/awn227

Bishop, D. 2003. *Test for reception of grammar (TROG-2)*. New York, NY: Pearson.

Bohlmann, N. L., Maier, M. F., & Palacios, N. 2015. Bidirectionality in self-regulation and expressive vocabulary: Comparisons between monolingual and dual language learners in preschool. *Child Development* 86, 1094–1111. https://doi.org/10.1111/cdev.12375

Böhm, B., Smedler, A., & Forssberg, H. 2004. Impulse control, working memory and other executive functions preterm children when starting school. *Acta Paediatrica* 93(10), 1363–1371. https://doi.org/10.1111/j.1651-2227.2004.tb02938.x

Carlson, S. M. 2005. Developmentally sensitive measures of executive function in preschool children. *Developmental Neuropsychology* 28(2), 595–616. https://doi.org/10.1207/s15326942dn2802_3

Blencowe, H., Cousens, S., Chou, D., Oestergaard, M., Say, L., Moller, A.-B., . . . Lawn, J. 2013. Born too soon: The global epidemiology of 15 million preterm births. *Reproductive Health* 10(Suppl. 1), S2, 1–16. https://doi.org/10.1186/1742-4755-10-S1-S2

Brancal, M., Alcantud, F., Ferrer, A., & Quiroga, M. 2005. *E.D.A.F. Evaluación de la discriminación auditiva y fonológica*. Madrid: TEA Ediciones.

Cattani, A., Bonifacio, S., Fertz, M., Iverson, J. M., Zocconi, E., & Caselli, M. C. 2010. Communicative and linguistic development in preterm children: A longitudinal study from 12 to 24 months. *International Journal of Language & Communication Disorders* 45(2), 162–173. https://doi.org/10.3109/13682820902818870

Caldwell, B., & Bradley, R. 1984. *Home observation for measurement of the environment. Administration manual* (Rev. ed.). Little Rock, AR: University of Arkansas at Little Rock.

D'Odorico, L., Assanelli, A., Franco, F., & Jacob, V. 2007. A follow-up study on Italian late talkers: Development of language, short-term memory, phonological awareness, impulsiveness, and attention. *Applied Psycholinguistics* 28(1), 157–169. https://doi.org/10.1017/S0142716406070081

Dunn, L. M., Dunn, L. M., & Arribas, D. 2005. *PEABODY. Test de vocabulario en imágenes*. Madrid: TEA Ediciones.

Duvall, S. W., Erickson, S. J., MacLean, P., & Lowe, J. R. 2015. Perinatal medical variables predict executive function within a sample of preschoolers born very low birth weight. *Journal of Child Neurology* 30, 735–740. https://doi.org/10.1177/0883073814542945

Farrell-Pagulayan, K., Busch, R. M., Medina, K. L., Bartok, J. A., & Krikorian, R. 2006. Developmental normative data for the Corsi Block-Tapping Task. *Journal of Clinical and Experimental Neuropsychology* 28(6), 1043–1052. https://doi.org/10.1080/13803390500350977

Foster-Cohen, S., Edgin, J. O., Champion, P. R., & Woodward, L. J. 2007. Early delayed language development in very preterm infants: Evidence from the MacArthur-Bates CDI. *Journal of Child Language* 34(3), 655–675. https://doi.org/10.1017/S0305000907008070

Foster-Cohen, S. H., Friesen, M. D., Champion, P. R., & Woodward, L. J. 2010. High prevalence/low severity language delay in preschool children born very preterm. *Journal of Developmental and Behavioral Pediatrics* 31(8), 658–667. https://doi.org/10.1097/DBP.0b013e3181e5ab7e

Fuhs, M. W., & Day, J. D. 2011. Verbal ability and executive functioning development in preschoolers at Head Start. *Developmental Psychology* 47, 404–416. https://doi.org/10.1037/a0021065

Gathercole, S. E. 2007. Working memory and language. In M. G. Gaskell (Ed.), *The Oxford handbook of psycholinguistics* (pp. 757–769). Oxford: Oxford University Press.

Gathercole, S. E., & Baddeley, A. D. 1990. The role of phonological memory in vocabulary acquisition: A study of young children learning new names. *British Journal of Psychology* 81, 439–454. https://doi.org/10.1111/j.2044-8295.1990.tb02371.x

Gathercole, S. E., Service, E., Hitch, G. J., Adams, A. M., & Martin, A. J. 1999. Phonological short-term memory and vocabulary development: Further evidence on the nature of the relationship. *Applied Cognitive Psychology* 13, 65–77. https://doi.org/10.1002/(SICI)1099-0720(199902)13:1<65::AID-ACP548>3.0.CO;2-O

Guarini, A., & Sansavini, A. 2012. Language, executive functions, short-term memory and literacy in preterm children: A longitudinal study. *Rivista Di Psicolinguistica Applicata* 12(3), 101–115.

Hodel, A. S., Senich, K. L., Jokinen, C., Sasson, O., Morris, A. R., & Thomas, K. M. 2017. Early executive function differences in infants born moderate-to-late preterm. *Early Human Development* 113, 23–30. https://doi.org/https://doi.org/10.1016/j.earlhumdev.2017.07.007

Howard, K., Roberts, G., Lim, J., Lee, K. J., Barre, N., Treyvaud, K., et al. 2011. Biological and environmental factors as predictors of language skills in very preterm children at 5 years of age. *Journal of Developmental and Behavioral Pediatrics* 32(3), 239–249. https://doi.org/10.1097/DBP.0b013e31820b7882

Ibbotson, P., & Kearvell-White, J. 2015. Inhibitory control predicts grammatical ability. *PLoS One* 10(12), e0145030. https://doi.org/10.1371/journal.pone.0145030

Im-Bolter, N., Johnson, J., & Pascual-Leone, J. 2006. Processing limitations in children with specific language impairment: The role of executive function. *Child Development* 77(6), 1822–1841. https://doi.org/10.1111/j.1467-8624.2006.00976.x

Kern, S., & Gayraud, F. 2007. Influence of preterm birth on early lexical and grammatical acquisition. *First Language* 27(2), 159–173. https://doi.org/10.1177/0142723706075790

Kessels, R. P. C., van Zandvoort, M. J. E., Postma, A., Kappelle, L. J., & de Haan, E. H. F. 2000. The Corsi Block-Tapping Task: Standardization and normative data. *Applied Neuropsychology* 7(4), 252–258. https://doi.org/10.1207/S15324826AN0704_8

Lowe, J., MacLean, P. C., Shaffer, M. L., & Watterberg, K. 2009. Early working memory in children born with extremely low birth weight: Assessed by object permanence. *Journal of Child Neurology* 24, 410–415. https://doi.org/10.1177/0883073808324533

Luciana, M., Lindeke, L., Georgief, M., Mills, M., & Nelson, C. A. 1999. Neurobehavioural evidence for working memory deficits in school-aged children with histories of prematurity. *Developmental Medicine and Child Neurology* 41, 521–533. https://doi.org/10.1017/S0012162299001140

Luoma, L., Herrgard, E., Martikainen, A., & Ahonen, T. 1998. Speech and language development of children born at <= 32 weeks' gestation: A 5-year prospective follow-up study. *Developmental Medicine and Child Neurology* 40(6), 380–387. https://doi.org/10.1111/j.1469-8749.1998.tb08213.x

Luu, T. M., Ment, L., Allan, W., Schneider, K., & Vohr, B. R. 2011. Executive and memory function in adolescents born very preterm. *Pediatrics* 127, e639–e646. https://doi.org/10.1542/peds.2010-1421

Marlow, N., Hennessy, E. M., Bracewell, M. A., Wolke, D., & Grp, E. P. S. 2007. Motor and executive function at 6 years of age after extremely preterm birth. *Pediatrics* 120(4), 793–804. https://doi.org/10.1542/peds.2007-0440

Marton, K., Kelmenson, L., & Pinkhasova, M. 2007. Inhibition control and working memory capacity in children with SLI. *Psychologia* 50(2), 110–121. https://doi.org/10.2117/psysoc.2007.110

Marton, K., Campanelli, L., Eichorn, N., Scheuer, J., & Yoon, J. 2014. Information processing andproactive interference in children with and without specific language impairment. *Journal of Speech Language and Hearing Research* 57(1), 106–119. https://doi.org/10.1044/1092-4388(2013/12-0306)

Menyuk, P., Liebergott, J., Schultz, M., Chesnick, M., & Ferrier, L. 1991. Patterns of early lexical and cognitive development in premature and full-term infants. *Journal of Speech and Hearing Research* 34(1), 88–94. https://doi.org/10.1044/jshr.3401.88

Mendoza, E., Carballo, G., Muñoz, J., & Fresneda, D. 2005. *CEG: Test de Comprensión de Estructuras Gramaticales*. Madrid: TEA Ediciones.

Mikkola, K., Ritari, N., Tommiska, V., Salokorpi, T., Lehtonen, L., Tammela, O., et al. 2005. Neurodevelopmental outcome at 5 years of age of a national cohort of extremely low birth weight infants who were born in 1996-1997. *Pediatrics* 116(6), 1391–1400. https://doi.org/10.1542/peds.2005-0171

Miyake, A., Friedman, N. P., Emerson, M. J., Witzki, A. H., & Howerter, A. 2000. The unity and diversity of executive functions and their contributions to complex "frontal lobe" tasks: A latent variable analysis. *Cognitive Psychology* 41, 49–100. https://doi.org/10.1006/cogp.1999.0734

Montgomery, J. W. 2003. Working memory and comprehension in children with specific language impairment: What we know so far. *Journal of Communication Disorders* 36, 221–231. https://doi.org/10.1016/S0021-9924(03)00021-2

Moreno, C. 1992. *Escala H.O.M.E. (Home Observation for Measurement of the Enviroment; Caldwell y Bradley, 1984) y C.V.C. Cuestionario de la Vida Cotidiana)*. Sevilla: University of Sevilla.

Mulder, H., Pitchford, N. J., & Marlow, N. 2011. Processing speed mediates executive function difficulties in very preterm children in middle childhood. *Journal of the International Neuropsychological Society* 17, 445–454. https://doi.org/10.1017/S1355617711000373

Mulder, H., Pitchford, N. J., Hagger, M. S., & Marlow, N. 2009. Development of executive function and attention in preterm children: A systematic review. *Developmental Neuropsychology* 34, 393–421. https://doi.org/10.1080/87565640902964524

Newborg, J., Stock, J. R., & Wnek, L. 1996. *Batelle, inventario de desarrollo*. Madrid: TEA Ediciones.

Ni, T. L., Huang, C. C., & Guo, N. W. 2011. Executive function deficit in preschool children born very low birth weight with normal early development. *Early Human Development* 87(2), 137–141. https://doi.org/10.1016/j.earlhumdev.2010.11.013

Nigg, J. T. 2006. *What causes ADHD? Understanding what goes wrong and why*. New York, NY: Guilford.

Noort-van der Spek, I. van Franken, M., & Weisglas-Kuperus, N. 2012. Language functions in preterm-born children: A systematic review and meta-analysis. *Pediatrics* 129(4), 745–754. https://doi.org/10.1542/peds.2011-1728

Pérez-Pereira, M., & Cruz, R. 2018. A longitudinal study of vocabulary size and composition in low risk preterm children. *First Language*, 38(1), 72–94. https://doi.org/10.1177/0142723717730484

Perez-Pereira, M., Fernandez, P., Luisa Gomez-Taibo, M., & Resches, M. 2014. Language development of low risk preterm infants up to the age of 30 months. *Early Human Development* 90(10), 649–656. https://doi.org/10.1016/j.earlhumdev.2014.08.004

Pérez Pereira, M., Peralbo, M., & Veleiro, A. 2017 Executive functions and language development in pre-term and full-term children. In A. Auza-Benavides & R. G. Schwartz (Eds.), *Language development and disorders in Spanish-speaking children* (pp. 91–112). New York, NY: Springer. https://doi.org/10.1007/978-3-319-53646-0_4

Réveillon, M., Borradori Tolsa, C., Monnier, M., Hüppi, P. S., & Barisnikov, K. 2015. Response inhibition difficulties in preterm children aged 9–12 years: Relations with emotion and behavior. *Child Neuropsychology* 22(4), 420–422. https://doi.org/10.1080/09297049.2014.994486

Ritter, B. C., Perrig, W., Steinlin, M., & Everts, R. 2014. Cognitive and behavioral aspects of executive functions in children born very preterm. *Child Neuropsychology* 20, 129–144. https://doi.org/10.1080/09297049.2013.773968

Roello, M., Ferretti, M. L., Colonnello, V., & Levi, G. 2015. When words lead to solutions: Executive function deficits in preschool children with specific language impairment. *Research in Developmental Disabilities* 37, 216–222. https://doi.org/10.1016/j.ridd.2014.11.017

Rueda, M. R., Fan, J., McCandliss, B. D., Halparin, J. D., Gruber, D. B., Lercari, L. P., et al. 2004. Development of attentional networks in childhood. *Neuropsychologia* 42(8), 1029–1040. https://doi.org/10.1016/j.neuropsychologia.2003.12.012

Saavalainen, P., Luoma, L., Bowler, D., Määttä, S., Kiviniemi, V., Laukkanen, E., et al. 2007. Spatial span in very prematurely born adolescents. *Developmental Neuropsychology* 32, 769–785. https://doi.org/10.1080/87565640701539535

Sansavini, A., Guarini, A., Alessandroni, R., Faldella, G., Giovanelli, G., & Salvioli, G. 2006. Early relations between lexical and grammatical development in very immature Italian preterms. *Journal of Child Language* 33(1), 199–216. https://doi.org/10.1017/S0305000905007208

Sansavini, A., Guarini, A., Alessandroni, R., Faldella, G., Giovanelli, G., & Salvioli, G. 2007. Are early grammatical and phonological working memory abilities affected by preterm birth? *Journal of Communication Disorders* 40(3), 239–256. https://doi.org/10.1016/j.jcomdis.2006.06.009

Scott, M. N., Taylor, H. G., Fristad, M. A., Klein, N., Espy, K. A., Minich, N., & Hack, M. 2012. Behavior disorders in extremely preterm/extremely low birth weight children in Kindergarten. *Journal of Developmental and Behavioral Pediatrics* 33, 202–213. https://doi.org/10.1097/DBP.0b013e3182475287

Taylor, J. 2002. *Cognitive grammar*. Oxford: Oxford University Press.

Ullman, M. T. 2001. A neurocognitive perspective on language: The declarative/ procedural model. *Neuroscience* 2, 717–725.

Vissers, C., Koolen, S., Hermans, D., Scheper, A., & Knoors, H. 2015. Executive functioning in preschoolers with specific language impairment. *Frontiers in Psychology* 6. https://doi.org/10.3389/fpsyg.2015.01574

Weiland, C., Barata, M. C., & Yoshikawa, H. 2014. The co-occurring development of executive function skills and receptive vocabulary in children enrolled in an urban preschool program. *Infant and Child Development* 23, 4–21. https://doi.org/10.1002/icd.1829

Vugs, B., Hendriks, M., Cuperus, J., & Verhoeven, L. 2014. Working memory performance and executive function behaviors in young children with SLI. *Research in Developmental Disabilities* 35(1), 62–74. http://dx.doi.org/10.1016/j.ridd.2013.10.022

White, L. J., Alexander, A., & Greenfield, D. B. 2017. The relationship between executive functioning and language: Examining vocabulary, sintax and language learning in preschoolers attending Head Start. *Journal of Experimental Child Psychology* 164, 16–31. http://dx.doi.org/10.1016/j.jecp.2017.06.010. https://doi.org/10.1016/j.jecp.2017.06.010

Woodward, L. J., Edgin, J. O., Thompson, D., & Inder, T. E. 2005. Object working memory deficits by early brain injury and development in the preterm infant. *Brain* 128, 2578–2587. https://doi.org/10.1093/brain/awh618

Woodward, L. J., Clark, C. A. C., Bora, S., & Inder, T. E. 2012. Neonatal White Matter abnormalities an important predictor of neurocognitive outcome for very preterm children. *PloS One* 7(12), e51879. https://doi.org/10.1371/journal.pone.0051879

Risk for language delay in healthy preterm and full-term children

A longitudinal study from 22 to 60 months

Mariela Resches,[1] Miguel Pérez-Pereira,[2]
Raquel Cruz Guerrero[2] and Montse Fernández Prieto[2]
[1]National Scientific and Technical Research Council (CONICET), Argentina / [2]Universidad de Santiago de Compostela

This study analysed the *Risk for Language Delay* (RLD) in a sample of healthy preterm children and a full-term control group. We collected direct and indirect measures of language development from 10 to 60 months, and we examined the influence of biomedical, cognitive and environmental variables over the RLD at 22, 30, and 60 months. While at the early ages there were not significant differences in the prevalence of RLD between preterm and full-term children, at 60 months receptive grammar delay was more frequent in the preterm group. Also, preterm children showed a higher instability in the prevalence of RLD over time. Lastly, cognitive development, maternal education and early expressive vocabulary were the most important factors to predict RLD.

Keywords: language delay, preterm children, lexical development, grammatical development

Introduction

A large number of previous studies show that preterm birth (< 37 weeks of gestational age) represents a risk condition for language development (Foster Cohen, Edgin, Champion & Woodward, 2007; Guarini et al., 2010; Stolt et al., 2007; Stolt et al., 2016). Some research focused on early lexical and grammatical development suggests that preterm children (PR) have a smaller and more immature lexicon, and significantly more reduced MLU's than full-term (FT) children. Those differences tend to be greater as gestational age (GA), and birth weight (BW) are lower (Adams-Chapman, Bann, Carter, & Stoll, 2015; Kern & Gayraud, 2007; Foster

https://doi.org/10.1075/z.223.04res

Cohen et al., 2007; Stolt et al., 2007). Similar results were obtained when longer-term language outcomes of PR and FT children were compared (Barre, Morgan, Doyly, & Anderson, 2011; Foster-Cohen, Friesen, Champion, & Woodward, 2010; Wolke & Meyer, 1999; Woodward et al., 2009).

However, these results are far from being conclusive. Some works did not find significant differences between FT and PR children's language development, at least at the early ages (Cattani et al., 2010; Pérez Pereira, Fernández, Resches, & Gómez Taibo, 2013; Pérez Pereira, Fernandez, Gómez Taibo, & Resches, 2014; Sansavini et al., 2006; Stolt et al., 2007). Sample selection issues may partially explain such discrepancies. Most of the studies carried out on the PR population have focused on very low BW (< 1000gr.) and/or extremely low GA (<28 weeks) children. Also, exclusion criteria have not been clearly established in many studies, some of them including some subjects with associated medical complications. Even though most of the PR children (around 80%) are over 32 weeks of GA and a mean BW of 2000 gr. (Blencowe et al., 2012), those research findings have been easily generalised to the whole PR population. There are some other factors which might also contribute to different results among studies. Some authors suggest that direct measures of language skills may be more sensitive than indirect measures in detecting language delays in moderate-to-late PR children (Stolt et al., 2009). However, given the wide variability and the context-dependent nature of very young children's linguistic behaviour, sensitivity remains a common issue both for direct and indirect approaches to language assessment at early ages (Law & Roy, 2008). Other sources of variation among results obtained with language development in PR children are differences both in the age of assessment and on the kind of language abilities evaluated (i.e. expressive/receptive; vocabulary/grammar).

Moreover, the relative scarcity of long-term, longitudinal studies about language development of healthy, moderate-to-late PT children from different approaches of assessment makes it difficult to conclude the stability of their results over time. Also, this lack of studies may hinder the identification of those factors influencing PR children's language outcomes at each stage of development.

Pérez-Pereira et al. (2014) assessed the early language and communicative development of an initial sample of 150 healthy PR children (mean $GA = 32.62$; mean $BW = 1{,}727.57$gr.), and 49 FT children between 10 and 30 months of age. They did not find significant differences between the PR and FT groups in communicative lexical or grammatical development at any of the age points analysed. They found that cognitive development at 22 months together with the lexical size at the same age were the most important variables for predicting language development at 30 months. More recently, Pérez-Pereira and Cruz (2018) analysed the vocabulary growth and composition of this same PR sample. Again, they found that when biomedical complications associated with prematurity are excluded, GA did not contribute to explaining the longitudinal changes in these variables.

Based on a more immature, although healthy PR sample (mean $GA = 30.4$; BW ≥1200 gr.), Sansavini et al. (2006) pointed to partially similar results. These authors did not find a lower lexical or grammatical development in the PR group, as compared to a FT sample at 30 months. Nevertheless, they observed a wider range of individual variability within the PR group, showing a tendency for a higher incidence of *Risk for Language Delay* (RLD; Language outcomes ≤10th percentile or ≤ −1.25 SD in the absence of sensorial or neurological impairment). Interestingly, those preterms at RLD were males with a $BW \leq 1000$ gr and ≤ 31 weeks GA. Therefore, for this subgroup of PR children other biological factors, like gender, might interact with prematurity to amplify the risk for language difficulties. In contrast, contextual variables such as low maternal education did not represent a risk factor, at least at 30 months of age. In a later study, Sansavini et al. (2010) analysed the evolution of RLD in this same PR sample. They compared the percentage of children at RLD at 30 months with that found one year later, at 42 months of age. At 30 months, the incidence of children at RLD was not significantly higher for the PR than for the FT group. At 42 months, in turn, there was a significant increase in the number of PR children at RLD, with more than 30% of them at −1.25 SD in morphosyntactic production, compared with a 7.5% for the FT children. This rate of RLD among the PR children was similar to findings from other studies (Briscoe, Gathercole & Marlow, 2001; Singer et al., 2001; Woodward et al., 2009). Sansavini et al. (2010) also showed that both poorer language and cognitive skills at 30 months were the best candidates for predicting a preterm's risk status one year later. Also, this time, maternal education contributed increasing the prediction of RLD. This last finding agrees with others suggesting that, as development progresses, for immature but healthy PR children, biomedical risk factors tend to lose strength in favour of environmental variables.

A few studies have provided information about the later evolution of the RLD in PR children. Stolt et al. (2014), for example, analysed the prevalence of *weak language skills* (defined as language scores under the 10th percentile of the control group) between 2 and 5 years old in a group of very low birth weight (VLBW mean $BW = 1066$ gr.) children. They found that, despite being a VLBW sample, when children with neurological impairment (NI) were excluded from this group, the percentage of PR children with weak expressive language skills at 2 years of age was not significantly different from the full-term controls (15% vs 9% respectively). However, at 5 years of age, the prevalence of weak language skills among the VLBW group increased by as much as 23%, even after excluding children with NI. In contrast, this percentage remained stable in the FT group. Stolt et al. (2014) also showed that low expressive language scores at 2 years predicted a poor performance on a group of measures of complex language abilities at 5 years of age. In sum, both Sansavini et al.(2010) and Stolt et al. (2014, 2016) informed that the rate of PR children at RLD increased significantly throughout time. These findings contradict some others suggesting that very preterm children catch up to their peers regarding their language development (Luu, Vohr, Allan, Schneider & Ment, 2011; Ment et al., 2003). These discrepancies may be related to different factors affecting the stability of results over time.

Recently, Putnick, Bornstein, Eryigit-Madzwamuze & Wolke (2017) compared the long-term stability of language performance of PR children. Their results revealed a stronger stability in very PR children than in moderate-to-late PR and term children, although those differences are attenuated when the effect of family SES and non-verbal intelligence were controlled. Other studies suggest that the stability of language outcomes depends on the assessed language functions. According to a recent meta-analysis (van Noort-van der Spek, Franken & Weisglas-Kuperus, 2012), while for simple language functions (vocabulary and short sentence processing) differences between PR and FT children remained stable over time, for complex language functions (understanding and production of complex grammatical structures), group differences increased significantly from 3 to 12 years of age.

Furthermore, several other factors may increase the PR children's probability of being at RLD. First, there are a number of biomedical risk factors: low APGAR score (Pérez-Pereira et al., 2013), length of stay in Neonatal Intensive Care Unit (NICU) (Marston et al., 2007; Perez Pereira et al., 2013;), and some medical complications derived from brain or lung immaturity (Foster Cohen et al., 2010; Singer et al., 2001). Second, a good number of previous studies indicate that RLD in PR children does not seem to be specific but rather associated to more general cognitive difficulties (Adams-Chapman et al., 2015; Foster Cohen et al., 2010; Sansavini et al., 2010; Putnik et al., 2017). Finally, these and other studies also point out that certain environmental variables may increase the RLD among these children: low SES (Wolke & Meyer, 1999), low maternal education (Sansavini et al., 2010) and other variables which may affect communicative interactions: risk for maternal depression (McManus & Poehlmann, 2012) or a low quality of the social and material stimuli coming from the home environment (Molfese, Holcomb & Helwig, 1994).

This study has two goals: (1) To analyse the prevalence of RLD in a group of healthy, low-risk PR children, at 22, 30 and 60 months of age, as compared to a FT control group, and (2) To identify which biomedical, contextual or individual variables may increase the probability of RLD on this sample, and whether their predictive value changes over time. Results are intended to provide a non-biased perspective about the evolution, stability, and change in some factors influencing the RLD in a PR sample probably more representative than others from previous studies.

Methodology

Participants

This study is part of a follow-up, longitudinal study where the effects of numerous variables on preterms' language development were examined. The initial sample was recruited just after birth from four different hospitals in Galicia (Spain). There were 150 PR children (79 boys, 71 girls; mean *GA* = 32.60, *SD* = 2.43; range 26–36) and 49 FT children (25 boys, 24 girls; mean *GA* = 39.84; *SD* = 1.44; range 37–42). Parents' consent and approval by the Galician Ethics Committee of Clinical Research were obtained before the beginning of the research.

To distinguish between the effect of premature birth and other confounding variables, the following exclusion criteria were applied: cerebral palsy (as diagnosed up until 9 months of age), periventricular leukomalacia, intraventricular hemorrhage < grade II, hydrocephalus, encephalopathy, genetic malformations, chromosomal syndromes, metabolic syndromes associated to mental retardation, or important motor or sensorial impairments. Newborn children with Apgar scores below 6 at 5 min were also excluded.

Children were assessed at 10, 22, 30, 48 and 60 months old. Given that the prevalence of RLD will be examined at 22, 30 and 60 months, the main biomedical and demographic characteristics of the sample at 22 and 60 months are presented (Table 1). As can be observed, both at 22 and 60 months PR and FT children were not different regarding gender distribution, Apgar score, or maternal education. Also, if we consider their general characteristics and composition regarding GA and BW (with a 70% of moderate-to late PR children), this sample may be considered a low risk, representative PR sample.

Both at 22 and 30 months, children were identified as presenting RLD if their language outcomes were below the 10th percentile of the normative sample from indirect, parent report measures (IDHC). At 60 months, when direct measures of morphosyntactic development were applied, children at RLD were those whose language scores were lower than 1.25 SD of the mean for the FT sample.

Measures and instruments

Given the complex and multivariate nature of this study, it was not reasonable to collect repeated measures of all of the variables at all age points. Instead, some ages were selected as more proper than others to measure the different linguistic, cognitive and environmental variables.

Table 1. Biomedical and demographic data of the PR and FT groups at 22 and 60 months

Variable	PR		FT	
	22 m	60 m	22 m	60 m
	Mean (SD)		Mean (SD)	
GA (weeks)	32.62 (2.41)	32.57 (2.29)	39.70 (1.48)	39.70 (1.53)
BW (gr.)	1,721 (435)	1,708 (427)	3,373 (433)	3,340 (440)
Apgar score (1′)	7.94 (1.30)	7.90 (1.31)	8.13 (1.20)	8.18 (1.31)
	n (%)		n (%)	
Gender (girls)	65 (47.1)	44 (42.3)	20 (46.9)	15 (45.5)
Stay in NICU				
No stay	36 (26.2)	28 (26.9)	40 (93.1)	30 (90.9)
1–15 days	58 (42.3)	42 (40.4)	2 (4.6)	2 (6.1)
> 15 days	43 (31.3)	34 (32.7)	1 (2.3)	1 (3.0)
Mother's Education				
Basic Educ.	34 (24.8)	23 (22.1)	17 (39.5)	12 (36.4)
High sch./Tech.	56 (40.8)	46 (44.2)	10 (23.2)	10 (30.3)
Higher Ed.	47 (34.3)	35 (33.7)	16 (37.2)	11 (33.3)

Note: *GA* = Gestational Age; *BW* = Birth Weight; NICU = Neonatal Intensive Care Unit; *m* = months

Linguistic measures

Ten months (corrected age for PR children) was selected as a crucial point to observe the emergence of the first pre-linguistic abilities. Early receptive vocabulary and communicative development were assessed through the *Inventario do Desenvolvemento de Habilidades Comunicativas*, Form I: *Palabras e Xestos*, "Words and Gestures" (IDHC; Perez Pereira & García Soto, 2003). The IDHC is the Galician version of the Mac Arthur-Bates Communicative Development Inventory, CDI (Fenson et al., 2007). Two measurements were considered: Total receptive vocabulary (From the section "Vocabulary understanding") and Total Gestures (From the section "Gestures and actions").

At 22 and 30 months (corrected age for the PR group), the IDHC, Form II: *Palabras e Oracións*, "Words and Sentences" was applied (Perez Pereira & Resches, 2011). This range of ages is especially important to establish the point at which the rapid growth of the first vocabulary begins. The section "Word production" was used as a measure of expressive vocabulary both at 22 and 30 months. At 30 months, when the first combination of words in most toddlers is expected, parent responses to the section "Sentence Complexity" were taken as a measure of children's early grammatical development.

At 60 months, when basic language abilities are expected to be consolidated, two measures of expressive and receptive grammar were applied. These measures represent what some authors called *complex language functions* (see van Noort-van der Spek et al., 2012). Both the production and understanding of complex sentences involve the integration across multiple language components and other basic processes for language development, like memory. So, they were considered proper and reliable measurements of a 5-year-old's language skills.

Morphosyntactic production was evaluated through the expressive subscale of the *Test de desarrollo de la morfosintaxis en el niño* (TSA; Aguado, 2000). The TSA-expressive has 34 items. In the first 29 items, the child is shown a card with two drawings, and the examiner says one sentence for each of the drawings. Then, the child is asked to say the sentence matching the picture the examiner points to (i.e., *La chica mira a los perros*; "The girl looks at the dogs"). The last five items the child is asked to conclude a sentence started by the examiner (i.e *Cuando hace frío…*; "When it's cold…"; max. Score = 68).

Grammatical comprehension was assessed through the *Test de Comprensión de Estructuras Gramaticales* (CEG; Mendoza, Carballo, Muñoz & Fresneda, 2005). The CEG consists of 80 items displaying the most representative Spanish grammatical structures. A card presents each item with four drawings. The child is asked to choose the drawing representing the sentence said by the examiner (i.e. *El ratón persigue al gato;* "The mouse chases the cat"; max. Score = 80).

Cognitive and other contextual measures

At 22 and 60 months the Spanish version of the *Battelle Developmental Inventory* (BDI; Newborg, Stock, & Wnek, 1996) was applied. The BDI is composed of five subscales: adaptive, personal-social, communication, motor, and cognitive. At 22 months, the sum of the raw scores in four of the five subscales was considered as a good measure of early cognitive development, which is non-symbolic but mainly practical at the first ages. The score from the communication subscale was excluded to avoid spurious associations with the language measures taken as dependent variables (DV). At 60 months, only the raw score from the cognitive scale was used, since at this age that scale represents a proper measurement of non-verbal intelligence.

As for environmental variables, besides the maternal education, the risk for maternal depression was assessed. Maternal depression might affect the first mother-infant interactions, as well as the quality of family linguistic input and experiences at the preschool age. The Spanish version of the CES-D scale (Radloff, 1977) was applied both at children's 10 months and 60 months. CES-D is a 20-item screening questionnaire aimed to evaluate the presence of symptoms associated with depression among caregivers (max score = 60). Scores ≥16 denote risk for clinical depression. Also, the quality of the stimulation provided by the home environment was assessed through the Spanish adaptation of *The Home Observation for the Measurement of the Environment* scale (HOME; Caldwell & Bradley, 1984). The HOME scale has different versions depending on the child's age since the resources and experiences required for identifying a stimulating environment are different for toddlers than preschoolers. When the children were 22 months, the infant and toddlers' scale was applied (max score: 45). At 48 months children's home environment was reassessed through the version for preschoolers (max. Score: 50).

Procedure

When participants entered the study (15 days), their mothers participated in an interview to gather data on the family's sociodemographic characteristics and children's health. At 10 months, mothers filled out checklists both on child's language development (IDHC-Form I) and her risk for depression (CES-D). Completed forms were sent by mail within the first week after receiving them. At 22 months, the children's cognitive development (BDI), and the quality of their home environments (HOME) were directly assessed by a trained psychologist, who visited their homes. We were informed of their linguistic abilities through the IDHC-Form II, which the mothers filled out a few days before the visit, or sent within the first week after the visit. At 30 months, the IDHC-Form II was completed and mailed again. At 48 and 60 months, the former trained evaluator made two home visits. At 48 months she collected information about the home environment (HOME), and at 60 months, children's cognitive (BDI) and receptive and expressive morphosyntactic abilities (CEG and TSA) were assessed through direct testing. Children were individually evaluated in a quiet room of their homes.

Analyses performed

Firstly, to identify those children at RLD, cut-offs to language scores at 22, 30 and 60 months were applied. According to the previous literature about language delay in PR and non-PR populations, at 22 and 30 months, we used the 10th percentile from the normative sample of the IDHC "Word Production" and "Sentence complexity" sections. At 60 months, both for grammatical comprehension (CEG) and morphosyntactic production (TSA) a cut-point of ≤ −1.25 SD of the mean from the FT sample was used.

In response to the first of our goals, at each age mean scores and the percentage of children at RLD in the PR and FT groups were compared using independent-samples *t* test and Chi^2 test. Also, for both groups, changes in the rate of prevalence of RLD throughout time were examined through the *McNemar's Chi*[2] test for related samples. Considering previous results with this sample and the low number of individuals at RLD, comparisons were made with the whole PR sample instead of dividing it into groups of GA.

Regarding our second goal (see above), a series of stepwise logistic regression models were performed. The DV's were the 22, 30 and 60 month lexical and grammatical measures, dichotomised regarding the RLD. For each DV, four consecutive models were performed. A step forward method was applied to retain the previously selected independent variables. In the first model, the following biomedical risk-variables were entered: PR/FT birth; APGAR-risk (cut-point = ≤ 7); Stay in NICU (3 groups, see Table 1) and sex. For the second model, a number of environmental risk-variables were considered: Mother's education (3 groups, see Table 1); risk for maternal depression at 10 months for DV's at 22 and 30 months, or at 60 months for DV's at that age (cut-point = ≥ 16); HOME-risk at 22 months or at 48 months for DV's at 60 months (cut-point = ≤ 2nd Quartile according to norms). In a third model, scores from the BDI at 22 or 60 months were entered, together with the biomedical or environmental variables selected on the previous models. Finally, for the fourth model, earlier language scores were summed up to the selected variables from the former model.

Results

Descriptive language, cognitive and environmental measures in PR and FT children

First, PR and FT mean lexical and grammatical scores at 22, 30 and 60 months were compared (Table 2). As shown in previous studies, we did not find significant differences between PR and FT children in the IDHC language measurements up to 30 months of age. However, at 22 months PR children got significantly lower scores in cognitive abilities than the FT children (BDI; $PR = 215.20$ (16.08); $FT = 224.32$ (17.45); $t\,(117) = -3.13$, $p = .001$). In turn, contextual variables at early age – risk for maternal depression at 10 months or the quality of the family environment at 22 months – were not significantly different between groups (CES-D; $PR = 10.3$ (8.80); $FT = 11.1$ (7.54); $t\,(194) = -0.53$, $p = .58$; HOME Scale; $PR = 38.2$ (4.33); $FT = 38.7$ (3.97); $t\,(178) = -0.62$, $p = .53$).

At 60 months of age, grammatical comprehension abilities (CEG) were significantly lower among the PR children. In contrast, PR and FT mean scores in morphosyntactic production (TSA) were not significantly different (Table 2). There were no significant differences between PR and FT children's performance on

Table 2. Language outcomes of the PR and FT groups at 22, 30 and 60 months: Means (SD) and number (percentage) of children at RLD at each age

Outcome	PR	FT	t/X^2	p
22 months	n = 137	n = 43		
Expressive Vocabulary (M (SD))	158.6 (147.28)	173.8 (137.19)	−.59	.55
RLD (≤10th Perc.) (n (%))	37 (27.0)	8 (18.6)	1.23	.26
30 months	n = 115	n = 37		
Expressive Vocabulary (M (SD))	419.5 (175.44)	411.9 (173.76)	.23	.81
RLD (≤10th Perc.) (n (%))	19 (16.5)	7 (19.4)	.16	.68
Syntactic Complexity (M(SD))	20.9 (14.35)	20.5(13.32)	.16	.87
RLD (≤10th Perc.) (n (%))	22 (19.8)	5 (14.2)	.54	.46
60 months	n = 104	n = 33		
Receptive Grammar (M(SD))	47.8 (8.97)	52.1 (7.33)	2.23	.027*
RLD (−1.25 SD) (n (%))	27 (25.9)	4 (12.1)	2.74	.074§
Expressive Grammar (M (SD))	42.1(11.21)	43.6 (8.17)	.68	.49
RLD (−1.25 SD) (n (%))	12 (12)	2 (6.2)	.84	.35

* $p < .05$; § $p < .10$
Note: RLD = Risk for Language Delay;

the BDI's cognitive scale (*PR* = 84.0 (11.30); *FT* = 85.9 (3.18); *t* (136.25) = −1.56 *p* = .11). No significant differences were found neither for the HOME scale at 48 months (*PR* = 48.9 (3.57); *FT* = 49.9 (2.46); *t* (143) = −1.61, *p* = .10) nor for the risk for maternal depression at children's 60 months old (*PR* = 9.10 (6.32); *FT* = 10.73 (8.81), *t* (121) = −1.11, *p* = .268).

PR and FT children's RLD from 22 to 60 months

Second, the prevalence of RLD along time, both for PR and FT children, was compared. At 22 months, almost 30% of the PR children had an expressive vocabulary below the 10th percentile, compared to 18% from the FT group. Those differences, however, did not reach statistical significance (see Table 2). At 30 months, while the percentage of RLD remained stable for the FT group (*McNemar's* $X^2(1) = 1.00$), that percentage significantly decreased for the PR group, (McNemar's X^2 $(1) = .011$). At 60 months of age, in turn, PR children's prevalence of RLD in grammatical comprehension increased to 26%, while that percentage slightly decreased to 12% for the FT group. Between-group differences were marginally significant. Nevertheless, percentages of RLD from 30 to 60 months significantly increased for the PR children (*McNemar's* $X^2(1) = .021$) while not for the full terms (*McNemar's*

$X^2(1) = .453$). About the prevalence of RLD in morphosyntactic production (TSA), there were no significant differences between PR and FT groups, with percentages around the expected values for the general population.

Predicting RLD at 22, 30 and 60 months

To identify those factors predicting RLD for the whole sample, four stepwise logistic regression models were performed (see above). For the first model, among the biomedical variables, in this low-risk sample only being male was significantly related to a higher probability of RLD at 22 months ($OR = .432, p = .021$; *Nagelkerke's* $R^2 = .046$); and at 30 months for syntactic complexity ($OR = .338$, $p = .024$; *Nagelkerke's* $R^2 = .064$). The second model assessed the predictive value of some environmental variables on the RLD. Results showed that maternal education was a significant predictor of RLD at 22 months ($OR = 1.60, p = .037$; *Nagelkerke's* $R^2 = .079$), at 30 months for a poor performance in syntactic complexity ($OR = 1.90, p = .027$; *Nagelkerke's* $R^2 = .056$) and at 60 months of age for grammatical comprehension ($OR = 2.41, p = .006$; *Nagelkerke's* $R^2 = .108$). The third model assessed the predictive role of children's cognitive performance in interaction with the previously selected biomedical and contextual variables. While a lower level of cognitive development was a significant predictor of RLD at all ages and for all DV's, maternal education was the only variable which remained in the model increasing the total explained variance at 22 months (*Nagelkerke's* $R^2 = .320$), at 30 months for risk for delay in syntactic complexity (*Nagelkerke's* $R^2 = .250$), and at 60 months for grammatical comprehension (*Nagelkerke's* $R^2 = .212$). Finally, the fourth model evaluated the predictive capacity of the former linguistic variables, after considering the influence of cognitive development and maternal education on the corresponding DV's. Table 3 shows the model's selected variables at each age. As can be observed, at 22 months the risk for lexical delay increased not only because of a poor cognitive performance or a lower level of maternal studies, but children's prelinguistic abilities at 10 months (gestures and receptive vocabulary) contributed in a modest, although significant, way to increase the model's total explained variance (44.8%). In contrast, at 30 months, once former language abilities entered the model, expressive vocabulary at 22 months became the only significant predictor of both risk for lexical and syntactic delay, accounting for 36.5% and 42.7% of the variance. Last, at 60 months of age, non-verbal cognitive development, maternal education and early vocabulary size at 22 months were significant predictors of risk for delay in grammatical comprehension, accounting for 28.3% of explained variance. In turn, non-verbal cognitive skills and lexical development at 30 months explained only 13% of the variance in the prediction of risk for delay in morphosyntactic production.

Table 3. Stepwise logistic regression analyses: Selected contextual, cognitive and linguistic variables as predictors of RLD at different ages

Dependent variables	Nagelkerke's R^2	OR	95% CI	p
RLD-Exp.Vocabulary-22 m.	.448			
BDI-Total score		.907	.871–.943	.000
Maternal education		2.14	1.21–3.78	.009
Total gestures-10 m.		.894	.833–.961	.002
Word understanding-10 m.		1.01	1.00–1.02	.005
RLD-Exp.Vocabulary-30 m.	.365			
Exp.Vocabulary-22 m		.979	.968–.990	.000
RLD- Sent. Complexity-30 m.	.427			
Exp.Vocabulary-22 m		.974	.960–.988	.000
RLD- Recep. Grammar- 60 m	.283			
BDI-Cognitive scale-60 m		.861	.767–.967	.011
Exp.Vocabulary-22 m		.995	.990–1.00	.037
Maternal education		1.88	.997–3.57	.051
RLD-Exp. Grammar-60 m	.135			
BDI-Cognitive scale-60 m		.868	.757–996	.044
Exp. Vocabulary- 30 m		.997	.993–1.00	.055

Notes: RLD = Risk for Language Delay; BDI = Battelle Developmental Inventory; OR = Odds Ratio; CI = Confidence Interval

Discussion

The first goal of this study was to examine the prevalence of RLD in a group of healthy, low-risk PR children from 22 to 60 months of age, as compared to a FT sample. As previous studies with healthy, and even more immature PR children have shown (Sansavini et al., 2010; Stolt et al., 2014), in this work we did not find significant differences between PR and FT children in the prevalence of RLD at 22 and 30 months old. Our results were similar to those informed by Sansavini et al. (2010), who found 16 to 24% of their PR children performing under the 10th percentile in lexical and grammatical development at 30 months. However, results from Stolt et al. (2014) showed that, when children with NI were excluded from their VLBW sample at 24 months, there were only 15% of PR children with weak language skills. Our study differs from Stolt et al. (2014) not only in the criteria for defining early language delay, but mainly because we collected measures of early expressive language at two age-points. When PR's vocabulary production at

22 and 30 months was compared to that of the FT group, PR children showed a higher prevalence of RLD before 24 months, and a significant reduction after eight months. In contrast, those percentages remained stable for the FT group and within the expected epidemiological values (Zubrick, Taylor, Rice, & Seglers, 2007).

At 5 years of age, for a more complex language function like grammatical comprehension, PR children performed significantly lower than FT children. Between-group differences in the prevalence of RLD were only marginally significant. Nevertheless, the percentage of PR children at risk for delay in grammatical comprehension at 5 years significantly increased regarding the observed at 30 months for expressive vocabulary. Our low-risk PR results showed similar values to those informed by Stolt and collaborators at 5 years old (Stolt et al., 2014, 2016). In their studies, language skills at 5 years of age were assessed through the language subscale from the NEPSY II test. When Stolt et al. (2016) analysed the scores from the five subtests conforming the NEPSY-Language score they found that the VLBW group only showed significant differences to controls on the "Comprehension of Instructions" subtest. This subtest requires an understanding of grammatically complex sentences and working memory, both the same abilities required for good performance in our Comprehension of Grammatical Structures Test (CEG).

As for morphosyntactic production (TSA), no significant differences were found between PR and FT groups. The prevalence of RLD on this measure was slightly lower than the observed for grammatical comprehension. On the one hand, these differences could be explained by differences in the complexity of the grammatical structures presented on each test. On the other hand, demands on working memory probably are higher for the CEG than for the TSA test.

In general, these results are in line with previous studies which highlight the importance of considering both the sample selection (Pérez Pereira et al., 2014; Pérez Pereira & Cruz, 2018) and the kind of assessed language abilities (van Noort-van der Spek et al., 2012). During the early ages, and when simple language functions like vocabulary or early grammar were assessed, the prevalence of RLD among PR children without associated medical complications was not significantly different from the FT children. In fact, the percentage of PR children at risk for lexical delay significantly decreased from 22 to 30 months. In contrast, when performance in grammatical comprehension at 5 years was assessed, the prevalence of PR children at RLD increased again. These results follow those obtained through meta-analysis by van Noort-van der Spek et al. (2012) who found that as PR children grow up, they may have increasing difficulties with complex language function.

Nevertheless, considering results from other studies (Stolt et al., 2009), the direct or indirect nature of the linguistic measures applied at different ages (parent report vs. standardised tests) might be a third, non negligible factor – besides the sample selection and the kind of language abilities – influencing results from the present study.

In any case, this pattern of results suggests that among healthy, moderate to late PR children, language growth could be quite unstable, with more children with poor vocabulary at the beginning, but who tend to catch up in a short time. In turn, language difficulties might reemerge at later ages because of the higher processing demands from more complex language abilities. Future studies should carefully analyse the individual pathways of those PR children with persistent language delay before those who recover either at middle or long-term.

The second goal of this study was to identify those biomedical, individual and environmental factors, which could be accurate predictors of RLD across time. As was referred to in previous studies analyzing the mean language performance of this healthy PR sample (Pérez Pereira et al., 2013; 2014), in the present study those biomedical variables associated with prematurity did not contribute to the prediction of RLD. In line with Sansavini et al. (2006; 2011), we found that male gender made a modest, although significant contribution to the prediction of RLD, but only up to 30 months. However, this association between gender and risk for early language difficulties disappeared when general cognitive abilities were taken into account. Therefore, this study confirms the importance of cognitive development as a predictor of RLD both at early and later ages, and even after considering maternal education and former language abilities. These results extend those previously obtained with this sample, and at the same time support findings from other studies with healthy, although more immature, PR children. RLD did not seem to be specific but associated to subtle, more general cognitive difficulties (Adams-Chapman et al. 2015; Foster Cohen et al., 2010; Putnik et al., 2017; Sansavini et al., 2010). Unlike previous studies assessing the predictive value of maternal education on PR children's early language abilities (Pérez-Pereira et al., 2014), we found that a low level in the mother's education made a unique contribution to predicting which children may be at RLD both at 22 and 5 years. It is probable that the maternal level of education is not a good predictor of the vocabulary growth from the PR group as a whole. However, it may become an important variable in predicting which children could fall in the lowest end of the distribution. At 22 months, perhaps more than at 30, the rapid growth of expressive vocabulary is an especially challenging task because it is affected by certain environmental risk factors, such as a low level of education in the mother.

With regards to the predictive value of former language abilities on later RLD, this study supports previous results with the until-30-months sample but also shows the important role of early expressive vocabulary for the long-term prediction of RLD. As in Pérez-Pereira et al. (2014), a low receptive vocabulary and a few gestures at 10 months were significant predictors of risk for expressive vocabulary delay only at 22 months. In turn, a poor lexical development at 22 months helped to predict the risk for a lexical and grammatical delay not only in the short term, at 30 months, but also at a longer-term, for grammatical comprehension at 5 years of age. Also, a low expressive vocabulary at 30 months increased the prediction of risk for morphosyntactic production delay two and a half years later. These results are in agreement with those found by Stolt et al. (2014) who highlighted the predictive value of VLBW children's expressive vocabulary at 2 years on their weak language skills at 5 years of age.

In sum, this study demonstrates the need for following the pathways of language development among healthy, low-risk PR children, beyond the early ages. As other previous studies suggest, this may be especially true in the case of those children with histories of late language emergence (Rice, Taylor, & Zubrick, 2008). Even though PR children's language delays may not become evident from the beginning, when demands on language processing are higher and involve other capacities, like working memory or cognitive control, subtler language difficulties may appear. Those difficulties, in turn, might affect other domains of later development, including scholarly learning abilities.

Among these low-risk PR children, even though the biomedical variables do not seem to help the early detection of those individuals at a higher RLD, the assessment of the first expressive vocabulary and the early cognitive development together with the evaluation of the familiar risk associated with a low educational level may be useful. Considering these other variables would allow us to implement early intervention strategies addressed to those most vulnerable PR children.

References

Adams-Chapman, I., Bann, C., Carter, S. L., & Stoll, B. J. 2015. Language outcomes among ELBW infants in early childhood. *Early Human Development* 91, 373–379. https://doi.org/10.1016/j.earlhumdev.2015.03.011

Aguado G. 2000. *El desarrollo de la morfosintaxis en el niño: TSA*. Madrid: CEPE.

Barre, N., Morgan, A., Doyly, L., & Anderson, P. 2011. Language abilities in children who were very preterm and/or very low birth weight: a meta analysis. *The Journal of Pediatrics* 158(5), 766–774. https://doi.org/10.1016/j.jpeds.2010.10.032

Blencowe, H., Cousens, S., Oestergaard, M. Z., Chou, D., Moller, A. B., Narwal, R., Adler, A., Vera Garcia, C., Rohde, S., Say, L,, & Lawn, J. E. 2012. National, regional, and worldwide estimates of preterm birth rates in the year 2010 with time trends since 1990 for selected countries: A systematic analysis and implications. *The Lancet* 379, 2162–2172. https://doi.org/10.1016/S0140-6736(12)60820-4

Briscoe, J., Gathercole, S., & Marlow, N. 2001. Everyday memory and cognitive ability in children born very prematurely. *The Journal of Child Psychology and Psychiatry and Allied Disciplines* 42(6), 749–754. https://doi.org/10.1111/1469-7610.00771

Caldwell, B. M., & Bradley, R. H. 1984. *Home observation for measurement of the environment* (rev. ed.). Little Rock, AR: University of Arkansas at Little Rock. [Spanish version: Moreno C. (1992). *Escala HOME y cuestionario de la vida cotidiana*. Sevilla: University of Sevilla].

Cattani, A., Bonifacio, S., Fertz, M., Iverson, J. M., Zocconi, E., & Caselli, M. C. 2010. Communicative and linguistic development in preterm children: A longitudinal study from 12 to 24 months. *International Journal of Language & Communication Disorders* 45, 162–173. https://doi.org/10.3109/13682820902818870

Fenson, L., Marchman, V. A., Thal, D., Dale, P. S., Reznick, J. S. & Bates, E. 2007. *The MacArthur Bates communicative development inventories: User's guide and technical manual* (second edition). Baltimore, MD: Paul H. Brookes.

Foster-Cohen, S. H., Friesen, M. D., Champion, P. R., & Woodward, L. J. 2010. High prevalence/low severity language delay in preschool children born very preterm. *Journal of Developmental & Behavioral Pediatrics* 31(8), 658–667. https://doi.org/10.1097/DBP.0b013e3181e5ab7e

Foster-Cohen, S., Edgin, J. O., Champion, P. R. & Woodward, L. J. 2007. Early delayed language development in very preterm infants: Evidence from the MacArthur-Bates CDI. *Journal of Child Language* 34, 655–675. https://doi.org/10.1017/S0305000907008070

Guarini, A., Sansavini, A., Fabbri, C., Savini, S., Alessandroni, R., Faldella, G., et al. 2010. Longterm effects of preterm birth on language and literacy at eight years. *Journal of Child Language* 37, 865–885. https://doi.org/10.1017/S0305000909990109

Kern, S., & Gayraud, F. 2007. Influence of preterm birth on early lexical and grammatical acquisition. *First Language* 27,159–173. https://doi.org/10.1177/0142723706075790

Law, J., & Roy, P. 2008. Parental report of infant language skills: A review of the development and application of the communicative development inventories. *Child and Adolescent Mental Health* 13, 198–206. https://doi.org/10.1111/j.1475-3588.2008.00503.x

Luu, T., Vohr, B., Allan, W., Schneider, K., & Ment, L. 2011. Evidence for catch-up in cognition and receptive vocabulary among adolescents born very preterm. *Pediatrics* 128, 313–322. https://doi.org/10.1542/peds.2010-2655

Marston, L., Peacock, J. L., Calvert, S. A., Greenough, A., & Marlow, N. 2007. Factors affecting vocabulary acquisition at age 2 in children born between 23 and 28 weeks' gestation. *Developmental Medicine & Child Neurology* 49(8), 591–596. https://doi.org/10.1111/j.1469-8749.2007.00591.x

McManus, B. M., & Poehlmann, J. 2012. Maternal depression and perceived social support as predictors of cognitive function trajectories during the first 3 years of life for preterm infants in Wisconsin. *Child: Care, Health and Development* 38(3), 425–434.

Mendoza, E., Carballo, G., Muñoz, J., & Fresneda, M. D. 2005. *CEG: Test de comprensión de estructuras gramaticales*. Madrid: TEA

Ment, L. R., Vohr, B., Allan, W., Katz, K. H., Schneider, K. C., Westerveld, M., Duncan, C. C., & Makuch, R. W. 2003. Change in cognitive function over time in very low-birth-weight infants. *JAMA* 289(6), 705–711. https://doi.org/10.1001/jama.289.6.705

Molfese, V. J., Holcomb, L., & Helwig, S. 1994. Biomedical and socioenvironmental influences on cognitive and verbal abilities in children 1 to 3 years of age. *International Journal of Behavioral Development* 17, 271–287. https://doi.org/10.1177/016502549401700203

Newborg, J., Stock, J. R., & Wnek, L. 1996. *Batelle, inventario de desarrollo* [The Batelle Developmental Inventory] Madrid: TEA

Pérez Pereira, M., & García Soto, X. R. 2003. El diagnóstico del desarrollo comunicativo en la primera infancia: Adaptación de las escalas MacArthur al gallego. *Psicothema* 15(3), 352–361.

Pérez-Pereira, M., & Cruz, R. 2018. A longitudinal study of vocabulary size and composition in low risk preterm children. *First Language* 38(1), 72–94. https://doi.org/10.1177/0142723717730484

Pérez-Pereira, M., & Resches, M. 2011. Concurrent and predictive validity of the Galician CDI. *Journal of Child Language* 38(1), 121–140. https://doi.org/10.1017/S0305000909990262

Pérez-Pereira, M., Fernández, P., Gómez-Taibo, M. L., & Resches, M. 2014. Language development of low risk preterm infants up to the age of 30 months. *Early Human Development* 90, 649–656. https://doi.org/10.1016/j.earlhumdev.2014.08.004

Pérez-Pereira, M., Fernández, P., Resches, M., & Gómez-Taibo, M. 2013. Determinants of early language and communication in preterm and full term infants: A comparative study. *Enfance* 65(1), 59–76. https://doi.org/10.4074/S0013754513001079

Putnick, D. L., Bornstein, M. L., Eryigit-Madzwamuse, S., & Wolke, D. 2017. Long-term stability of language performance in very preterm, moderate-late preterm, and term children. *The Journal of Pediatrics* 181, 74–79. https://doi.org/10.1016/j.jpeds.2016.09.006

Radloff, L. S. 1977. The CES-D scale: A self-report depression scale for research in the general population. *Applied Psychological Measurement* 1(3), 385–401. https://doi.org/10.1177/014662167700100306

Rice, M., Taylor, C., & Zubrick, D. 2008. Language outcomes of 7-year-old children with or without a history of late language emergence at 24 months. *Journal of Speech, Language, and Hearing Research* 51, 394–407. https://doi.org/10.1044/1092-4388(2008/029)

Sansavini, A., Guarini, A., Alessandroni, R., Faldella, G., Giovanelli, G., & Salvioli, G. 2006. Early relations between lexical and grammatical development in very immature Italian preterms. *Journal of Child Language* 33, 199–216. https://doi.org/10.1017/S0305000905007208

Sansavini, A., Guarini, A., Justice, L. M., Savini, S., Broccoli, S., Alessandroni, R., & Faldella, G. 2010. Does preterm birth increase a child's risk for language impairment? *Early Human Development* 86(12), 765–772. https://doi.org/10.1016/j.earlhumdev.2010.08.014

Singer, L. T., Siegel, A. C., Lewis, B., Hawkins, S., Yamashita, H., & Baley, J. 2001. Preschool language outcomes of children with history of bronchopulmonary dysplasia and very low birthweight. *Developmental and Behavioral Pediatrics* 22(1), 19–26. https://doi.org/10.1097/00004703-200102000-00003

Stolt, S., Haataja, L., Lapinleimu, H., & Lehtonen, L. 2009. Early lexical development of prematurely born very-low-birth-weight children, and its relations to language skills at 2;0. *Journal of Communication Disorders* 42, 107–123. https://doi.org/10.1016/j.jcomdis.2008.10.002

Stolt, S., Klippi, A., Launonen, K., Munck, P., Lehtonen, L., Lapinleimu, H., et al. 2007. Size and composition of the lexicon in prematurely born very-low-weight and full-term Finnish children at two years of age. *Journal of Child Language* 34, 283–310. https://doi.org/10.1017/S0305000906007902

Stolt, S., Lind, A., Matomäki, J., Haataja, L., Lapinleimu, H., & Lehtonen, L. 2016. Do the early development of gestures and receptive and expressive language predict language skills at 5; 0 in prematurely born very-low-birth-weight children? *Journal of Communication Disorders* 61, 16–28. https://doi.org/10.1016/j.jcomdis.2016.03.002

Stolt, S., Matomäki, J., Lind, A., Lapinleimu, H., Haataja, L., & Lehtonen, L. 2014. The prevalence and predictive value of weak language skills in children with very low birth weight–a longitudinal study. *Acta Paediatrica* 103(6), 651–658. https://doi.org/10.1111/apa.12607

van Noort-van der Spek, I, Franken, M.-C., & Weisglas-Kuperus, N. 2012. Language functions in preterm-born children: a systematic review and meta-analysis. *Pediatrics* 129, 745–754. https://doi.org/10.1542/peds.2011-1728

Wolke, D., & Meyer, R. 1999. Cognitive status, language attainment, and prereading skills of 6-year-old very preterm children and their peers: The Bavarian longitudinal study. *Developmental Medicine & Child Neurology* 41(2), 94–109. https://doi.org/10.1017/S0012162299000201

Woodward, L. J., Moor, S., Hood, K. M., Champion, P. R., Foster-Cohen, S., Inder, T. E. & Austin, N. C. 2009. Very preterm children show impairments across multiple neurodevelopmental domains by age 4 years. *Archives of Disease in Childhood – Fetal and Neonatal Edition* 94, 339–344. https://doi.org/10.1136/adc.2008.146282

Zubrick, S., Taylor, C., Rice, M., & Seglers, D. 2007. Late language emergence at 24 months: An epidemiological study of prevalence, predictors and covariates. *Journal of Speech, Language, and Hearing Research* 50, 1562–1592. https://doi.org/10.1044/1092-4388(2007/106)

Word segmentation and mapping in early word learning

Differences between full term and moderately preterm infants

Laura Bosch,[1,2] Maria Teixidó[1] and Thais Agut[2,3]
[1]Universitat de Barcelona / [2]Institut de Recerca Sant Joan de Déu /
[3]Neonatology Unit Hospital Sant Joan de Déu

Comparative study with infants differing in gestational age at birth, tested on a dual word segmentation and mapping task with natural language passages and visual cues to facilitate word extraction and word-referent association, two abilities linked to vocabulary building. Infants were tested at 9 months corrected age for gestation, with preterm infants having longer language experience than full-terms, but similar maturational age. Only full terms succeeded on the word mapping test. While visual cues were expected to facilitate word extraction, unsuccessful mapping is possibly related to the cognitive demands of the task, requiring simultaneous processes for the young learner. Differences in language development levels were also identified, suggesting a complex interplay of factors behind preterm infants' early language learning skills.

Keywords: speech segmentation, word mapping, dual task, cognitive demands, moderately preterm, word learning mechanism

Introduction

An important milestone in the early stages of native language learning is the building of a first receptive vocabulary. Recent research has revealed that already by 6 months of age infants begin to recognize some familiar words, i.e. common words frequently used in their environment to refer to food and body parts (Bergelson & Swingley, 2012). This early process to connect words and referents is favoured in home environments where noun labels can be repeatedly heard for objects infants are looking at and attending to (Bergelson & Aslin, 2017). This early skill to form

https://doi.org/10.1075/z.223.05bos

word-referent mappings, together with the capacity to attribute referential value to those frequently experienced sound patterns adults produce in the presence of specific objects, set the ground for word comprehension development, triggering successful word learning and the building of a first receptive vocabulary.

While it is certainly true that in some instances the words infants hear in the presence of specific referents are produced in isolation, several studies have reported that this situation is usually limited to around 10% of the utterances they are exposed to (Brent and Siskind, 2001; Bergelson & Aslin, 2017). Thus, one "problem" to be solved by the young language learner concerns the extraction of possible word-forms from fluent speech, either before or simultaneously with the mapping process. In what follows a short review of the available data on these skills will be reviewed.

Research on the emergence of word segmentation in young infants has revealed that around seven months of age this ability is already in place for monosyllabic elements or for two-syllable items that follow the predominant stress pattern of the language (Juskzyk & Aslin, 1995; Jusczyk, Houston, & Newsome, 1999). After the seminal work by P. W. Jusczyk in the field of word segmentation in infancy, research expanded with studies involving languages other than English, differing in rhythm and lexical stress properties, and describing a hierarchy of cues, statistical and prosodic in nature, that mostly contribute to successful word segmentation (see Saffran, 2001; Seidl & Johnson, 2006; Johnson & Jusczyk, 2001, for different perspectives on the topic). Evidence of word segmentation skills at an earlier age has also been gathered, showing that by 6 months of age this skill is already present, especially for short elements or word-forms located in favourable positions within the sentences (e.g. at the end of the sentence or at a phonological-phrase boundary position) or for those that are preceded by already familiar nouns which can serve as anchors and simplify the segmentation demands (Bortfeld, Morgan, Golinkoff, & Rathbun, 2005; Bosch, Figueras, Teixidó, & Ramon-Casas, 2013; Johnson, Seidl, & Tyler, 2014; Nishibayashi, Goyet, & Nazzi, 2015). More recent data from French-learning infants seem to indicate that the skill could be in place even before 6 months of age, at least for short elements that match the rhythm unit of the language, i.e. the syllable in syllable-timed languages such as French (Berdasco-Muñoz, Nishibayashi, Baud, Biran, Nazzi, 2018).

From all this work on early word segmentation it can be concluded that there are mainly two types of strategies young infants can exploit to extract word-forms from the speech they hear, i.e. lexically guided and non-lexically guided strategies. Considering the limited number of words in young infants' receptive vocabularies by 6–9 months of age, non-lexically guided strategies are the ones more likely to be exploited at early ages. As already mentioned, these strategies are based on infant's sensitivities to regularities and distributional information in the input.

Regularities that can be easily detected by the naive listener are related to prosody or to segmental information. Predominant word stress patterns (e.g. syllable-initial word stress in disyllabic words) can favour extraction of trochaic word-forms. Frequently occurring adjacent syllables are likely to be grouped together forming a unit, a possible word-form. In a similar way, syllables that are frequently repeated in the speech stream can be easily detected and isolated. Finally, phonotactic and allophonic cues can also guide word extraction, depending on how regular the languages are at these levels and also depending on the number of units already available to the infant, as a minimum amount of elements is needed for regularities to be captured. Thus, several cues are available to word segmentation, starting by those related to prosody and distributional properties of syllables and segments, to which more fine-grained cues will gradually be added, eventually outweighing the initial ones (Mattys, White, & Melhorn, 2005). Outside the lab, in natural environments and contexts of interaction, parents address their infants using a speech register termed infant-directed-speech (IDS), which emphasizes prosodic features, increases the saliency of specific words, places them at phrase or sentence boundary and includes many repetitions of elements (usually nouns) in the presence of their referents. This linguistic and communicative behaviour favours speech segmentation processes, as it involves producing those cues infants are sensitive to. But also, when adults point to specific objects while naming them or move an object they are holding while repeating its name, either in isolation or most frequently in short sentences, they are actually favouring not only segmentation, but, crucially, the association between a word-form unit and its possible referent. It is in this sense that these early processes, taking place before the end of the first year of life, must be considered as a first step leading towards later and more sophisticated word learning processes that will be fundamental in the second year of life.

A review of the literature, thus, suggests that word segmentation demands, at least for short elements or for those that adhere to the most frequent lexical stress patterns of the language, can possibly be handled by infants early in their second semester of life. Less information is available, though, about infants' capacity to both segment and successfully map the extracted items to possible referents, objects or entities in their environment. Assuming that early word segmentation skills have been positively linked to later language outcomes (Newman, Ratner, Jusczyk, Jusczyk, & Dow, 2006; Singh, Reznick, & Xuehua, 2012), this connection should also involve the mapping process, the ability to associate the segmented word-forms to referents. There is experimental evidence that in their second year of life toddlers more readily connect recently extracted word-forms to novel objects when successively tested on word segmentation and word learning (Estes, Evans, Alibali, & Saffran, 2007), but research addressing simultaneous segmentation and mapping in the first year of life is still scarce.

Evidence of an early ability to solve the demands of a dual task (i.e. simultaneously extracting a word-form unit from connected speech and mapping the segmented unit to a referent) comes from a first study with 6-month-old infants, using short artificial language utterances and testing for successful segmentation and mapping of a single word supported by prosodic information (Shukla, White, & Aslin, 2011). The finding about the relevant contribution of prosodic cues to facilitate both word-form extraction and label-referent mapping sets the basis for studies addressing the emergence of this more sophisticated skill and its constraints at an early age. Some limitations have been recently identified in behavioural ongoing studies in our lab involving 6-month-old infants, but not slightly older infants, using natural language utterances and testing for simultaneous segmentation and mapping of two, not just one, monosyllabic elements (Teixidó, 2017; Teixidó & Bosch, 2016). While simultaneous segmentation and mapping might be facilitated in certain contexts and positive evidence of this skill can be obtained in highly controlled lab settings (see also recent electrophysiological evidence of segmentation and mapping in 6-month-olds, by Männel, Teixidó, Bosch, Friederici, & Friedrich, 2017), we adopt here a more parsimonious position, considering that simultaneous segmentation and mapping, as a word learning mechanism, might initially be cognitively too demanding for the young learner and, thus, not a useful strategy until the infant gains more expertise with language and word learning.

From this perspective, and taking into account previous results in our lab, the aim of the present research is to gain greater insight on the cognitive demands of a simultaneous segmentation and mapping task and explore whether this skill is well established by the age of 9 months to serve as an efficient word learning mechanism that might accelerate the building of a receptive vocabulary. To do so, we designed an audiovisual segmentation and mapping task and compared the results from two different populations tested at a similar maturational age: infants born at term and healthy preterm infants, who are nevertheless considered to be at a certain risk for cognitive and language delays (Aylward, 2014; Caravale, Tozzi, Albino, & Vicari, 2005; Putnick, Bornstein, Eryigit-Madzwamuse, & Wolke, 2017; Wolke & Meyer, 1999). More specifically, we report data from a sample of moderately preterm infants, those born with gestational ages within the range of 33–36 weeks and tested at 9 months of age (corrected for gestation). The comparison between full term and moderately preterm infants can shed light on the cognitive demands of a dual task and the ability to cope with those demands by 9 months of age, when successful segmentation and mapping, as separate skills, should no longer be a problem.

The focus on moderately preterm infants was motivated by previous results in our lab testing preterm infants of different gestational ages on a classical word segmentation task using the familiarization-preference procedure (Bosch, 2011;

Bosch, Solé, Teixidó, Arca, & Agut, 2013). In this task, adapted from Jusczyk & Aslin, 1995, infants were first familiarized with two short passages presented in alternation involving repetitions of two different words. After 1 minute and a half of attention time to those passages, infants were then tested on four word lists, two involving the words from the familiarization passages and the other two containing novel words. A preference for the familiar words over the novel ones is usually interpreted as evidence of successful word segmentation. Note that in this task no objects are presented, no mapping is involved. It is a purely auditory word segmentation task in which word extraction can only be reached by relying on prosodic information and distributional properties of syllables in the speech stream, as no visual cues are available. When this experimental procedure was applied to different groups of 9-month-old infant participants differing in gestational age at birth, reliable evidence of word segmentation could only be gathered from full term and moderately preterm participants, while very preterm infants were still lagging behind the positive results of the other two groups. It must be acknowledged that available data on word segmentation (as a single task) in preterm infants remains controversial, with positive results having been obtained at a very early age in a sample of French-learning preterm participants extracting syllables from natural speech utterances (Berdasco-Muñoz et al., 2018), while less positive outcomes were obtained in our studies with Spanish-learning and Catalan-learning preterm participants extracting monosyllabic word-forms (Bosch, 2011). Differences might be attributed to the characteristics of the participants, the implementation of the experimental tasks, the nature of the testing material or even the language properties, as suggested by Berdasco-Muñoz et al., 2018. But this debate is out of the scope of the present research. Our priority in designing this research about infants' ability to simultaneously segment and map two words from natural speech utterances was to select an age at which word segmentation, as a separate skill, was likely to be available in the population under study.

The inclusion of a sample of moderately preterm participants has the additional value of targeting a population whose early speech perception and word learning skills remain rather unexplored (but see Nazzi, Nishibayashi, Berdasco-Muñoz, Baud, Biran, & Gonzalez-Gomez, 2015). These infants are generally considered to have low or no risk for neurocognitive disorders and they are less frequently involved in follow-up programs after discharge from hospital. Recent studies from a clinical perspective, however, have begun to highlight the relevance of a regular follow-up for these infants, who might also be at a certain risk for neurocognitive delays or negative outcomes once they reach school (Caravale, Mirante, Vagnoni, & Vicari, 2012; see also Perez-Pereira, Fernández, Gómez-Taibo, & Resches, 2014, for a different result).

To sum up, taking into account our previous research signalling differences between preterm and full term infants on word segmentation skills (Bosch, 2011; Bosch et al., 2013), as well as data from moderately preterm populations revealing the presence of suboptimal outcomes in neuropsychological assessment (Caravale et al., 2012; de Jong et al., 2015), and also considering the cognitive demands of a dual task involving simultaneous segmentation and mapping of two different word-forms to be associated to two novel distinct objects, we first hypothesized that while full term infants would succeed at the dual task by 9 months of age, preterm infants might not show a similar result, failing to successfully map the two novel words to their referents or differing from full terms in their mapping strategies. However, because preterm infants would be tested at age corrected for gestation, being almost two months older than the full term counterparts, they would have had additional exposure and experience with language, a factor that might compensate for the initial differences in brain maturation between these two groups. In this case, the alternative hypothesis would predict similar outcomes in the dual task by both groups. This result would highlight the positive role of language experience when maturational age is equated. To obtain a better perspective about the role played by cognitive and language factors on the results from the experimental task, independent measures of the levels attained in cognitive and language/communication development would be obtained in both groups at the tested age. We were expecting no differences in these measures between groups, especially because moderately preterm infants constitute a low risk group and testing was done at corrected age for gestation. Alternatively, finding significant between-group differences in any of these developmental measures could also be informative about the role that these variables might play in infants' capacity to cope with the cognitively demanding dual segmentation and mapping task.

Methodology

Participants

Thirty-four 9-month-old infants, corrected age for gestation in preterm infants, from the Barcelona area formed the final sample. They were divided into two groups of 17 infants, the full-term group (FT, 8 boys) and the moderately preterm group (MP, 10 boys). Mean age of the FT group was 274 days ($SD = 5.02$), mean birth weight was 3473 g (SD = 564) and mean gestation weeks were 39.7 ($SD = 1.3$). Regarding the MP group, mean age corrected for gestation was 277 days ($SD = 8.5$), mean birth weight was 2144 g (SD = 359) and mean gestation weeks were 33.8 ($SD = 1.01$). Statistical comparison of these variables revealed no significant between-group differences in age when corrected for gestation ($t_{(32)} = -1.18$; $p = 0.25$), although chronological age differences were obviously significantly different ($p < 0.0001$). As expected, highly significant differences in birth weight and weeks of gestation were found ($t_{(32)} = 8.19$; $p < 0.0001$; $t_{(32)} = 14.31$; $p < 0.0001$, respectively). Nine additional participants were tested but excluded from the final sample due to non-completion of the task or very low fixation on the objects displayed on the screen (2), low attention time (<650 ms) to test trials (6), side bias (1) and technical problems (1). Infants in both groups were growing up in monolingual or bilingual homes having either Catalan or Spanish as their predominant language in their input, according to the language questionnaire that was used (Bosch & Sebastián-Gallés, 2001). Infants were always tested with material in their native or dominant language (similar versions of the auditory stimuli had been prepared). The educational level of their parents was also measured, revealing no significant between-group differences (45% of the mothers had attained secondary educational levels and 55% had a university degree). This distribution was slightly different for fathers, but similar in both groups: 73% had attained secondary educational levels and 26% were university graduates. Groups were thus found to be comparable regarding parental educational levels.

Materials

We designed an audiovisual task. Auditory material consisted of a selection of passages and words from a previous word segmentation study (Bosch et al., 2013). Two four-sentence passages ([gol] and [tren] passages), containing repetitions of these two target words in either initial or final-sentence position, were used in the familiarization phase (see Appendix 1). In the test phase, word lists containing eight different tokens of the target words were used, adjusting trial duration to fifteen seconds. Measures comparing the acoustic properties of the cognate target words in the Catalan and Spanish versions of the material confirmed that they were equivalent. As visual referents, two distinct geometrical shapes were used, a bright orange diamond and a green square.

Four different videos were created by merging audio and visual stimuli. Each video consisted in a familiarization phase of 150 seconds playing both passages in alternation, each passage being presented five times which resulted in twenty opportunities to hear each target word. To enhance word segmentation and mapping during this phase, the target object loomed aligned to target word onset. There were four trials in the test phase, two for each target word. Both objects were statically displayed on the screen while word lists were played (Figure 1). Word-object association, side location on the screen and order of presentation were carefully counterbalanced.

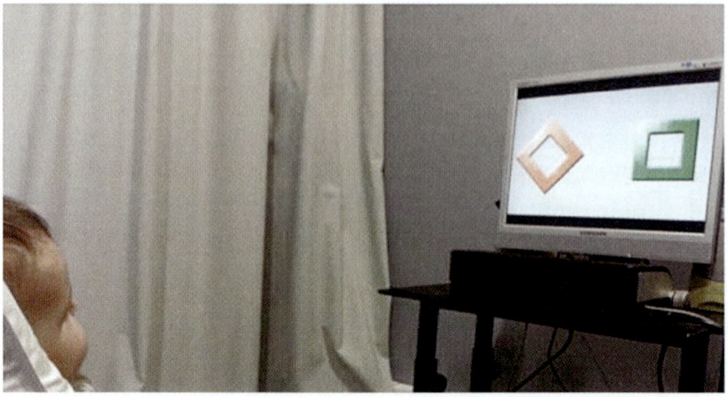

Figure 1. Outline of the experimental procedure and visual stimuli used in the task. Passages containing repetitions of the two target words were presented in alternation during the familiarization, followed by a short test phase to assess word extraction and word-object association

Procedure

Infants were seated on a high chair at 65 cm from the screen, while parents sat behind the infant and were encouraged to avoid interference. A Tobii X120 eye tracker recorded the infants' gaze at a sampling rate of 60 Hz. A five-point calibration procedure was used before the experiment began. Two areas of interest (AOI) around the shapes (visual referents for the target words) were established and infants' gaze was monitored by the eye tracker.

After the audiovisual segmentation and mapping task, infants were tested on their cognitive and language developmental levels using the Bayley Scales of Infant and Toddler Development (BSID-III, Bayley, 2006). Only the Cognitive and Language/Communication subscales were administered.

Measures

In the *familiarization phase*, total accumulated fixation time to each object was first obtained and percentage was computed ([total fixation time to object A and B * 100]/total familiarization time). A second measure was the percentage of attention time to the looming objects, corresponding to a window of analysis of 800 ms from word onset. These measures were taken in order to verify that performance between groups was comparable and that participants had had similar opportunities to see the visual cue signaling word onset and favoring word-referent mapping. In the *test phase*, Proportion of Total Looking Time (PTLT) to each target object was first obtained (target / [target + distracter]). Then, a difference score was calculated using the mean PTLT value to objects when they were target minus the mean PTLT value when they were distracters. Positive values would be considered as an indication of successful mapping.

Regarding BSID-III measures, composite scores were obtained for the Cognitive and Language subscales. Within the latter, scalar scores for Receptive and Expressive communication were first computed.

Results

Familiarization phase

Total accumulated attention time during familiarization was similar between groups (43.5% and 44% for FT and MP groups, respectively) with no significant differences ($t < 1$). Total attention time to the looming objects was 53.1% and 52% for the FT and MP groups respectively; again no significant differences were found ($t < 1$). The distribution of attention between the two passages and the two target words was also similar in both groups, suggesting that their behavior was comparable during familiarization.

Test phase

PTLT to target objects was first computed in each group (PTLT to distracters being complementary). This value in the FT group was 0.57 ($SD = 0.11$), while it was 0.48 ($SD = 0.11$) in the MD group. The former was significantly different from chance [$t_{(16)} = 2.44$; $p = 0.02$], while the latter was not ($t < 1$). The critical dependent variable was the difference score based on the mean PTLT to objects when they were target minus the mean PTLT to those objects when they were distracters. The FT group had a mean difference score of 0.13 ($SD = 0.22$), and the MP group had a mean difference score of −0.04 ($SD = 0.20$) (see Figure 2). A one-way ANOVA comparing both groups showed a significant difference [$F_{(1, 32)} = 5.98$, $p = 0.02$]. Thirteen of the 17 FT infants had a positive PTLT difference score value, while only 7 of the 17 MD infants had a positive value.

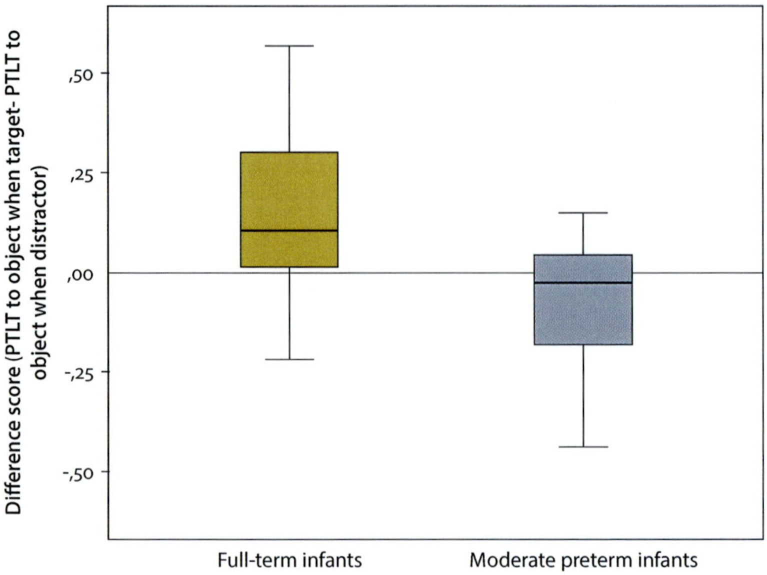

Figure 2. Boxplots representing the median, Q1 and Q3, maximum and minimum values of the distribution of the difference PTLT score measure for each group of participants (full term and moderately preterm infants). Positive values indicate higher fixation values to the object when target compared to when it was a distracter, thus, suggesting successful mapping

BSID-III measures of cognitive and language development

Composite scores from the administered subscales were obtained and compared between groups. Mean scores on the Cognitive subscale were within the normal range: 100.9 ($SD = 6.9$) for the FT group and 96.2 ($SD = 8.4$) for the MP group. This difference did not reach statistical significance [$F_{(1, 32)} = 3.19$, $p = 0.084$]. Regarding the Language/Communication subscale, mean composite scores were also within the normal range: 103.2 ($SD = 7.7$) for the FT group and 96.5 ($SD = 9.1$) for the MP group, but in this case the difference reached significance [$F_{(1, 32)} = 5.21$, $p = 0.029$]. An additional comparison based on the scalar scores corresponding to the receptive and expressive subscales revealed a highly significant difference only in receptive communication [$F_{(1, 32)} = 8.13$, $p = 0.008$], but not in expressive communication [$F_{(1, 32)} = 2.33$, $p = 0.14$].

To further analyze the possible link between these developmental levels and the difference PTLT score from the dual task, correlation analyses were undertaken for each group. No significant results were obtained. Correlations between the dependent variable and neonatal characteristics such as birth weight and weeks of gestation did not reach significance.

Discussion

Results from the audiovisual dual task in our study indicate that by 9 months of age full term infants can successfully extract and link novel word-forms to their referents, a precursor skill setting the ground for later word learning, Data reveal that they can simultaneously segment these word-forms from fluent speech and map them onto different objects. But the same strategy might not yet be available for infants born preterm tested at a similar age (corrected for gestation), even in the case of moderately preterm infants. Although their ability to segment words from fluent speech might not be impaired, this ability alone is not related to mapping processes. Their skill mapping labels to referents might not be delayed (but see Gogate, Maganti, & Perenyi, 2014, for evidence of a delayed emergence of the ability to link syllable-object pairings in two-month-old moderately preterm infants), but the high demands of a task requiring simultaneous segmentation and mapping seem to constrain the possibility to use this strategy as a mechanism in early word-to-world mapping, considered as a precursor step to early word learning processes. This limitation might have consequences on the speed at which novel words will be gradually incorporated in the initial phases of vocabulary building. We did not obtain general measures of receptive vocabulary in our sample of moderate preterm infants, but the fact that receptive language scores from the BSID-III were lagging behind the scores from the full term group seem to support this tentative interpretation.

The dual task we have used required segmentation and mapping of monosyllabic elements. Considering previous research in our lab (Bosch, 2011), and also recent data from syllabic segmentation in French-learning preterm infants tested as early as by 4 months of age (Berdasco-Muñoz et al., 2018), it seems plausible to suggest that segmentation *per se* is not the problem, but rather the higher demands imposed by a dual task were. Unsuccessful results from the moderately preterm group cannot be attributed to lower cognitive levels of development, as their results from the Cognitive subscale of the BSID-III did not significantly differ from those obtained by the full term group. Their difficulties might instead reveal less expertise in each of the activities involved in the task (i.e. segmenting word-forms and mapping them onto distinct objects), thus limiting the possibility to use this strategy as a word learning mechanism. Attention and memory constraints need also to be considered as relevant factors. The fact that the task required extracting and mapping *two* different elements adds higher levels of complexity to the task, such that only more experienced early word learners, i.e. those with higher receptive vocabularies, would manage to successfully cope with these taks demands.

Certainly, no significant correlation could be obtained between preterm infants' cognitive scores on the BSID-III and the PTLT difference score in the task. Future research, with an extended sample of participants, covering different gestational ages, and using different and more specific measures of cognitive skills beyond a general developmental score, might shed light on the origin of the disadvantage found in the moderately preterm group. Different methodological approaches can also be relevant to better understand the underlying mechanisms in this dual task and how they might be affected in preterm participants. An approach using electrophysiological measures might prove useful to compare populations of full term and preterm infants, as revealed by a first attempt to identify the processes and underlying mechanisms in a simultaneous segmentation, mapping and categorization task in typically developing participants at the age of six months (Männel et al., 2017).

The additional language experience moderately preterm infants had (recall that they were tested at an older chronological age compared to full term participants) did not seem to enhance their capacity to solve the task. Mean scores from the language/communication subscale of the BSID-III were found to be significantly different between the full term and preterm groups. In spite of the chronological age difference, receptive communication measures were not equivalent to those in the full term group. Thus it can also be argued that preterm's slightly lower levels of development identified by the BSID-III language/communication subscales reveal a less optimal achievement that might have a parallel in their difficulties to cope with the demands of our dual task. All in all, a complex interplay between language and cognitive factors sems to be behind preterm infants' early word-to-world mapping skills as revealed by the present results.

An open question, relative to preterm infants' abilities in early segmentation and word-referent mapping, would be to know whether other preterm groups, born with lower gestational ages, would show similar difficulties in the dual segmentation and mapping task. It could be argued that, if tested at age corrected for gestation, very preterm infants (i.e. those born within the range of 28–32 weeks of gestation), who would have had longer exposure to the language and might have experienced different language learning contexts, might benefit from this additional experience and show better results than those obtained by moderately preterms in this task. This seems counterintuitive, but the interplay between maturational and experience factors is far from simple. Some research has suggested somewhat "positive" effects of preterms' earlier exposure to the native language input, at least in some areas of speech perception involving low-level processing in which preterm infants have not shown delays compared to their full term counterparts (González-Gómez & Nazzi, 2012a; 2012b). Other research, however, has considered that no acceleration of processes, such as perceptual narrowing, is present in preterm infants (Jansson-Verkasalo, et al., 2010; Peña, Werker, & Dehaene-Lambertz, 2012). In this context, and considering the nature of the dual task and its cognitive demands, we would hypothesize similar difficulties in very preterm infants, compared to moderate preterm infants, when tested at the age of nine months (corrected for gestation). This still remains an open question, but preliminary data from ongoing research in our lab seem to indicate that the task is equally demanding for very preterm infants.

Finally, it is important to indicate that failure to succeed in the segmentation and mapping task should not be viewed as a severe limitation in the early stages of vocabulary building. Words can be linked to their referents, especially when the context and the social environment favours this process, most frequently by reducing the demands of speech segmentation (i.e. extracting words from fluent speech when they are located in final sentence position, or often produced in isolation and frequently heard in the communicative interaction between the adult and the infant). The restricted access to using the simultaneous segmentation and mapping strategy might instead limit or disfavour its use in less controlled contexts, possibly hampering a rapid vocabulary growth in preterm infants compared to their full term counterparts. Future research will reveal if this hypothesis is confirmed.

The present finding about the differences between full term and moderately preterm infants needs to be highlighted. It suggests that even in low risk moderately preterm populations, born between 33–36 gestation weeks, regular follow-up should be considered in order to detect early developmental delays and prevent later difficulties in language acquisition and learning.

Acknowledgments

Research supported by the Spanish MINECO (project PSI-2014-55105P). We thank Jorgina Solé and Jessica Sánchez-Galán for their help in recruiting and testing participants. We are also grateful to the families of the participants in this research.

References

Aylward, G. P. 2014. Neurodevelopmental outcomes of infants born prematurely. *Journal of Developmental & Behavioral Pediatrics* 35(6), 394–407. https://doi.org/10.1097/01.DBP.0000452240.39511.d4

Bayley, N. 2006. *Bayley scales of infant and toddler development: BSID-III.* New York, NY: Harcourt Assessment, Psych. Corporation.

Berdasco-Muñoz, E., Nishibayashi, L. L., Baud, O., Biran, V., & Nazzi, T. 2018. Early segmentation abilities in preterm infants. *Infancy* 23(2), 268–287. https://doi.org/10.1111/infa.12217

Bergelson, E., & Aslin, R. N. 2017. Nature and origins of the lexicon in 6-mo-olds. *Proceedings of the National Academy of Sciences* 114(49), 12916–12921. https://doi.org/10.1073/pnas.1712966114

Bergelson, E., , & Swingley, D. 2012. At 6–9 months, human infants know the meanings of many common nouns. *Proceedings of the National Academy of Sciences*, 109(9), 3253–3258. https://doi.org/10.1073/pnas.1113380109

Bortfeld, H., Morgan, J. L., Golinkoff, R. M., & Rathbun, K. 2005. Mommy and me: Familiar names help launch babies into speech-stream segmentation. *Psychological Science* 16(4), 298–304. https://doi.org/10.1111/j.0956-7976.2005.01531.x

Bosch, L. 2011. Precursors to language in preterm infants: speech perception abilities in the first year of life. In O. Braddick, J. Atkinson, & G. Innocenti (Eds.), *Gene expression to neurobiology and behavior: Human brain development and developmental disorders* (Progress in Brain Research, Vol., 189) (Ch. 14, pp. 239–257). https://doi.org/10.1016/B978-0-444-53884-0.00028-2

Bosch, L., & Sebastián-Gallés, N. 2001. Evidence of early language discrimination abilities in infants from bilingual environments. *Infancy* 2(1), 29–49. https://doi.org/10.1207/S15327078IN0201_3

Bosch, L., Figueras, M., Teixidó, M., & Ramon-Casas, M. 2013. Rapid gains in segmenting fluent speech when words match the rhythmic unit: evidence from infants acquiring syllable-timed languages. *Frontiers in Psychology*, 4. https://doi.org/10.3389/fpsyg.2013.00106

Bosch, L., Solé, J., Teixidó, M., Arca, G., & Agut, T. 2013. Delayed ability to segment words from fluent speech in infants born preterm. Paper presented at the 16th European Conference on Developmental Psychology (ECDP, Lausanne, Switzerland).

Brent, M. R., & Siskind, J. M. 2001. The role of exposure to isolated words in early vocabulary development. *Cognition* 81(2), B33-B44. https://doi.org/10.1016/S0010-0277(01)00122-6

Caravale, B., Mirante, N., Vagnoni, C., & Vicari, S. 2012. Change in cognitive abilities over time during preschool age in low risk preterm children. *Early Human Development* 88(6), 363–367. https://doi.org/10.1016/j.earlhumdev.2011.09.011

Caravale, B., Tozzi, C., Albino, G., & Vicari, S. 2005. Cognitive development in low risk preterm infants at 3–4 years of life. *Archives of Disease in Childhood-Fetal and Neonatal Edition* 90(6), F474-F479. https://doi.org/10.1136/adc.2004.070284

de Jong, M., Verhoeven, M., Lasham, C. A., Meijssen, C. B., & van Baar, A. L. 2015. Behaviour and development in 24-month-old moderately preterm toddlers. *Archives of Disease in Childhood* 100(6), 548–553. https://doi.org/10.1136/archdischild-2014-307016

Estes, K. G., Evans, J. L., Alibali, M. W., & Saffran, J. R. 2007. Can infants map meaning to newly segmented words? Statistical segmentation and word learning. *Psychological Science* 18(3), 254–260. https://doi.org/10.1111/j.1467-9280.2007.01885.x

Gonzalez-Gomez, N., & Nazzi, T. 2012a. Phonotactic acquisition in healthy preterm infants. *Developmental Science* 15(6), 885–894. https://doi.org/10.1111/j.1467-7687.2012.01186.x

Gonzalez-Gomez, N., & Nazzi, T. 2012b. Acquisition of nonadjacent phonological dependencies in the native language during the first year of life. *Infancy* 17(5), 498–524. https://doi.org/10.1111/j.1532-7078.2011.00104.x

Gogate, L., Maganti, M., & Perenyi, A. 2014. Preterm and term infants' perception of temporally coordinated syllable–object pairings: Implications for lexical development. *Journal of Speech, Language, and Hearing Research* 57(1), 187–198. https://doi.org/10.1044/1092-4388(2013/12-0403)

Jansson-Verkasalo, E., Ruusuvirta, T., Huotilainen, M., Alku, P., Kushnerenko, E., Suominen, K., & Hallman, M. 2010. Atypical perceptual narrowing in prematurely born infants is associated with compromised language acquisition at 2 years of age. *BMC neuroscience* 11(1), 88. https://doi.org/10.1186/1471-2202-11-88

Johnson, E. K., & Jusczyk, P. W. 2001. Word segmentation by 8-month-olds: When speech cues count more than statistics. *Journal of Memory and Language* 44(4), 548–567. https://doi.org/10.1006/jmla.2000.2755

Johnson, E. K., Seidl, A., & Tyler, M. D. 2014. The edge factor in early word segmentation: utterance-level prosody enables word form extraction by 6-month-olds. *PloS One* 9(1), e83546: https://doi.org/10.1371/journal.pone.0083546

Jusczyk, P. W., & Aslin, R. N. 1995. Infants' detection of the sound patterns of words in fluent speech. *Cognitive Psychology* 29(1), 1–23. https://doi.org/10.1006/cogp.1995.1010

Jusczyk, P. W., Houston, D. M., & Newsome, M. 1999. The beginnings of word segmentation in English-learning infants. *Cognitive Psychology* 39(3), 159–207. https://doi.org/10.1006/cogp.1999.0716

Männel, C., Teixidó, M. Bosch, L, Friederici, A., & Friedrich, M.2017. Sentence prosody cues object category learning by 6 months. Potser presented at the 9th meeting of the Society for the Neurobiology of Language (Baltimore, MD. 8–10 November 2017).

Mattys, S. L., White, L., & Melhorn, J. F. 2005. Integration of multiple speech segmentation cues: A hierarchical framework. *Journal of Experimental Psychology: General* 134(4), 477. https://doi.org/10.1037/0096-3445.134.4.477

Nazzi, T., Nishibayashi, L. L., Berdasco-Muñoz, E., Baud, O., Biran, V., & Gonzalez-Gomez, N. 2015. Language acquisition in preterm infants during the first year of life. *Archives de Pediatrie: Organe Officiel de la Societe Francaise de Pediatrie* 22(10), 1072–1077. https://doi.org/10.1016/j.arcped.2015.07.002

Newman, R., Ratner, N. B., Jusczyk, A. M., Jusczyk, P. W., & Dow, K. A. 2006. Infants' early ability to segment the conversational speech signal predicts later language development: A retrospective analysis. *Developmental Psychology* 42(4), 643. https://doi.org/10.1037/0012-1649.42.4.643

Nishibayashi, L. L., Goyet, L., & Nazzi, T. 2015. Early speech segmentation in French-learning infants: Monosyllabic words versus embedded syllables. *Language and Speech* 58(3), 334–350. https://doi.org/10.1177/0023830914551375

Pena, M., Werker, J. F., & Dehaene-Lambertz, G. 2012. Earlier speech exposure does not accelerate speech acquisition. *Journal of Neuroscience* 32(33), 11159–11163. https://doi.org/10.1523/JNEUROSCI.6516-11.2012

Pérez-Pereira, M., Fernández, P., Gómez-Taibo, M. L., & Resches, M. 2014. Language development of low risk preterm infants up to the age of 30 months. *Early Human Development* 90(10), 649–656. https://doi.org/10.1016/j.earlhumdev.2014.08.004

Putnick, D. L., Bornstein, M. H., Eryigit-Madzwamuse, S., & Wolke, D. 2017. Long-term stability of language performance in very preterm, moderate-late preterm, and term children. *The Journal of Pediatrics* 181, 74–79. https://doi.org/10.1016/j.jpeds.2016.09.006

Saffran, J. R. 2001. Words in a sea of sounds: The output of infant statistical learning. *Cognition* 81(2), 149–169. https://doi.org/10.1016/S0010-0277(01)00132-9

Seidl, A., & Johnson, E. K. 2006. Infant word segmentation revisited: Edge alignment facilitates target extraction. *Developmental Science* 9(6), 565–573. https://doi.org/10.1111/j.1467-7687.2006.00534.x

Shukla, M., White, K. S., & Aslin, R. N. 2011. Prosody guides the rapid mapping of auditory word forms onto visual objects in 6-mo-old infants. *Proceedings of the National Academy of Sciences* 108(15), 6038–6043. https://doi.org/10.1073/pnas.1017617108

Singh, L., Steven Reznick, J., & Xuehua, L. 2012. Infant word segmentation and childhood vocabulary development: A longitudinal analysis. *Developmental Science* 15(4), 482–495. https://doi.org/10.1111/j.1467-7687.2012.01141.x

Teixidó, M. 2017. *Constraints on early word segmentation and mapping* (Unpublished doctoral dissertation). University of Barcelona.

Teixidó, M., & Bosch, L. 2016. Exploring simultaneous word segmentation and word-referent mapping: Can pupil dilation explain differences between 6- and 9-month-old infants? AttLis workshop, Potsdam, Germany.

Wolke, D., & Meyer, R. 1999. Cognitive status, language attainment, and prereading skills of 6-year-old very preterm children and their peers: the Bavarian Longitudinal Study. *Developmental medicine and child neurology*, 41(2), 94–109. https://doi.org/10.1111/j.1469-8749.1999

Appendix 1.

Passages used in the familiarization phase of the segmentation and mapping task (selected from the material in Bosch et al., 2013). Target words are in bold and they were located either at a phrase boundary or in sentence-final position to facilitate extraction. Comparable, but not literal translations of the sentences were created in Spanish (left) and Catalan (right). Target words were cognates and similar length in syllables of the sentences was prioritized over meaning.

Tren passage:

Un **tren** tiene seis vagones.	Un **tren** té set vagons.
En la foto hay un **tren**.	A la foto hi ha aquell **tren**.
El **tren** está parado.	El **tren** no s'atura mai.
!Mira ese coche junto al **tren**!	Mira el cotxe a prop del **tren**!

Gol passage:

Un **gol** llega de repente.	Un **gol** va venir de sobte.
Esperan otro **gol**.	Esperava el primer **gol**.
El **gol** no era bueno.	El **gol** no era massa bo.
Soñaré con este **gol**.	Sommiaré amb el meu **gol**.

PART II

Specific Language Impairment

The influence of maternal education on the linguistic abilities of monolingual Spanish-speaking children with and without Specific Language Impairment

Alejandra Auza-Benavides,[1,2] Christian Peñaloza C.[3] and Chiharu Murata[4]
[1]Hospital General Dr. Manuel Gea González / [2]Instituto Mexicano para la Atención del Desarrollo del Niño (IMAD, A.C.) / [3]Universidad Nacional Autónoma de México / [4]Instituto Nacional de Pediatría

Many Spanish-speaking children from low socioeconomic status grow in families with low maternal education (ME), which may reflect differences in quality and quantity of children's input. Lexical and grammatical abilities from these children are frequently confused with those of children with Specific Language Impairment (SLI). The aim of this research was to compare lexical and grammatical abilities in 400 monolingual children with and without SLI (aged 4;0 to 6;11) classified in ME groups. Analyses of variance revealed differences between ME groups. Regression analyses revealed that ME and age contributed to the greatest amount of variance in lexical but not grammatical abilities. The discussion is centered on the importance of considering ME as a distal factor that affects linguistic abilities.

Keywords: maternal education, grammatical measures, lexical measures, specific language impairment

Overview

Language development and language difficulties have been studied from different perspectives. One of the most salient considers different social, economic and cultural factors. It has been observed that language difficulties can be caused by distal factors from the social environment such as economy and education; intermediate factors like school, home or family; or child's inherent proximal factors as

https://doi.org/10.1075/z.223.06ale

psychological or biological features (Coreil, 2009). Nevertheless; distal, intermediate or proximal factors have been under or overestimated and direct causal relations have been established between these factors and language in children. One possible approach to study language development and its difficulties is to consider the particular characteristics of a given population. In Mexico, many Spanish-speaking children from low socioeconomic status are raised in families with low maternal education (ME), which may reflect differences in the quality and quantity of language input and output of the children. Lexical and grammatical abilities of these children are frequently confused as Specific Language Impairment (SLI). The aim of this research was to compare lexical and grammatical abilities in 392 Mexican monolingual children with and without SLI considering the effect of ME.

Family and socioeconomic status

Socioeconomic status of the families has been largely considered in literature as an important factor in child development given that families are the main conduct of influence in children's development (Conger & Conger, 2002; Repetti, Taylor & Seeman, 2002). Families with social and economic disadvantages are at a higher risk of developing physical and psychological problems (Berkman & Kawachi, 2000, Bradley & Corwyn, 2002; Oakes & Rossi, 2003). More specifically, they are at risk of developing mental and cognitive problems including language difficulties (Ackerman, Brown, & Izard, 2004; Dearing, McCartney & Taylor 2001).

Family and language development

A Family Investment Model (Conger & Donellan, 2007) proposes that the more educated the parents are, the better the children's development is. When families promote interactions with their children, they can learn and use different social and neuropsychological mechanisms that involve attention, affection and stimulation (Keller, Kartner, Borke, Yovsi, & Kleis, 2005). Moreno Manso, García-Baamonde Sánchez, & Blázquez (2010) stated that family interactions are a "natural linguistic contribution" where a diverse linguistic repertoire starts to be productive. Since the age of two, children are able to start conversations about present and past events (Sparks, Carmiol, & Ríos, 2013). Parents need to be sensitive about these and other important communicative interactions in order to promote the best natural linguistic settings. Previous studies have found significant correlations between parental sensitivity and ME. Mothers who have higher levels of school education are more prone to cognitively stimulate their children. It has also been found that positive and significant interactions with children are established when parents are highly educated and earn high salaries (Bradley &

Corwyn, 2005; Raviv, Kessenich, & Morrison, 2004; Tamis-LeMonda, Shannon, Cabrera, & Lamb, 2004).

Risk factors associated to language difficulties

Family members who live in socioeconomically restricted situations spend more time outside their homes, usually because they live far away and dedicate extra hours to work (Evans, Gonnella, Marcynyszyn, Gentile, & Salpekar, 2005; Evans & Wachs, 2010). Consequently, they have fewer opportunities to significantly interact with their children (Bradley & Corwyn, 2005; Brody & Flor, 1997; Hart & Risley, 1995). Given that family members are stressed by economical and everyday situations, they do not have enough time to spend on developing efficient parental strategies and this may contribute to poor cognitive, social and school abilities in the children (Conger & Conellan, 2007). Unfortunately, this holds true in Mexico where half of the population (more than 53 million people) lives in poverty (CONEVAL, 2012). Low ME has been associated to poverty, which is considered a distal social factor that defines the family's educational profile (Desai & Alva, 1998). Moreover, ME has been associated to neurodevelopment in children (Koutra et al., 2012) and more specifically, to communicative outcomes, such as grammar and lexical abilities (Hart & Risley, 1995; Hoff, 2003, 2006; Law, McBean, & Rush, 2011). Results of some studies have shown differences in the quality and quantity of communicative input of children whose mothers have less education as compared to more educated mothers who also practice more talking (Gathercole & Hoff, 2008). Also, low ME has been linked to an increase in the percentage of grammatical errors in children with and without language disorders (Law, McBean, & Rush, 2011; Le Normand, Parisse, & Cohen, 2008).

Studies have privileged ME as an associated variable within a wide spectrum of health phenomena on child development. However, there is evidence that the father also influences the child's growth during the first months of life, especially in the area of emotional and linguistic development (Cabrera, Shannon, & Tamis-LeMonda, 2007). In fact, it has been noted that the level of education of both the mother and the father interacts in different ways and in different moments along a child's life (Erola, Jalonen, & Lehti, 2016). Particularly within linguistic development, studies have shown that the vocabulary of an infant, younger than three years of age and living in a rural context, is associated to the educational level of the parents. Interestingly, the correlation is even stronger with the paternal vocabulary rather than the maternal (Pancsofar, Vernon-Feagans, & The Family Life Project Investigators, 2010). Nevertheless, in Latinoamerica, paternal education is not always adequately possible to measure, due to sociological situations. Currently in Mexico, 17.5% of homes are classified as single-parent. These families may be particularly vulnerable, especially when this condition is combined with the economic precariousness and laboral instability (INEGI, 2015). Along this research work 28% of the questionnaires were not filled out when information regarding the father's background and education level were sought for. The assumption we arrived from this is that in many of these homes, the father is absent. This is the reason why in this study, the data processed were only those of the mother.

In nutshell, ME has been commonly used as an indicator of socio-environmental status of the family. There is sufficient evidence that its variation allows us to explain, along with other factors, differences in the cognitive and linguistic development of a child. Therefore, a low ME level represents family vulnerability and inadequate child development alert signal. Presently, studies on linguistic abilities in children with and without SLI that include ME as a study variable are scarce, since SLI by definition excludes any socio-environmental remarks (Bishop, 2014). Hence, it is relevant to know if there is an interaction between ME level and clinical diagnosis of SLI and how this relates to a set of linguistic measures. In case of an existing interaction, it is relevant to explore how it happens.

Goals

The first goal of this study is to observe the influence of ME on a set of linguistic measures obtained from narrative samples. The second goal is to observe the effect of interaction between the ME and the clinical diagnosis of SLI on these linguistic measures.

Specifically, the current study examined the following research questions:

1. **Is ME a factor that influences the lexical and grammatical measures obtained from narrative samples?** It was hypothesized that ME will contribute to differentiate, at least the lexical measures, but not the grammatical ones.
2. **If so, is there an interaction between ME and the diagnosis of SLI?** It was hypothesized that there is an interaction between ME and diagnosis of SLI, which explains the variation in lexical measures, but not in the grammatical ones.

Methodology

Participants

A total of 415 monolingual Spanish-speaking children, aged between 4;0 and 6;11 years ($M = 5;3$), from Central Mexico participated in the study. Of them, information was collected on the years of education of 392 mothers (final sample). 162 (41.3%) of the participants were girls. SLI diagnosis were made in 136 (34.7%)

of the total sample. The most relevant descriptive characteristics of the children classified by language diagnosis are presented in Table 1.

Table 1. Descriptive characteristics of children in the study

Variables	SLI (n = 136)	TLD (n = 256)	P-value
Age [in months mean (SD)]	62.4 (10.1)	64.9 (10.3)	0.15[¥]
Female gender [N (%)]	51 (38%)	111 (43%)	0.26[£]

SLI = Specific Language Impairment; TLD = Typical Language Development. [¥]Student's t test; [£]χ^2 test.

Selection criteria

Each participant with SLI met the following criteria: existence of parental and/or teacher concern about language development, no background of motor-skill, hearing and emotional or neurological problems and a nonverbal cognitive scale score over 85 in Kaufman Assessment Battery for Children 2 (KABC-2, Kaufman & Kaufman, 2004). When children were between 4;0 and 4;11 years of age, the Spanish morphosyntax BESA subtest (Peña, Gutiérrez-Clellen, & Iglesias, 2014) was applied (minimum score = 50). For children aged between 5;0 and 6;11, the Spanish version of the Clinical Evaluation of Language Fundamentals 4 (SCELF-4, Semel, Wiig, & Secord, 2006) was applied and for this, the score to be obtained must be at least one standard deviation below the mean in the Word Structure and Sentence Repetition Subtests.

For the children with Typical Language Development (TLD) the following criteria were met: there was no explicit parental and/or teacher concern regarding the child's language development; no background of motor skill, hearing, emotional or neurological problems and a score greater than 85 in the nonverbal inventory in the cognitive test of KABC-2 (Kaufman & Kaufman, 2004). Children between the ages of 4;0 and 4;11 years obtained a score higher than the cut-off point (50) on the morphology Spanish subtest BESA (Peña et al., 2014) while children between the ages of 5;0 and 6;11 must get a score above the mean in the two subtests (Word Structure and Sentence Repetition) of the Spanish version of the SCELF-4 (Semel et al., 2006).

Instruments

Clinicians and researchers working with monolingual Spanish-speaking children in Mexico and other Latin countries commonly use converging evidence from a variety of methods of assessment: standardized normed referenced tests, such as the Bilingual English-Spanish Assessment (BESA; Peña et al., 2014) and the

Spanish Clinical Evaluation of Language Fundamentals – Fourth Edition, Spanish (CELF-4 Spanish; Semel, et al., 2006); language sample analyses (e.g., Bedore & Leonard, 2001; 2005; Gutiérrez-Clellen, Restrepo, Bedore, Peña, & Anderson, 2000); and parent interviews (Restrepo, 1998). Although BESA and CELF-4 Spanish were normed on a bilingual Hispanic population (62% of the children were of Mexican ascend on the CELF-4) living in the U.S. whose first language was Spanish, these are two commonly used Spanish standardized norm-referenced tests. One reason is because there are no available standardized tests for monolingual Spanish-speaking children in Mexico. Second, because according to their manuals, these tests demonstrate very good diagnostic accuracy: BESA is reported to have 87.5% sensitivity and 100% specificity, and CELF-4 Spanish 96% sensitivity and 87% specificity. In previous studies with monolingual children, these tests have been helpful on the identification of monolingual children with SLI (Auza, Kapantzoglou, & Murata, 2018; Morgan, Restrepo & Auza, 2009; 2013).

Bilingual English- Spanish language test (BESA). BESA (Peña et al., 2014) was designed to identify Spanish-speaking children with SLI. The morphosyntactic subtest was used because it has demonstrated to have good sensitivity (87.5) and specificity (100) in children aged between 4;0 and 5;11 years, both in monolingual and bilingual native Spanish-speaking children (Gutiérrez-Clellen et al., 2006). In this subtest, the cut-off score for these ages was 50% and this means that any individual who scores 50% or less is considered as having SLI. Although the sensitivity and specificity of BESA morphology subtest for these ages are high, in children older than 6;0, the specificity is higher, nevertheless, the sensitivity is not adequate to detect children with SLI. Because of this, the *Spanish Clinical Evaluation of Language Fundamentals – 4 (*SCELF-4) was applied to older children.

Spanish Clinical Evaluation of Language Fundamentals – 4 (SCELF-4). SCELF-4 (Semel *et al.*, 2006) is designed to identify Spanish-speaking children with SLI. The technical manual indicates that this test is valid and demonstrates a high sensitivity (96%) and specificity (87%) for children over 5 years of age. The test–retest reliability is equal or higher than 0.80 for all the subtests. In this research, two subtests (Word Structure and Sentence Repetition) were used.

Parent's questionnaire. The objectives of this were to obtain information on the child's life (weight at birth, presence of hearing infections during first year of life, age of first words, preschool attendance or not, among others) and on the family (age and level of education of the parents). Furthermore, some questions adapted from the Parent's questionnaire of Restrepo (1998) were included in order to know if the parents showed any explicit concern regarding their child's language development.

Experimental task

Language sample. A children's book with drawings and without text was used to perform a retell task. The selected book was "One Frog Too Many" (Mayer & Mayer, 1975), for which a script was read to the child. A narrative task was selected, because evidence has shown that these types of tasks allow to obtain more complex and varied information concerning linguistic abilities, rather than conversational interactions in children over 4 years of age (Pavez, Coloma, Araya, Maggiolo, & Peñaloza, 2015; Southwood & Rusell, 2004; Wagner, Nettelbladt, Sahlen, & Nilholm, 2000). In addition, frog stories have been widely used in different contexts and populations to obtain spontaneous language samples. Also, the linguistic measurements obtained seem to be a valid and ecological method for detecting children with and without language difficulties (Castilla & Eriks, 2011; Gutiérrez-Clellen & Simón-Cereijido, 2007; Restrepo, 1998; Westby, Van Dongen, & Maggart, 1989).

Procedure

Parents of the children were contacted through school teachers or health center professionals. All parents signed an informed consent approved by the Institutional Review Board (IRB), where the study was accepted. The parent's questionnaire was given to the parents of the children that met the inclusion criteria and was answered at home.

Children who participated in this research were evaluated through two or three individual sessions, each lasting approximately 20 minutes. Neither the clinical instruments of identification nor the story retells had a fixed order of procedure. Some of the children received the clinical tools first, while others received it last. If the participant was tired, the session was interrupted and continued another day during the same week.

Regarding the narrative retell task, first, the examiner read the script of the story to the child while he/she observed the illustrations. Subsequently, the child was asked to retell the story supporting on the illustrations. Each sample was audio-recorded and transcribed with SALT (*Systematic Analysis of Language Transcripts*, Miller & Iglesias, 2010).

Analysis

Language samples were segmented in TUs, according to SALT's system criteria. Every TU was classified as grammatical or ungrammatical depending on the presence or not of errors, such as substitutions or omissions of any morphosyntactic element (e.g. article substitution, verbal omission).

According to the segmentation and codification of the narrative retell, the following linguistic measures were obtained for each sample: mean length of utterance (MLU), total number of words (TNW), number of different words (NDW), number of TUs and number of TUs with %UGS. These linguistic measures were registered in a database along with the Parent questionnaire answers. The statistical analysis was carried out with JMP program, version 11.0.0.

Distribution of children according to the SLI diagnosis and educational level was characterized and the fitness of the model ($\chi 2$) was assessed. Also, all the obtained linguistic measure values were contrasted for each factor, applying Student's *t* test and variance (ANOVA) test.

To answer the first and second research questions, a least squares regression was used to model the effect of the diagnosis of SLI, the level of ME and the interaction between the two factors on MLU, TNW, NDW and %UGS. The values of the measurements were adjusted through the Box-Cox transformation, to meet the assumption of normality. The overall model evaluation was followed up to assess the fitness of the model. Likewise, the effect of each parameter and its interaction on variables was observed. In case of direct effects, a *p*-value of <0,05 was considered significant; in case of interactions effects, a *p*-value <0,2, according to Selvin's suggestions (Selvin, 1996). Moreover, to answer the second research question, an ANOVA was applied. In this case, a *p*-value was considered significant at the <0,05 level. In case of statistical significance, Tukey's HSD test was run.

Results

First, information regarding ME, both in complete years of education and educational level achieved are presented. Values are shown depending on the linguistic diagnosis of the child.

In Table 2, it can be observed that the mean of ME is greater in children with TLD than in children with SLI. A *t* test was conducted (*t* 2,65), with a significant difference ($p = 0{,}008$), although with a small effect size. Consequently, mothers of children with TLD had significantly more years of education than mothers of children with SLI.

Table 2. Years and level of maternal education, according to the clinical diagnosis of SLI

	SLI (n = 136)	TLD (n = 256)	Effect size	p-value
Years of education [mean (SD)]	10.5 (4.0)	11.6 (4.0)	0.28$	0.009¥
Educational level			0.15¶	0.030£
Primary [n (%)]	29 (21.3)	31 (12.1)		
Secondary [n (%)]	43 (31,6)	68 (26,6)		
High school [n (%)]	27 (19.9)	67 (26.2)		
College [n (%)]	37 (27.2)	90 (35.2)		

SLI = Specific Language Impairment; TLD = Typical Language Development. $Cohen's d; ¶ Cramer's V; ¥Student's t test; £χ^2 test.

Next, values of language measures can be observed in Table 3. Means are presented following the language status of children.

Table 3. Mean values of linguistic measures, according linguistic condition

	SLI (n = 136)	TLD (n = 256)	Effect size	p
MLU [mean (SD)]	6.73 (3.1)	8.39 (3.0)	0.54$	< 0.001¥
TNW [mean (SD)]	142.77 (71.5)	185.41 (78.4)	0.55$	< 0.001¥
NDW [mean (SD)]	58.27 (20.1)	74.63 (19.7)	0.79$	< 0.001¥
%UGS [mean (SD)]	43.4 (25.0)	13.15 (10.4)	1.47$	< 0.001¥

SLI = Specific Language Impairment; TLD = Typical language development; MLU = mean length of utterance; TNW = total number of words; NDW = number of different words; %UGS = percentage of ungrammatical sentences; $Cohen's d; ¥Student's t test.

In Table 3 it can be observed that children with TLD were significantly higher than children with SLI on MLU and on lexical measures. On the other hand, the %UGS was significantly lower in children with TLD.

Finally, values of language measures can be observed in Table 4, following level of Maternal Education.

Table 4. Mean values of linguistic measures, according level of maternal education

	Primary	Secondary	High School	College	Effect size	p
MLU [mean (SD)]	7.1 (2.5) ^{a}	7.4 (2.8)^{ab}	8.5 (3.5)^{b}	8.2 (3.3)^{ab}	0.30	0.022
TNW [mean (SD)]	172.7 (79.1)	163.7 (70.6)	184.0 (77.9)	171.1 (85.3)		0.407
NDW [mean (SD)]	67.1 (20.3)	67.1 (21.5)	71.9 (21.2)	71.2 (21.2)		0.304
%UGS [mean (SD)]	28.2 (24.5)	23.7 (22.7)	21.4 (19.4)	20.2 (21.3)		0.154

MLU = mean length of utterance; TNW = total number of words; NDW = number of different words; %UGS = percentage of ungrammatical sentences; p = value of significance of ANOVA. The groups that share letters a b form homogeneous groups, according to Tukey's HSD test.

In Table 4 it can be observed that the unique significantly different linguistic measure was MLU, when maternal education is taken as an isolated factor. Children whose mothers have an educational level of primary school produce shorter sentences than children whose mothers have high school, but there are not differences between other groups.

Interaction between clinical diagnosis of SLI and ME level

The effect of diagnosis of SLI and ME (primary, secondary, high school or college) on linguistic measures was modeled. Also, the interaction of SLI and ME was explored. Results of models explored for the four linguistic measures are presented in Table 5.

Table 5. Effect of clinical diagnosis of SLI, ME level and interaction among both factors in linguistic measures

	MLU ($R^2 = 0.09$)		TNW ($R^2 = 0.11$)		NDW ($R^2 = 0.15$)		%UGS ($R^2 = 0.36$)	
	F ratio	*p*	*F* ratio	*p*	*F* ratio	*p*	*F* ratio	*p*
Total model	68.12	<0.001*	80.76	<0.001*	65.71	<0.001*	16.57	<0.001*
SLI	20.47	<0.001*	25.64	<0.001*	43.26	<0.001*	31.15	<0.001*
ME	1.31	0.270	1.74	0.159	1.74	0.159	0.45	0.717
SLI*ME	2.34	0.073*	5.02	0.002*	3.48	0.016*	0.08	0.969

MLU = mean length of utterance; TNW = total number of words; NDW = number of different words; %UGS = percentage of ungrammatical sentences; SLI = Specific Language Impairment; ME = maternal education; * $p < .001$

It is observed that the values of each measures can be associated to the presence or absence of SLI. In contrast, ME by itself is not associated with the variation in any of the measures. However, in MLU and both lexical measures, the interaction between SLI and ME was significant (*p*-values <0,2 level). The variance observed on these linguistic measures can be explained by the interaction of both factors, specifically by the co-ocurrence of the diagnosis of SLI and a low ME. In other words, the effect of ME is different according to whether SLI is present or not in three of the four measures; only in %UGS ME does not generate any effect, either as an isolated factor or as an interaction.

Given that the "diagnosis of SLI" factor showed an interaction with ME on MLU and the lexical measures, it was necessary to observe how interaction occurred. For this, two ANOVA were applied; one, for the group with TLD, and one for the group with SLI. In case of statistical significance, Tukey's HSD test was run. Results are shown in Table 6.

Table 6. Analysis of variance for each linguistic measure with interaction effect observed

	Primary	Secondary	High School	College		
	mean (SD)	mean (SD)	mean (SD)	mean (SD)	*F*	*p*
With TLD						
MLU	6.9 (2.1)[a]	8.1 (2.9)[ab]	9.0 (3.3)[b]	8.6 (3.1)[ab]	3.36	0.020
TNW	165.6 (60.6)	187.9 (65.9)	198.6 (75.7)	180.0 (91.7)	1.27	0.285
NDW	70.2 (16.1)	75.3 (16.6)	76.4 (20.5)	74.2 (22.2)	0.62	0.603
With SLI						
MLU	7.3 (2.9)	5.9 (2.0)	7.1 (3.6)	6.8 (3.8)	1.03	0.382
TNW	178.8 (97.8)[a]	111.1 (48.9)[b]	139.4 (68.0)[ab]	144.8 (55.8)[ab]	4.59	0.005
NDW	64.0 (23.8)[a]	49.2 (20.3)[b]	58.2 (17.2)[ab]	62.5 (15.4)[ab]	3.28	0.024

TLD: typical language development; SLI: specific language impairment; MLU = mean length of utterance; TNW = total number of words; NDW = number of different words. The groups that share letters *a b* form homogeneous groups, according to Tukey's HSD test.

On Table 6, it can be observed that the effect of interaction is different on MLU *versus* lexical measures. The effect of ME influences on the MLU produced by children with TLD, but not on MLU produced by children with SLI. This effect is observed when primary and high school are contrasted. This result should not be interpreted as primary level being not different than high school, but statistical differences were not showed (please see Figures 1 and 2 in the Appendix).

In the case of the two lexical measures, it was observed than the effect of ME influences on the performance of children with SLI, but not on children with TLD. More specifically, the difference was observed when contrasting the performance of children with mothers with primary versus secondary. Surprisingly, in both cases, the contrast favored children with mothers with primary education (complementary information can be observed in Figures 3, 4, 5 and 6 in the Appendix).

Discussion

Maternal education (years of schooling plus educational level) is related in a complex way to language production in children. In fact, it was observed that maternal education by itself does not explain the variation reached on linguistic measures. However, significant interactions with presence or absence of SLI was observed. This allows analyze different phenomena.

First, the presence of a language disorder, in isolation, allows us to explain the variation in the values reached in the four linguistic measures in study. This agrees with previous reports, since children with SLI commonly demonstrate deficits in areas such as morphosyntax and lexical diversity (e.g., Conti-Ramsden & Jones, 1997; Leonard, 2014; Leonard, Miller, & Gerber, 1999; Scott & Windsor, 2000; Swanson, Fey, Mills, & Hood, 2005; Wright & Newhoff, 2001). Nevertheless, variations on lexical measures can also be explained by the co-ocurrence of the SLI diagnosis and the low maternal education. This result means that children with a language impairment, already known to be low in their linguistic abilities, their low performance deepens when their educational background precarious.

This raises the question on the level of impact that a disadvantaged context can generate in some language skills. There is abundant information that children who come from contexts of high social vulnerability can present deficient outcomes (e.g. Ackerman, Brown, & Izard, 2004; Bradley & Corwyn, 2002; Hoff, 2006). However, the linguistic condition of the children in these reports is not always accurate. In fact, it is not clear if the poor performance places them in the lower part of the normal curve or if they are similar to children with language disorders.

Second, it is observed that children with SLI from mothers with secondary education have a marked decrease in the total number of words as well as in the different number of words produced in their retells when compared with children from mothers with higher education and those with only primary education. This contradicts the linear idea of a bigger vulnerability by a lower maternal education (Hart & Risley, 1995), which makes us to rethink the ways in which this factor is interpreted. Even at the lexical level, it has not always been possible to establish a clear relationship (Black, Peppé, & Gibbon, 2008). From an ecological perspective, it is very likely that the phenomenon needs to be explained considering other variables that are impacting on the quantity and quality of the interaction with children with and without SLI. Other variables in the cultural context might be, for example, the level of parental stress, preschool non-attendance, or some other cultural factors that may propitiate an impoverished lexicon. However, the fact that there are differences between mothers with just primary education and mothers with secondary education in relation to their perceptions and expectations on their own parenting skills and the potential development of their child should not be ruled out (Rodríguez & Olswang, 2003), and such impacts on the quality and quantity of verbal interaction. All the above mentioned draw a panorama in which the interaction between maternal education and the child's linguistic abilities does not occur in a homogeneous way. In other words, both SLI condition and typical language development are diverse phenomena with a high heterogeneity and dynamism interacting with environmental factors (Conger & Donellan, 2002; Parise & Maillart, 2009; Petersen & Gardner, 2011).

Finally, the percentage of ungrammaticality of the children does not seem to depend on maternal education. This seems to corroborate the idea that morphosyntax-related abilities are more independent from child's environmental context, although evidence is still contradictory (Law, McBean, & Rush, 2011; Le Normand, Parisse, & Cohen, 2008). Moreover, this result is important, because it confirms the validity of the percentage of ungrammaticality to detect children with SLI, regardless of the socio-environmental and educational condition of the child.

If maternal education is taken as an indicator of socio-environmental level, our results depict the impact of this factor on children's language in the contexts of high vulnerability (Conger & Donellan, 2002). Although the grammatical abilities differ mainly by the presence or absence of the disorder, especially the percentage of ungrammatical utterances, the rest of the language skills seem to suffer a clear impoverishment in children with a marked social disadvantage, either in the absence of SLI, in terms of the mean length of utterance, or in the presence of the disorder, with regard to lexical measures. Previously, the linguistic measures such as the mean length of utterances and the percentage of ungrammatical utterances were useful in detecting children with language disorders (Simon-Cereijido & Gutiérrez-Clellen, 2007). In Spanish, however, these measures have rarely been associated with non-linguistic factors interacting with them and their consideration is usually restricted to sample description or as an inclusion / exclusion criterion that is not always well justified.

In recent years, however, research on the causes of SLI has led to a reconsideration of the role played by environmental factors in this disorder. Currently, it is recognized that SLI is a disorder (see Bishop, 2014) that can be related to both internal (genetic and / or cognitive) factors and child's environment (conditions of social vulnerability that impact on the linguistic quality of interaction and linguistic stimulation). This makes us to rethink on the way in which SLI is addressed and characterized, particularly on how these environmental factors may intervene. Maternal education is a variable that has been widely used in studies on typical development, but not in studies on SLI; and a variable like this may explain differences in language skills within the group of children with SLI. However, it would be ideal to have some sort of family educational index, not only conformed by maternal education, but also by other factors that account for an educational level. This would be ideal to raise the emotional stability of the main caregivers, increase their sensitivity and knowledge on the child's cognitive and communicative development, provide support networks, etc. Gender-role considerations must also be taken into account, so that this factor does not imply attribution of a mother-centered responsibility or a naturalization of the woman as the main caregiver (Hernández, 2014). Also, it would be beneficial too, to develop methods that assess the influence of other adult figures as parents, grandparents or others that are around the child during their development.

Limitations

Some external factors might be interacting and have not been contemplated. One is whether children with SLI have already attended speech therapy or not. It is likely that regardless of the context of vulnerability, maternal sensitivity to identify language difficulties in children may promote the search for language services for children with a disorder, or even in children who seem to lag behind in language development. Thus, other variables that may be influencing the quantity and quality of the interaction of children with and without SLI may be family sensitivity and particularly, the effect of stress in families suffering vulnerable socioeconomic situations. Further research should focus on how some conditions of social vulnerability and psychological factors of the family are associated to language development. Future studies on SLI should explore how language interacts with other distal and intermediate factors such as the family environmental organization and structure, the time and quality of primary caregiver-child interaction, and the access to diverse contexts of language stimulation.

Conclusions

It should be thought that the relationship between maternal education and any linguistic phenomenon is permeated by the interaction with other environmental factors. In that sense, maternal education is an indirect distal factor of the child's development and linguistic richness. A significant number of studies (Pancsofar, Vernon-Feagans, Odom, & Roe, 2008; Pungello, Iruka, Dotterer, Mill-Koonce, & Reznick, 2009; Raviv, Kessenich, & Morrison, 2004; Vernon-Feagans et al., 2008; Vernon-Feagans, Garrett-Peters, Willoughby, Mills-Koonce, & The Family Life Project Investigators, 2012) have shown how children's language abilities can be explained by the interaction of a number of distal factors (average family income and maternal education); intermediate factors (organizational stability of families, level of knowledge about child development, life satisfaction of adults in a family); and proximal factors (practices of cognitive stimulation, maternal sensitivity in the interaction). Our study revealed the importance of maternal education, but more research is needed to estimate the impact of other distal factors. We believe that future research focusing on the multilevel interaction of these factors and the SLI condition of Spanish-speaking children may be a great challenge for different areas studying language development.

References

Ackerman, B. P., Brown, E. D., Izard, C. E. 2004. The relations between contextual risk, earned income, and the school adjustment of children from economically disadvantaged families. *Developmental Psychology* 40, 204–216. https://doi.org/10.1037/0012-1649.40.2.204

Auza, A., Kapanzoglou, M., & Murata, C. 2018. Two grammatical tasks for identifying Spanish-speaking children with language impairment. *American Journal of Language Pathology* 27(2), 690–705. https://doi.org/10.1044/2017_AJSLP-17-0052

Berkman, L., & Kawachi, I. 2000. *Social Epidemiology*. Oxford: Oxford University Press.

Bedore, L. M., & Leonard, L. B. (2001). Grammatical morphology deficits in Spanish-speaking children with specific language impairment. *Journal of Speech Language and Hearing Research*, 44, 905-924.

Bishop, D. V. M. 2014. Ten questions about terminology for children with unexplained language problems. *International Journal of Language and Communication Disorders* 49(4), 381–415. https://doi.org/10.1111/1460-6984.12101

Black, E., Peppé, S., & Gibbon, F. 2008. The relationship between socio-economic status and lexical development. *Clinical Linguistics & Phonetics* 22(4–5), 259–265. https://doi.org/10.1080/02699200801918887

Bradley, R. H., & Corwyn, R. F. 2002. Socioeconomic status & child development. *Annual Review of Psychology* 53, 371–399. https://doi.org/10.1146/annurev.psych.53.100901.135233

Bradley, R. H., Corwyn R. F. 2005. Productive activity and the prevention of behavior problems. *Developmental Psychology* 41, 89–98. https://doi.org/10.1037/0012-1649.41.1.89

Brody, G. H., & Flor, D. L. 1997. Maternal psychological functioning, family processes, and child adjustment in rural, single-parent, African-American families. *Developmental Psychology* 33, 1000–1011. https://doi.org/10.1037/0012-1649.33.6.1000

Cabrera, N., Shannon, J., & Tamis-LeMonda, C. 2007. Fathers' influence on their children's cognitive and emotional development: From toddlers to pre-k. *Applied Development Science* 11(4), 208–213. https://doi.org/10.1080/10888690701762100

Castilla, A., & Eriks, A. (2011). Medidas de evaluación de lenguaje espontáneo en niños hispanohablantes en edad preescolar. *Revista de Logopedia, Foniatría Y Audiología*, 32, e7–e19.

CONEVAL 2012. *Informe de pobreza en México*. Ciudad de México: Consejo Nacional de Evaluación de la Política de Desarrollo Social.

Conger, R. D., & Conger K. J. 2002. Resilience in Midwestern families: Selected findings from the first decade of a prospective, longitudinal study. *Journal of Marriage and Family* 64, 361–373. https://doi.org/10.1111/j.1741-3737.2002.00361.x

Conger, R. D., & Donellan, M. B. 2007. An interactionist perspective on the socioeconomic context of human development. *Annual Review of Psychology* 58, 175–199. https://doi.org/10.1146/annurev.psych.58.110405.085551

Conti-Ramsden, G., & Jones, M. 1997. Verb use in specific language impairment. *Journal of Speech, Language and Hearing Research* 40, 1298–1313. https://doi.org/10.1044/jslhr.4006.1298

Coreil, J. 2009. Why study social and behavioral factors in public health? In J. Coreil (Ed.), *Social and behavioral foundations of public health*. Thousand Oaks, CA: Sage.

Dearing E., McCartney K., Taylor B. A. 2001. Change in family income to needs matters more for children with less. *Child Development* 72(6), 1779–1793. https://doi.org/10.1111/1467-8624.00378

Desai, S., & Alva, S. 1998. Maternal education and child health: Is there a strong causal relationship? *Demography* 35(1), 71–81. https://doi.org/10.2307/3004028

Erola, J., Jalonen, S., & Lehti, H. 2016. Parental education, class and income over early life course and children's achievement. *Research in Social Stratification and Mobility* 44, 33–43. https://doi.org/10.1016/j.rssm.2016.01.003

Evans, G. W., & Wachs, T. D. 2010. *Chaos and its influence on children's development: An ecological perspective*. Washington, DC: American Psychological Association. https://doi.org/10.1037/12057-000

Evans, G., Gonnella, C., Marcynnyszyn, L., Gentile, L., & Salpekar, N. 2005. The role of chaos in poverty and children's socioemotional adjustment. *Psychological Science* 16(7), 560–565. https://doi.org/10.1111/j.0956-7976.2005.01575.x

Gathercole V., & Hoff, E. 2008. Input and the acquisition of language: Three questions. In E. Hoff & M. Shatz, M. (Eds.), *Blackwell handbook of language development*. Oxford: Blackwell. https://doi.org/10.1002/9780470757833.ch6

Gutiérrez-Clellen, V. F., Restrepo, M. A., Bedore, L., Peña, E., & Anderson, R. 2000. Language sample analysis in Spanish-speaking-children: Methodological considerations. *Language, Speech, and Hearing Services in Schools* 31, 88–98. https://doi.org/10.1044/0161-1461.3101.88

Gutiérrez-Clellen, V. F., Restrepo, M. A., & Simon-Cereijido, G. (2006). Evaluating the discriminant accuracy of a grammatical measure with Spanish-speaking children. *Journal of Speech Language and Hearing Research*, 49, 1209-1223.

Hart, B., & Risley, T. R. 1995. *Meaningful differences in the everyday experience of young American children*. Baltimore, MD: Paul H. Brookes.

Hernández, A. L. 2014. Madres desde la distancia: el cuidado infantil entre el "aquí" y el "allí". Guatemaltecas migrantes en Madrid. *En Periferias, Fronteras y Diálogos. Actas del XIII Congreso de Antropología de la Federación de Asociaciones de Antropología del Estado Español.* Tarragona, 2–5 de septiembre de 2014. Universitat Rovira i Virgili.

Hoff, E. 2003. The specificity of environmental influence: Socioeconomic status affects early vocabulary development via maternal speech. *Child Development* 74(5), 1368–1378. https://doi.org/10.1111/1467-8624.00612

Hoff, E. 2006. How social contexts support and shape language development. *Developmental Review* 26(1), 55–88. https://doi.org/10.1016/j.dr.2005.11.002

INEGI. 2015. Datos Hogares. <http://www.beta.inegi.org.mx/temas/hogares/> (4 October, 2017).

Keller, H., Kartner, J., Borke, J., Yovsi, R., & Kleis, A. 2005. Parenting styles and the development of the categorical self: A longitudinal study on mirror self-recognition in Cameroonian Nso and German families. *International Journal of Behavioral Development* 29, 496–504. https://doi.org/10.1177/01650250500147485

Kaufman, A. S., & Kaufman, N. L. 2004. *Kaufman assessment battery for children* (2nd ed.). Circle Pines, MN: American Guidance Service.

Koutra, K., Chatzi, L., Roumeliotaki, T., Vassilaki, M., Giannakopoulou, E., Batsos, C., Koutis, A., & Kogevinas, M. 2012. Socio-demographic determinants of infant neurodevelopment at 18 months of age: Mother–child cohort (Rhea study) in Crete, Greece. *Infant Behavior & Development* 35, 48–59. https://doi.org/10.1016/j.infbeh.2011.09.005

Law, J., McBean, K., & Rush, R. 2011. Communication skills in a population of primary school-aged children raised in an area of pronounced social disadvantage. *International Journal of Language and Communicative Disorders* 46(6), 657–664. https://doi.org/10.1111/j.1460-6984.2011.00036.x

Le Normand, M.-T., Parisse, C., & Cohen, H. 2008. Lexical diversity and productivity in French preschoolers: Developmental and biosocial aspects by developmental, gender and sociocultural factors. *Clinical Linguistics & Phonetics* 22(1), 47–58. https://doi.org/10.1080/02699200701669945

Leonard, L. 2014. *Children with specific language impairment* (2nd ed.). Cambridge, MA: The MIT Press.

Leonard, L., Miller, C., & Gerber, E. 1999. Grammatical morphology and the lexicon in children with specific language impairment. *Journal of Speech, Language, and Hearing Research* 42, 678–689. https://doi.org/10.1044/jslhr.4203.678

Mayer, M., & Mayer, M. 1975. *One frog too many*. New York, NY: Penguin Young Readers Group.

Miller, J. & Iglesias, A. 2010. *Systematic analysis of language transcripts (SALT)*, Research Version 2010 [Computer Software]. Madison, WI: SALT Software, LLC.

Moreno Manso, J. M., García-Baamonde Sánchez, M. E., & Blázquez Alonso, M. 2010. Desarrollo lingüístico y adaptación escolar en niños en acogimiento residencial. *Anales de Psicología* 26(1), 189–196.

Morgan, G., Restrepo, M. A., & Auza, A. 2009. Grammatical profile(s) of monolingual Spanish-speaking children with language disorders. In J. Grinstead (Ed.), *Hispanic child languages: Typical and impaired development*. Amsterdam: John Benjamins. https://doi.org/10.1075/lald.50.13mor

Morgan, G., Restrepo, M. A., & Auza, A. 2013. Comparison of Spanish morphology in monolingual and Spanish – English bilingual children with and without language impairment. *Bilingualism: Language and Cognition* 16, 578–596. https://doi.org/10.1017/S1366728912000697

Oakes, J. M., & Rossi, P. H. 2003. The measurement of SES in health research: Current practice and steps towards a new approach. *Social Science and Medicine* 56, 769–784. https://doi.org/10.1016/S0277-9536(02)00073-4

Parise, C., & Maillart, C. 2009. Specific language impairment as systemic developmental disorders. *Journal of Neurolinguistics* 22, 109–122. https://doi.org/10.1016/j.jneuroling.2008.07.004

Pancsofar, N., Vernon-Feagans, L., Odom, E., & Roe, J. (2008). Family relationships during infancy and later mother and father vocabulary use with young children. *Early Childhood Research Quarterly*, 23, 493–593.

Pavez, M. M., Coloma, C. J., Araya, C., Maggiolo, M., & Peñaloza, C. (2015). Gramaticalidad y complejidad en narración y conversación en niños con trastorno específico del lenguaje. *Revista de Logopedia, Foniatría y Audiología*, 35(4), 150–158. https://doi.org/10.1016/j.rlfa.2015.07.004

Peña, E. D., Gutierrez-Clellen, V., Iglesias, A., Goldstein, B., & Bedore, L. M. 2014. *BESA: Bilingual English-Spanish assessment manual*. San Rafael, CA: AR-Clinical publications.

Petersen, D., & Gardner, C. 2011. Trastorno específico del lenguaje: Una revisión. *Revista Chilena de Fonoaudiología* 10, 19–32. https://doi.org/10.5354/0719-4692.2011.17348

Pungello, E., Iruka, I., Dotterer, A., Mills-Koonce, R., & Reznick, J. S. (2009). The effects of socioeconomic status, race, and parenting on language development in early childhood. *Developmental Psychology*, 45(2), 544–557.

Raviv, T., Kessenich, M., & Morrison, F. 2004. A meantional model of the association between socioeconomic status and three-year-old language abilities: The role of parenting factors. *Early Childhood Research Quarterly* 19, 528–547. https://doi.org/10.1016/j.ecresq.2004.10.007

Repetti, R., Taylor, S., & Seeman, T. 2002. Risky families: Family social environments and the mental and physical health of offspring. *Psychological Bulletin* 128(2), 330–366. https://doi.org/10.1037/0033-2909.128.2.330

Restrepo, M. A. 1998. Identifiers of predominantly Spanish-Speaking children with language impairment. *Journal of Speech, Language, and Hearing Research* 41, 1398–1411. https://doi.org/10.1044/jslhr.4106.1398

Rodríguez, B., & Olswang, L. 2003. Mexican-American and Anglo-American mother's beliefs and values about child rearing, education, and language impairment. *American Journal of Speech-Language Pathology* 12, 452–462. https://doi.org/10.1044/1058-0360(2003/091)

Scott, C. M., & Windsor, J. 2000. General language performance measures in spoken and written narrative and expository discourse of school-age children with language learning disabilities. *Journal of Speech, Language, and Hearing Research* 43(2), 324–339. https://doi.org/10.1044/jslhr.4302.324

Selvin S. 1996. *Statistical analysis of epidemiologic data*. New York, NY: Oxford University Press.

Semel, E., Wiig, E. H., & Secord, W. A. 2006. *Clinical evaluation of language fundamentals* [Spanish version]. San Antonio, TX: Psycorp.

Simon-Cereijido, G., & Gutiérrez-Clellen, V. 2007. Spontaneous language markers of Spanish language impairment. *Applied Psycholinguistics* 28, 317–339. https://doi.org/10.1017/S0142716407070166

Southwood, F., & Russell, A. F. (2004). Comparison of Conversation, Freeplay, and Story Generation as Methods of Language Sample Elicitation. *Journal of Speech, Language, and Hearing Research*, 47, 366-376.

Sparks, A., Carmiol, A. M., & Ríos, M. 2013. High point narrative structure in mother-child conversations about the past and children's emergent literacy skills in Costa Rica [Número monográfico: Desarrollo narrativo en América Latina]. *Actualidades en Psicología* 27(115), 91–109. https://doi.org/10.15517/ap.v27i115.9868

Swanson, L. A., Fey, M., Mills, C. E., & Hood, L. S. 2005. Use of narrative-based language intervention with children who have specific language impairment. *American Journal of Speech-Language Pathology* 14, 131–141. https://doi.org/10.1044/1058-0360(2005/014)

Tamis-LeMonda, C. S., Shannon, J. D., Cabrera, N., & Lamb, M. E. 2004. Fathers and mothers at play with their 2- and 3-year-olds: Contributions to language and cognitive development. *Child Development* 75, 1806–1820. https://doi.org/10.1111/j.1467-8624.2004.00818.x

Vernon-Feagans, L., Pancsofar, N., Willoughby, M., Odom, E., Quade, A., & Cox, M. (2008). Predictors of maternal language to infants during a picture book task in the home: SES, child characteristics and the parenting environment. *Journal of Applied Developmental Psychology*, 29, 213–226.

Vernon-Feagans, Garrett-Peters, Willoughby, Mills-Koonce, & The Family Life Project Investigators (2012). Chaos, poverty, and parenting: Predictors of early language development. *Early Childhood Research Quarterly*, 27(3), 339–351.

Wright, H. H., & Newhoff, M. 2001. Narration abilities of children with language-learning disabilities in response to oral and written stimuli. *American Journal of Speech-Language Pathology* 10, 308–319. https://doi.org/10.1044/1058-0360(2001/027)

Wagner, C., Nettelbladt, U., Sahlén, B., & Nilholm, C. (2000). Conversation versus narration in pre-school children with language impairment. *International Journal of Language and Communication Disorders*, 35(1), 83–93.

A. Appendix

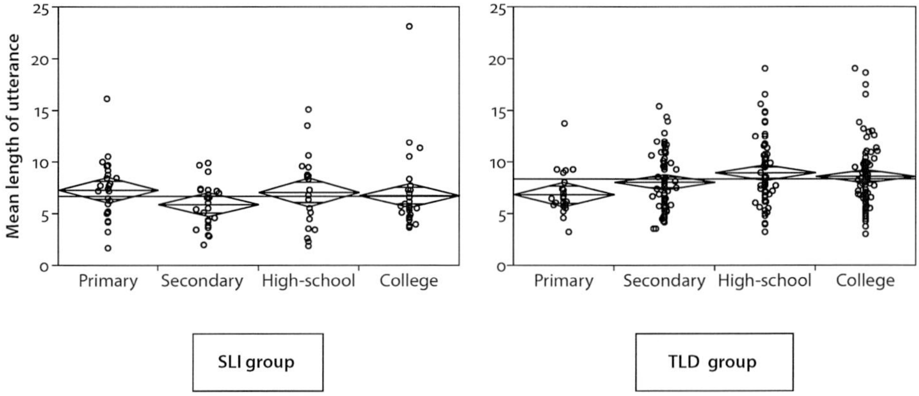

Graphic 1 and 2. Mean values of MLU in each level of ME, according linguistic condition

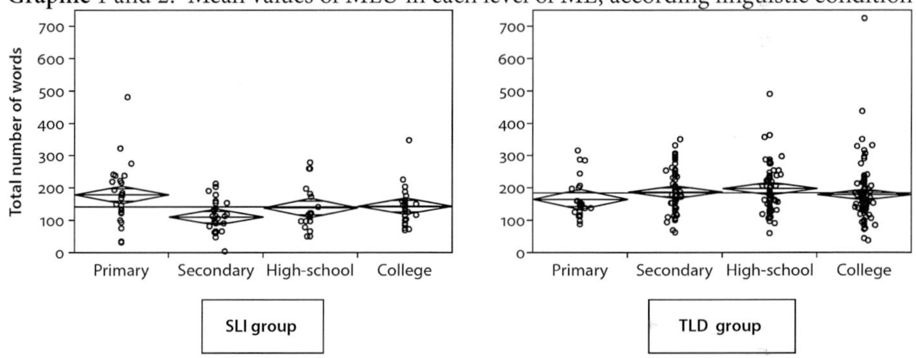

Graphic 3 and 4. Mean values of TNW in each level of ME, according linguistic condition

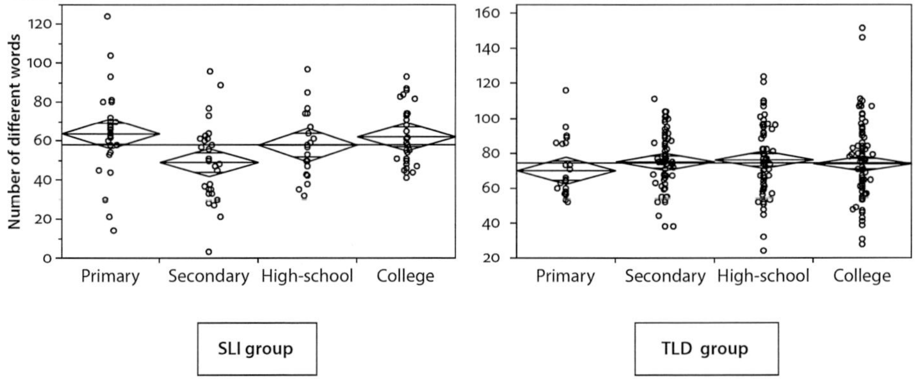

Graphic 5 and 6. Mean values of NDW in each level of ME, according linguistic condition

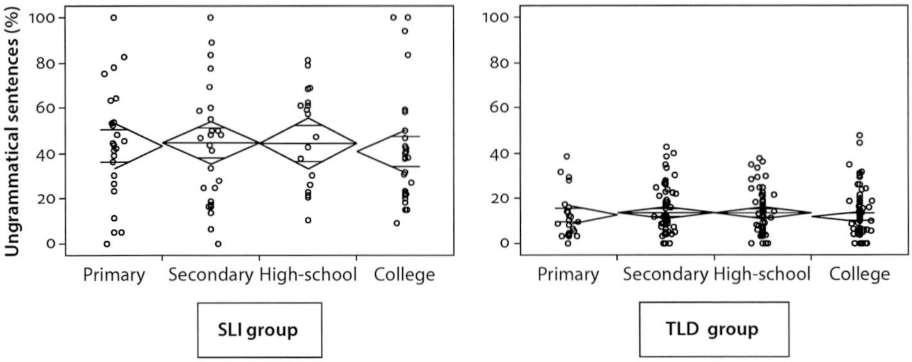

Graphic 7 and 8. Mean values of %UGS in each level of ME, according linguistic condition

Idiom understanding competence of Spanish children with Specific Language Impairment and Pragmatic Language Impairment

Clara Andrés-Roqueta and Rosa Ana Clemente
Universitat Jaume I

Children with pragmatic language impairment (PLI) have problems understanding idioms. However, whether similar difficulties are present in children with Specific Language Impairment (SLI), and which cognitive and linguistic factors are implied, is still not fully addressed. In this chapter the competence to understand idioms in Spanish children with SLI and PLI is compared to a typically developing group, using a verbal and a visual condition. Visual idioms challenged both children with SLI and PLI, but verbal indioms only challenged children with PLI. Also, their performance was related to their grammar and pragmatics skills, but not to the vocabulary ones. However, only children with PLI improved their competence on the visual condition. Practical implications for diagnosing and designing interventions are discussed.

Keywords: idioms, Specific Language Impairment (SLI), Pragmatic Language Impairment (PLI), pragmatics, figurative language, Social Communication Disorder (SCD)

Introduction

Figurative language and idiom understanding

Idioms are a kind of metaphorical language but with a high conventional component (Gernsbacher & Robertson, 1999). It is considered that there is a continuum of cases in peoples use of non-literal language: at one side are idioms (conventional ones), usually learned as lexemes, like "*it's raining cats and dogs*"; and at the other side are novel metaphors (usually made *ad hoc* at conversation), like "*my sister is a mosquito*" in a context were she is being very annoying (Pouscoulous, 2014). In this sense, idioms have a highly conventional component, and a child needs to

https://doi.org/10.1075/z.223.07and

hear it several number of times in different contexts to learn and fix their figurative meaning (Ackerman, 1982).

The ability to stress the figurative meaning of idioms and to inhibit their literal meaning improves throughout childhood until adulthood. There are two theoretical proposals that explain how this skill is developed in children:

The *Lexical representation hypothesis*, that considers idioms as "giant" lexical units (Ackerman, 1982). This approach highlights the importance of *context* and *social communication*, since as children get older they are more exposed to them in conversations with other people (Nippold & Duthie, 2003). Specifically, this competence has been related to communicative intention understanding (Levorato, Nesi, & Cacciari, 2004). Related to those findings, figurative language understanding has also been closely related to the *pragmatic* capacity to extract information from facial expressions and intonation (Winner & Leekam, 1991).

Meta-semantic theories state that the literal meaning of idioms can help to reduce their figurative meaning. According to these theories, *grammatical* and *semantic* analysis of the expression must give a good clue allowing the child to reject the literal option (Glucksberg, 2006).

Both theories are partially right, since not all idioms are acquired in the same way (Norbury, 2004). Although context plays a key role in their interpretation and learning, not all of them share the same characteristics. The extent to which the figurative sense can be deduced from the literal parts that make up the idiom is called the level of semantic transparency (Titone & Connine, 1994). Norbury (2004) showed how theory-of-mind and language competence correlated with the understanding of idioms, regardless of their semantic opacity.

Idiom understanding in children with SLI and PLI

Difficulties with pragmatics are reported in children with Specific Language Impairment (SLI).

SLI is a developmental disorder that affects to language acquisition and development, in the absence of other medical and psychological conditions. It is heterogeneous (different levels of language could be affected, and the deficits could be receptive or expressive); it is variable with time (different pictures observed across development); and it is non-exclusive, so a child could have different combinations of symptoms (Bishop, 2004).

Due to the heterogeneity observed within children with SLI, literature has described some children with predominant problems on the pragmatic skills. Classically, these children have been classified in different papers with a Pragmatic Language Impairment (PLI) (Bishop & Adams, 1989; Bishop & Norbury, 2002), because their pragmatic problems (e.g. poor conversational skills) are greater than their structural language problems. This question is central from a clinical perspective, because Social Communication Disorder (where a main characteristic is difficulties with pragmatics in excess of any structural language difficulties), has been proposed as a clinical category of its own, distinct from autism or Specific Language Impairment (SLI) (DSM-5; American Psychiatric Association, 2013).

In this sense, the extent of impairment understanding idioms within language disordered population, and the underlying causes are still under debate.

Research shows that children with SLI have greater problems than children with typical development (TD) in understanding different forms of non-literal language, including idioms. For example, Rinaldi (2000) found that teenagers with SLI who attended special schools displayed a bias towards literality in the understanding of idioms, because of an inability to use the context and choose an appropriate meaning.

Norbury (2004) analyzed the processing of non-familiar idioms in children with different communicative difficulties: SLI, autistic children with language disorder, autistic children without language disorder, and TD. Idioms were presented with and without context. It was found that the three clinical groups gave more literal responses than the TD group, but only the groups with language disorder (SLI and autism with language disorder), were less competent to use context in order to understand the idioms in comparison to the other groups.

Children with Pragmatic Language Impairment (PLI), which nowadays could be diagnosed as Social Communication Disorder, present an excessively literal understanding of language (Bishop & Rosenbloom, 1987). Following this premise, some studies have attempted to distinguish between the performance of groups of children with SLI and PLI. Vance and Wells (1994), compared the performance of 18 children with SLI (7 of whom were subjects with PLI) to 18 TD matched for linguistic age. Each child listened to 10 idioms and then chose among three drawings: literal meaning, figurative meaning, and a semantic distractor. No significant differences appeared between SLI and TD groups neither between the SLI and PLI, so authors attribute these difficulties to receptive language deficit general to the disorder. Nevertheless, it has been argued that no differences were found between the two clinical groups because of the simplification of the semantic and pragmatic demands of the task that was used, and understanding idioms in over-structured contexts is not the same as the skill of understanding them in normal conversation, where the speaker can refer to events that are not immediately deducible within the physical context.

In contrast, Kerbel and Grunwell (1998a, 1998b) compared groups of children with SLI, PLI and Asperger's syndrome, using realistic experimental contexts (dramatic works where the non-literal statements were uttered). Results showed that children with PLI presented more problems than the other groups, and they gave significantly fewer answers that were "appropriate to the context" and more that were "inappropriate to the context". However, this study has been criticised because they could have included some participants who would nowadays satisfy the criteria for high-performance autism in the PLI group (Norbury, 2004).

Among the works mentioned above, the study by Norbury (2004) is the one that includes the most representative sample of children with SLI. Nevertheless, despite this positive point, again not enough subjects with PLI were included in the sample to be able to establish differences with respect to the SLI group.

Aims and hypothesis

It is difficult to draw solid conclusions about results found in previous studies, since different samples, instruments and methodologies were used in the studies. In this sense, no agreement has been reached about whether there is a differentiated profile between SLI and PLI. Therefore, the present study has three aims:

1. To determine whether the lack of ability to understand idioms can be extended to SLI in general, or whether it is more related to subjects with SLI that have greater levels of pragmatic impairment.
2. To test if the competence to reach figurative meanings of idioms improves when a visual context is given.
3. To explore which language skills are related to idiom understanding within children with SLI.

Methodology

Participants

Thirty-five children diagnosed with Language Impairment (LI) were recruited (4;0 and 7;0 years old, 11 girls and 24 boys) from public and ordinary schools of Castellon (Spain). These children were being attended by speech and language therapists, but not presented other medical/psychiatric condition, or sensory deficits or learning difficulties or autistic traits. They were recruited when scored *1 SD* below the mean in at least one of the following grammar tests: a *Sentence Recall* subscale of a Spanish Children's Language Assessment Battery (Evaluación del Lenguaje Infantil, ELI – Saborit & Julian, 2005), and a Spanish receptive grammar test (Comprensión de Estructuras Gramaticales, CEG – Mendoza, Carballo, Munoz, & Fresneda, 2005).

Then, all the children with LI who scored 1 *SD* below the mean on the pragmatic subscale of the ELI were further classified as PLI. So, the initial LI group was divided into two subgroups: the SLI group (n = 19; 13 boys and 6 girls), and the PLI group (n = 16, 11 boys and 5 girls).

An age-matched control group consisting of thirty-five children with typical language development was created recruiting children of same gender and age (± 3 months) of each participant with LI.

Non-verbal intelligence of all participants was within the age-appropriate average as assessed by the Colored Progressive Matrix Test (Raven, Raven, & Court, 1998).

Materials

Language measures

Besides the linguistic profile of the subjects was assessed through the following tasks:

a. Grammar:
   Receptive measure: Understanding Grammar Structures (CEG).
   Expressive measure: Sentence Recall (from the ELI)
b. Vocabulary measures:
   Receptive measure: Naming (from the ELI).
   Expressive measure: Identification (from the ELI)
c. Pragmatic measure: the ELI pragmatic subscale.
   Receptive measure: gesture-speech integration (from the ELI).
   Expressive measure: defining non-literal language, and use of politeness (from the ELI).

Idiom understanding tasks

a. *Verbal condition*

A verbal condition was created to assess the ability to grasp figurative meanings of idioms through spontaneous oral language. Before administering the task to the sample, a pilot test was carried out with forty TD children aged between three and seven years, to select familiar idioms for children of these ages. Thus, from the initial set of forty-five Spanish idioms, the seven shown in Table 1 were chosen.

To evaluate the participant's understanding, the examiner introduced the task as follows: "*I am going to say some sentences that contain some funny expressions that people sometimes use. For example, like when people say "it's raining cats and dogs" and they don't mean there are pets falling out of the sky – they just mean that it's raining really hard. Don't worry if you've never heard them, just think about the words and what they might mean.*"

Table 1. List of the verbal idioms selected to design the verbal and visual condition

Spanish idiom	Figurative meaning
Ese niño come como un cerdo.	That boy eats in a dirty way or eats a lot.
Ese niño da mucha guerra.	That boy is behaving really badly.
Se llevan como el perro y el gato	They are always arguing
Estoy hecho polvo	I'm very tired.
Ese coche va a toda leche	That car is going very fast.
Échame una mano	Help me.
Se ha quedado en pelotas	He / She is undressed.

Then they were asked the following question "*What does it mean when we say…?*", together with the set phrase (e.g. "*I'm shattered*"). The selected expressions were presented one by one. Children who did not answer were encouraged to guess what was said and to say what they thought it meant, without being afraid of getting it wrong.

Their answers were scored with: 0 points (omissions or responses involving the literal meaning); and 1 point (answers involving the figurative meaning).

Visual condition

A visual condition was created using the same idioms of the verbal condition. These tasks have lower pragmatic demands as they offer a visual context, and also the literal meaning is presented among the choices.

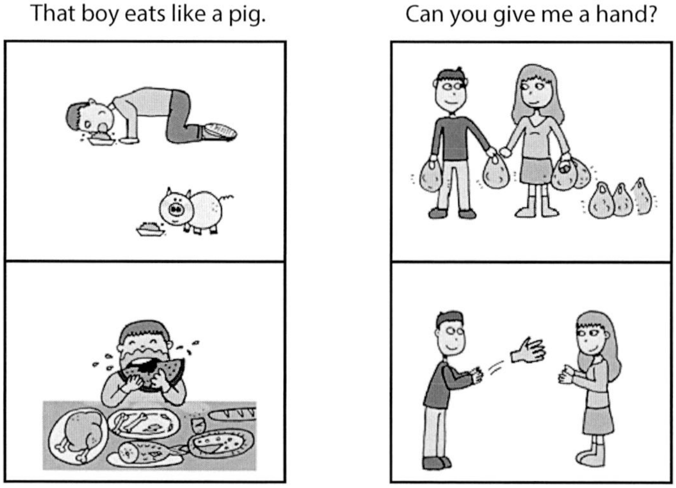
That boy eats like a pig.
Can you give me a hand?

Figure 1. Example of two idioms (visual condition)

In this condition, a card with two pictures accompanied each idiom: one of which contained the literal meaning of the phrase, while the other represented its figurative meaning (Figure 1).

Instructions were as follows: "*I am going to say some sentences containing some funny phrases that people sometimes use. Then I will show you some pictures, and you will have to say which of the two you think best matches what is being said*.". Then they were asked the following question: "*What does … mean?*" and shown the pictures.

The participants' answers were scored with: 0 points (drawing with a literal meaning), and 1 point (drawing with a figurative meaning).

Procedure

All children were assessed during school time in three sessions, after obtaining permission from government, parents and school. In the first two sessions, a study of their language profile was carried out. In the following sessions, the rest of the instruments related to the aims of the study were administered. The visual task was administered the last one, after the verbal one (4 weeks later), in order to prevent a learning effect on the expressions.

Results

When the LI sample was subdivided into two groups (SLI and PLI) the data failed the Shapiro–Wilk test of normality, showing several unequal variances across groups for idiom understanding measures. Therefore, non parametric tests were used to explore the data: Kruskal–Wallis test, Mann–Whitney U test, and Wilcoxon rank test.

I. Between-group comparisons on key and related measures

Descriptive data of groups on idiom understanding measures and language measures are detailed on Table 2. The Kruskal–Wallis test showed a main effect of group on the visual condition of the task ($X^2_{(2)} = 7.60$, $p = .006$), but not on the verbal one ($X^2_{(2)} = 2.31$, $p = .129$), indicating that the visual condition showed greater differences between groups.

With respect pairwise contrasts in the verbal condition, Mann–Whitney U test revealed no significant differences between SLI and TD groups ($U = 250$, $p = .129$), but between PLI and TD groups ($U = 92.5$, $p < .001$). Moreover, PLI group was also less competent that SLI one on this condition ($U = 77.5$, $p = .012$).

Table 2. Descriptive data on idiom understanding measures and language measures

	SLI (n = 19)		PLI (n = 16)		TD (n = 35)	
	M (SD)	*Mdn*	*M* (SD)	*Mdn*	*M* (SD)	*Mdn*
Age (months)	65.74 (16.83)	66	62.75 (12.45)	61	64.31 (7.52)	64
Grammar (receptive)	50.21 (13.55)	53	49.50 (6.60)	50.5	64.31 (7.52)	64
Grammar (expressive)	5.15 (1.97)	4	6.00 (1.96)	7	7.94 (1.21)	8
Vocabulary (receptive)	20.05 (7.09)	23	21.00 (4.73)	22	23.11 (5.19)	26
Vocabulary (expressive)	18.73 (7.63)	20	17.12 (5.86)	17	21.40 (6.60)	24
Pragmatics (receptive)	5.42 (0.83)	6	4.12 (1.66)	4.5	5.54 (0.78)	6
Pragmatics (expressive)	3.68 (2.16)	4	1.5 (1.03)	1.5	4.97 (1.72)	5
Idioms (Verbal)	3.26 (1.69)	4	1.75 (1.52)	1	4.17 (1.93)	4
Idioms (Visual)	2.78 (1.58)	3	2.73 (1.70)	2.5	4.31 (1.95)	4

Note: Age = chronological age in months; Language measures = raw scores

With respect to the visual condition, the pairwise analysis revealed significant differences between SLI and TD groups ($U = 182.5$, $p = .006$), between PLI and TD groups ($U = 172.5$, $p = .027$). However, on this condition PLI group showed similar competence SLI one ($U = 146.5$, $p = .857$).

II. Within-group comparisons between verbal and visual conditions

Within-group analyses were conducted to determine whether the presence of the figurative meaning would benefit the performance of groups (see Table 3). Wilcoxon rank test did not show significant differences within TD and SLI groups. However, it was shown that visual condition improved performance of the PLI group.

Table 3. Within-group comparisons between different conditions of the idiom comprehension task: Verbal and visual

	Verbal / Visual	
	Z	*p*
SLI (n = 19)	−1.08	.279
PLI (n = 16)	−2.19	.028
TD (n = 35)	−.491	.623

Table 4. Zero-order nonparametric spearman correlations between verbal condition and related measures within the LI and TD group

	LI (n = 35)		TD (n = 35)	
	Bivariate	**Partial (age)**	**Bivariate**	**Partial (age)**
Age (months)	.56**	–	.61**	–
Grammar (receptive)	.59**	.42*	.58**	.31
Grammar (expressive)	.32	.07	.58**	.36*
Vocabulary (receptive)	.45**	.16	.52**	.12
Vocabulary (expressive)	.57**	.28	.57**	.26
Pragmatics (receptive)	.54**	.39*	.23	–.19
Pragmatics (expressive)	.48**	.26	.58**	.33*

- Note 1: *$p < .05$; **$p < .01$
- Note 2: Age = chronological age in months; Language measures = raw scores

III. Correlations between idiom understanding (verbal condition) and language measures

Zero-order nonparametric correlations (Spearman) between idiom understanding (verbal condition) and language measures are presented in Table 4. For these analyses, SLI and PLI groups were taken together (LI, n = 35).

For children with LI, idiom understanding was positively correlated with age and most of the language measures. However, when the effect of age was partialled out, only the relation with grammar (receptive), pragmatics (receptive) remained significant. For children with TD, idiom understanding was also positively correlated with age and most of the language measures. However, when the effect of age was partialled out, only the relation with grammar (expressive) and pragmatics (expressive) remained significant.

Therefore, it seems that for children with LI receptive skills (grammar and pragmatics) are crucial to grasp figurative meanings of idioms.

Discussion

The present study had three aims regarding idiom understanding competence of children with LI.

The first aim was to determine whether the lack of ability to understand idioms could be extended to SLI in general, or whether it is more related to subjects with SLI that have greater levels of pragmatic impairment (that is in more cases, PLI). The data from the inter-group comparisons in the idioms tasks help to show that idiomatic expressions are a greater challenge for participants with PLI, since they differed from their TD peers in both the verbal and the visual conditions. In contrast, the group of SLI was seen to differ from TD peers only in the visual condition. In this sense, results reveal that children of PLI group must have greater difficulties than children of SLI group.

Moreover, SLI and PLI groups differed significantly on the verbal condition, but not on the visual one. This finding helps to unify and interpret the apparent disagreement found in the literature about whether children with SLI and PLI have a differentiated or similar profile. It is in line with the literature that found no differences among these populations with SLI when the pragmatic load was lower (Vance & Wells, 1994), and also in line with the works of Kerbel and Grunwell (1998a, 1998b), who found differences on a verbal task.

The second aim was to test if the competence to reach figurative meanings of idioms improves when a visual context is given. In this respect, within-group analysis comparing idioms in terms of their pragmatic simplification (visual versus verbal condition), showed that only a significantly better performance on the visual condition was observed within the PLI group. Therefore, a greater deficit in idiom understanding is present in children with PLI when comes to interpreting idioms in isolation.

Children with PLI must have smaller difficulties to understand idioms in structured contexts (or when the referents are visually accessible), but bigger ones to understand them in a spontaneous conversation, where the speaker refers to events that cannot readily be deduced from the physical context (Bishop & Rosenbloom, 1987).

These data are likely to be reflecting that when children hear a new idiom, the presence of the figurative meaning in the visual context is an advantage, above all when they face pragmatic problems to get the meaning from the linguistic context. Children with pragmatic difficulties may not believe that a figurative meaning is expected and therefore they do not start up the inferences and analogical processes required to reach it. This highlights the importance of exposure and social construction in the learning of figurative language, as is the case with learning vocabulary in general (Nippold & Duthie, 2003).

Finally, the last aim was to investigate which language skills are related to idiom understanding within children with SLI. In this sense, bivariate and partial correlations showed that idiom-understanding competence improves with age in children with LI and also in TD children. However, when the effect of age is ruled out, receptive structural language skills (especially grammar) and pragmatic receptive skills are crucial.

The relation of idiom understanding competence with structural language and pragmatics is in line with previous findings (Norbury, 2004). Our research suggests that structural language is important, but also pragmatic competence.

In a wider theoretical framework, this study provides the literature with more evidence from a Spanish sample of the existence of a differentiated profile between SLI and PLI using pragmatic measures (Kerbel & Grunwell, 1998a, 1998b). The study also helps to demonstrate that these difficulties are lower when the visual context is provided.

As a practical issue the present findings highlight the importance of evaluating the participants' pragmatic language competence with different tasks, in order to establish whether the pragmatic difficulties go beyond the overall structural language difficulties that a child with SLI presents. In this sense, it is important to prevent families, speech and language therapists, and the other professionals who work with children with LI that linguistic pragmatic problems are present within SLI (not only in PLI). Pragmatic problems co-occur with structural language problems (Andrés-Roqueta & Katsos, 2017).

Moreover, it has been stated that pragmatic problems can be solved or can improve (Conti-Ramsden, Botting, & Knox, 2001). So, the fact that some children with PLI improve in the visual tasks suggests that they are not "seriously" challenged by idioms. Indeed, the fact that the idiomatic expression is represented graphically must help children to generate global coherence to the speaker's utterance. Therefore, different visual contexts should be included when designing training materials to improve this competence with these children, to facilitate generalization of the new learning.

Acknowledgements

Authors want thank support from Grant GV/2015/092 Q5 by *Conselleria de Educación, Cultura y Deporte* of *Generalitat Valenciana* (Spain) and Grant UJI-PLI016-12 funded by *Universitat Jaume I de Castelló* (Spain).

References

Ackerman, B. P. 1982. On comprehending idioms: Do children get the picture? *Journal of Experimental Child Psychology* 33, 439–454. https://doi.org/10.1016/0022-0965(82)90058-3

American Psychiatric Association. 2013. *Diagnostic and statistical manual of mental disorders* (DSM- 5th ed.). Washington, DC: American Psychiatric Association. https://doi.org/10.1176/appi.books.9780890425596

Andrés-Roqueta, C., & Katsos, N. 2017. The contribution of grammar, vocabulary and Theory of Mind in pragmatic language competence in children with autistic spectrum disorders. *Frontiers in Psychology* 8, 996. https://doi.org/10.3389/fpsyg.2017.00996

Bishop, D. V. M. 2004. Diagnostic dilemmas in specific language impairment. In L. Verhoeven & J. van Balkom (Eds.), *Classification of developmental language disorders* (pp. 309–326). Mahwah, NJ: Lawrence Erlbaum Associates.

Bishop, D. V. M., & Adams, C. 1989. Conversational characteristics of children with semantic-pragmatic disorder, II: What features lead to a judgement of inappropriacy? *British Journal of Disorders of Communication* 24 (3): 241–263. https://doi.org/10.3109/13682828909019890

Bishop, D. V. M., & Norbury, C. F. 2002. Exploring the borderlands of autistic disorder and specific language impairment: A study using standardised diagnostic instruments. *Journal of Child Psychology and Psychiatry and Allied Disciplines* 43(7), 917–929. https://doi.org/10.1111/1469-7610.00114

Bishop, D. V. M., & Rosenbloom, L. 1987. Childhood language disorders: Classification and overview. In W. Yule & M. Rutter (Eds.), *Language development and disorders*. London: MacKeith Press.

Conti-Ramsden, G., Botting, N., & Knox, E. 2001. Follow-up of children attending infant language units: outcomes at 11 years of age. *International Journal of Language & Communication Disorders* 36(2), 207–219. https://doi.org/10.1080/13682820121213

Gernsbacher, M. A., & Robertson, R. R. W. 1999. The role of suppression in figurative language comprehension. *Journal of Pragmatics* 31, 1616–1630. https://doi.org/10.1016/S0378-2166(99)00007-7

Glucksberg, S. 2006. Beyond literal meanings: The psychology of allusion. *Psychological Science* 2(3), 146–152. https://doi.org/10.1111/j.1467-9280.1991.tb00122.x

Kerbel, D., & Grunwell, P. 1998a. A study of idiom comprehension in children with semantic-pragmatic difficulties, Part I: Task effects on the assessment of idiom comprehension in children. *International Journal of Language and Communication Disorders* 33, 1–22. https://doi.org/10.1080/136828298247901

Kerbel, D., & Grunwell, P. 1998b. A study of idiom comprehension in children with semantic-pragmatic difficulties, Part II: Between-groups results and discussion. *International Journal of Language and Communication Disorders* 33, 23–44. https://doi.org/10.1080/136828298247910

Levorato, M. C., Nesi, B., & Cacciari, C. 2004. Reading comprehension and understanding idiomatic expressions: A developmental study. *Brain and Language* 9, 303–314. https://doi.org/10.1016/j.bandl.2004.04.002

Mendoza, E., Carballo, G., Muñoz, J., & Fresneda, M. D. 2005. *Test de comprensión de estructuras gramaticales (CEG)*. Madrid: TEA Ediciones.

Nippold, M. A., & Duthie, J. K. 2003. Mental imagery and idiom comprehension: A comparison of school-age children and adults. *Journal of Speech, Language, and Hearing Research* 46, 788–799. https://doi.org/10.1044/1092-4388(2003/062

Norbury, C. F. 2004. Factors supporting idiom comprehension in children with communication disorders. *Journal of Speech, Language, and Hearing Research* 47, 1179–1193. https://doi.org/10.1044/1092-4388(2004/087

Pouscoulous, N. 2014. The elevator's buttocks. Metaphorical abilities in children. In D. Matthews (Ed.), *Pragmatic development in first language acquisition* (pp. 239–259). Amsterdam: John Benjamins.

Raven, J., Raven, J. C., & Court, J. H. 1998. *Coloured progressive matrices*. Oxford: Oxford Psychologists Press.

Rinaldi, W. 2000. Pragmatic comprehension in secondary school-aged students with specific developmental language disorder. *International Journal of Language and Communication Disorders* 35, 1–29. https://doi.org/10.1080/136828200247223

Saborit, C., & Julián, J. P. 2005. *L'avaluació del llenguatge infantil. ELI*. Universitat Jaume I de Castelló (UJI). Col·lecció: Educació.

Titone, D. A., & Connine, C. M. 1994. Descriptive norms for 171 idiomatic expressions: Familiarity, compositionality, predictability, and literality. *Metaphor and Symbolic Activity* 9, 247–270. https://doi.org/10.1207/s15327868ms0904_1

Vance, M., & Wells, B. 1994. The wrong end of the stick: Language-impaired children's understanding of nonliteral language. *Child Language Teaching and Therapy* 10, 23–46. https://doi.org/10.1177/026565909401000102

Winner, E., & Leekman, S. 1991. Distinguishing irony from deception: Understanding the speaker's second-order intention. *British Journal of Developmental Psychology* 9, 257–270. https://doi.org/10.1111/j.2044-835X.1991.tb00875.x

Evaluation of narrative skills in language-impaired children

Advantages of a dynamic approach

Ingrida Balčiūnienė[1,2] and Aleksandr N. Kornev[1]
[1]Saint-Petersburg State Pediatric Medical University / [2]Vytautas Magnus University

The chapter presents our findings on a complex experimental comparative study of the narrative analysis of language-impaired and typically-developing monolingual Russian children. The data of storytelling and retelling according to wordless picture sequences were collected from specifically language-impaired preschoolers, dyslexic school-age children, and typically-developing peers. Then, following the methodology of the dynamic approach to narrative assessment, an impact of such factors as session, story complexity, and story mode on the measures of narrative macrostructure, microstructure, linguistic dysfluency, and language errors was estimated. The study provides evidence that the given extralinguistic factors significantly influence the narrative measures; namely, the language-impaired children, contrary to the typically-developing peers, tended to be significantly sensitive to the experiment session and the story mode.

Keywords: narrative, dynamic approach, language impairment

Introduction

In a number of studies, a narrative has been analyzed as *a text* with the main focus on its linguistic and structural features in typically-developing (TD) and clinical populations. From this perspective, some age- and clinical-related limitations have been described (Duinmeijer et al., 2012; Fey et al., 2004; Fiestas et al., 2005; Thorne et al., 2007). It is known significantly less about the psycholinguistics of development of narrative programming skills. There is multiple evidence of a child's speech inter- and intra-individual variability presumably caused by limitations in language competence, a deficit of cognitive resources, and the influence

https://doi.org/10.1075/z.223.08bal

of the communicative context and the communication intention (Gonzalez et al., 2012; Holm et al., 2007; Kapa et al. 2017).

When producing an unprepared oral narrative, one has to develop a structure of events and to produce oral discourse almost in parallel. This is a high resource-demanding activity. The basic skills that a child has to acquire are the following: to plan a logically well-organized semantic design, to transform it into a structurally relevant propositional net, to generate a verbal and syntactically structured text, and to narrate it fluently to a listener. The narrator's skills in story-telling and his/her involvement in the narrative elicitation procedure influence narration results; this should be particularly taken into account when assessing clinical populations (Balčiūnienė & Kornev, 2016; Kornev & Balčiūnienė, 2015, 2017).

In the majority of narrative studies, the narrator's qualities are not taken into consideration, although his/her attitude to the assessment procedure and to the experimenter as well as his/her previous experience in similar tasks are the key source of variability in discourse production. For instance, the content of experiment sessions is a new learning experience for participants and, thus, the preceding tasks have an influence on the following ones. However, the distinctions in participants' learning abilities lead to different dynamic changes in their responses. In addition, this data might demonstrate learning and cognitive resources in TD and learning- or language-disordered children. Both TD and language-disordered children are usually rather sensitive to different circumstances of language assessment and, thus, clinical linguists and speech language pathologists need standardized evaluation tools (Petersen et al., 2008). Corpus-based evaluations of primary language-disordered and dyslexic children exemplify the difference between standardized language assessment and the data of discourse analysis (Ukrainetz & Blomquist, 2002). The former is more relevant to measuring language competence, while the latter is more valid in evaluating language performance. The specific language impairment (SLI), as a language delay "that cannot be attributed to problems of hearing, neurological status, nonverbal intelligence, or other known factors" (Leonard, 2000), affects language behaviour and discourse production (Bliss & McCabe, 2006). Similar evidence has been obtained in dyslexic (DYS) children (Mackie & Dockrell, 2004; Nippold et al., 2008; Puranik et al., 2007). The internationally agreed definition claims that dyslexia is "a specific learning disability that is neurobiological in origin. It is characterized by difficulties with accurate and/or fluent word recognition and by poor spelling and decoding abilities …" (Lyon et al., 2003). Although this general statement is universal for all languages and cultures, the ease and length of typical paths to reading acquisition vary dramatically depending on the features of the language in which the child is learning to read and the cultural environment in which this acquisition occurs. Russian orthography is rather transparent for reading; however, its high morphological richness and inflectional and word structure complexity impose heavy requirements to discourse processing and inference-making ability for reading comprehension. In this respect, narrative language proficiency has predictive value for reading acquisition. Comparative studies in narrative production and comprehension between DYS and SLI children are still lacking, especially concerning languages with transparent literacy. Previous studies in English-speaking populations have suggested that children with oral language deficits in preschool are often diagnosed with reading problems at school (Catts et al., 2001, 2008). Despite a long history of studies of language impairments and intervention in language-impaired populations, efficient and ecologically valid diagnostic tools are needed. They should also be sensitive to the dynamics and variations of the narration measures based on the condition of a participant's language and executive resources. In order to reach this aim, the *Russian Assessment for Narratives – RAIN* was developed (Balčiūnienė & Kornev, 2016; Kornev & Balčiūnienė, 2014, 2015, 2017). The main methodological sources for elaboration of the RAIN were Stein and Glenn (1975), Stein and Albro (1997), Schneider et al. (2005), Gagarina et al. (2012, 2015). The RAIN incorporates a dynamic assessment procedure and enables the evaluation of both a current state of the narrative language (the so-called "actual zone of development" according to Vygotsky, 1962) and a potential achievement influenced by a priming ("a zone of proximal development").

In this study, we have hypothesized that language-disordered (both SLI and DYS) children face difficulties in producing narrative discourse, and these difficulties arise as some specific limitations at both macro- and microstructural level. The limitations presumably are additionally provoked by some extralinguistic circumstances, such as story complexity, task mode (telling *vs.* retelling), and the order of task presentation (first vs. second session) in the experiment setting. In order to test the hypothesis, we have aimed at (a) assessing macro- and microstructural measures in SLI and DYS children; (b) comparing them to these in TD peers, and (c) evaluating an impact of the aforementioned extralinguistic factors on the main macro- and microstructural measures in the scope of a dynamic paradigm.

Methodology

Participants

The RAIN was piloted in two studies in monolingual Russian-speaking (1) typically-developing (TD) and specifically language-impaired (SLI) preschoolers and (2) 3–4-grade TD and dyslexic (DYS) students. In Table 1, the characteristics of the samples are provided.

Table 1. Characteristics of the samples

	Study 1		Study 2	
	TD	SLI	TD	DYS
N	12	12	12	12
Mean age (SD) in months	77.8 (3.8)	77.5 (4.3)	120.9 (8.3)	118.9 (8.7)
Language	Russian monolinguals			

In the first study, the SLI group consisted of 12 clinically-referred 6-year-old children (mean age 77.5 months, SD 4.3 months) who received a two-year-course of speech therapy. The control group consisted of 12 TD peers (mean age 77.8 months, SD 3.8 months) without any developmental disorders. Nonverbal IQ (according to *the Raven's Colored Progressive Matrices Test*) in both groups was at a normal range. In the second study, the DYS group consisted of 12 children (mean age 118.9 months, SD 8.7 months) with dyslexia, and the control group comprised 12 peers (mean age 120.9 months, SD 8.3 months) without any developmental disorders. The subjects with dyslexia were recruited for the current study from a large group of children with dyslexia formed in the previous study (Grigorenko et al., 2011), where 750 dyslexics were selected from 15,000 2nd-6th-form students by means of a standard reading assessment test (Kornev, 1995; Kornev & Ishimova, 2010). Inclusion criteria were a reading score below 6 percentiles of the whole distribution and normal nonverbal intelligence on the basis of the *Cattell Culture Fair Test*. Typically-developing (TD) peers (mean age 120.9 months) without any developmental disorders were randomly selected from an ordinary school. Both studies were conducted in Saint-Petersburg (Russia) at state kindergartens and schools. Before participation in the study, written informed consent was obtained from the parents. An approval from the Ethical Commission of Saint-Petersburg State Pediatric Medical University was received.

Material

In both studies, two picture sequences were employed for narrative elicitation. Each sequence consisted of six coloured pictures (10 x 10 cm) without text (see Picture 1).

The pictures have been developed in the framework of the COST Action IS0804 *Language Impairment in a Multilingual Society: Linguistic Patterns and the Road to Assessment*, <http://www.bi-sli.org>. Despite almost identical storylines and pictorial content, the *Baby-Goats* sequence is significantly more complex (Kornev & Balčiūnienė, 2014) to perceive because of the parallel development of two episodes.

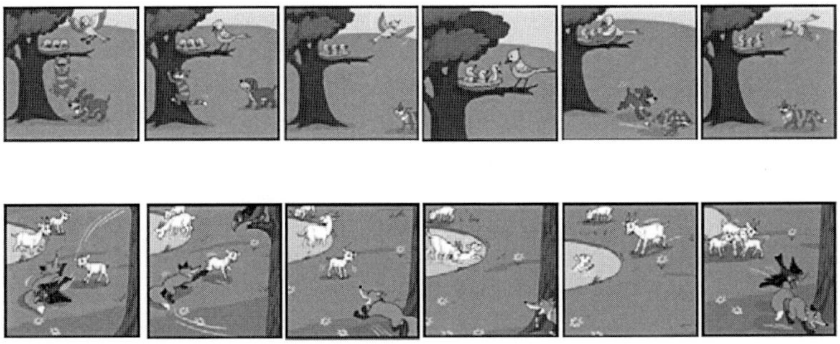

Picture 1. Visual stimuli: *The Baby-Birds* and *The Baby-Goats*

Procedure

Each participant performed two tasks, i.e. story-telling and retelling; both tasks were followed by ten comprehension questions. Each child was tested individually; the sessions were separated by a few minutes of spontaneous conversation between the interviewer and the child. In both studies, the order of the tasks was counterbalanced with regard to story complexity and the task mode; i.e. half of the samples started with story-telling, while the others started with retelling. Half of the samples performed story-telling according to the *Baby-Birds* sequence and retold the story according to the *Baby-Goats* sequence, while the others did the opposite.

All the stories were transcribed using the CHAT tools (MacWhinney, 2017a). The transcribers coded each word with morphological information, including the base form of a word and a set of tags expressing Russian morphological characteristics in order to perform automated morphological analysis, using the CLAN tools (MacWhinney, 2017b). The main macrostructural measures were coded with respect to the presence and accuracy of the structural elements.

Measures

The *macrostructural characteristics* examined were the following: (1) *story structure*, (2) *episode completeness*, and (3) *internal state terms*.

Story structure (SS) also called 'story grammar' (Stein & Glenn, 1979), 'narrative quality' (Fey et al., 2004), or a plotline (Duinmeijer et al., 2012) can be generally perceived as a set of structural elements that are logically connected to each other by temporal/causal means and, thus, create a coherent story (more on this, see Kornev & Balčiūnienė, 2017). Table 2 presents the set of structural elements of both, the *Baby-Birds* and the *Baby-Goats*, sequences.

Each of the structural elements (i.e. setting, goal, attempt, and outcome of each episode) was scored 1 point; thus the SS was scored 0–10 points in total.

Table 2. Macrostructural framework of the sequences

Episode	Element	*Baby-Birds*	*Baby-Goats*
	Setting	*One day...*	*Once upon a time...*
1	Goal	The mother bird wants to feed her chicks.	The mother goat wants to help her baby goat.
	Attempt	The mother bird flies away.	The goat runs into the water.
	Outcome	The mother bird brings a worm.	The goat saves the baby goat.
2	Goal	The cat wants to catch the chicks.	The fox wants to catch the other baby goat.
	Attempt	The cat starts climbing the tree.	The fox grabs the baby goat.
	Outcome	The dog stops the cat.	The bird stops the fox.
3	Goal	The dog wants to help the chicks.	The bird wants to help the baby goat.
	Attempt	The dog grabs the cat's tail.	The bird grabs the fox's tail.
	Outcome	The cat runs away.	The fox runs away.

Episode completeness (EC) is a relatively novel measure in narrative studies (Balčiūnienė & Kornev, 2016; Coggins et al., 1998; Gagarina et al., 2012, 2015; Kornev & Balčiūnienė, 2017). In the present study, all episodes were classified into complete and incomplete ones and scored on the basis of their inner structure (see Table 3).

Table 3. Scoring EC

Episode	Structure	Points
Complete	Goal-Attempt-Outcome	4
Incomplete	Goal-Outcome	3
	Goal-Attempt	2
	Attempt-Outcome	2
	Bare Goal/Attempt/Outcome	1

Since each picture sequence entails three episodes, the EC score can range from 0–12 points in total.

The *microstructural characteristics* examined included (1) *productivity*, (2) *lexical diversity*, and (3) *syntactic complexity*.

Productivity was measured by the *total number of utterances* and the *total number of word tokens without mazes*.

Lexical diversity was measured by the *lemma/token ratio* (LTR) of the content words and the so-called *narrativity index*, i.e. *verb/noun ratio*. Originally, the LTR was suggested for analyzing English language, but in the languages where affixation is typical, it is closely related to derivational morphology. The verb/noun ratio measured the development of the so-called 'true narrative,' i.e. a transition from a simple description of the pictures to a verbalized sequence of logically related events.

Syntactic complexity was measured by the *mean length of utterance in words* and *the number of clauses per utterance.*

Linguistic (dis)fluency was measured by the number of incomplete utterances, hesitations, repeats, revisions, and false starts per utterance. *Hesitations* included *silent pauses* and *fillers. Repeats* were grouped into repeated parts of a word, words, and strings of words. *Revisions* were classified into phonological, lexical, and grammatical modifications of speech. *False starts* were viewed as a separate type of linguistic disfluencies, which, in contrast to revisions and repeats, were neither revised nor repeated after dropping them. Finally, *incomplete utterances* were also considered as a separate type of linguistic dysfluencies.

Linguistic errors were categorized into lexical, grammatical, and stylistic ones.

In both studies, individual measures of narrative macro- and microstructure, linguistic dysfluencies, and linguistic errors were evaluated and compared between the groups by means of statistical analysis.

Finally, an impact of such variables as *group* (clinical vs. control), *session* (first vs. second), *story complexity* (*The Baby-Birds* vs. *The Baby-Goats*), and *mode* (telling vs. retelling) was evaluated on the dynamics of the narrative macro- and microstructure.

Results of Study 1

In contrast to numerous previous studies that have demonstrated many limitations in both macro- and microstructure of SLI children in comparison to their TD peers, we have observed only a few differences between the groups. This might be explained by an effect of a long remedial treatment course (1–2 years) provided for all SLI participants. However, the multivariate ANOVA analysis has revealed that various internal (personal) and external variables had a significant influence on the qualitative and quantitative measures of the narrative. To specify, in the SLI group, the narrative macrostructure (SS and EC) tended to be significantly sensitive to such variables as *session* and *mode,* while such a tendency was not observed in the TD group (see Table 4).

Additionally, the EC was analyzed from the perspective of the inner structure of each episode. Hence, the different structures (complete and incomplete) of each of the Goal-Attempt-Outcome sequences were estimated. In the telling mode, the SLI children produced a significantly smaller number of complete (GAO-GAO-GAO

Table 4. The impact of independent variables on the macrostructure in preschoolers

Independent variable	SLI children, $N = 12$			TD children, $N = 12$		
	F	Sig.	η^2	F	Sig.	η^2
	Dependent variable					
	SS			SS		
Session	8.02	0.047	0.67	–	–	–
Mode	5.00	0.089	0.56	–	–	–
	EC			EC		
Session	5.62	0.077	0.58	–	–	–

or GAO-GA-AO) episode structures than the TD peers ($F = 5.09$; $P < 0.038$). On the basis of the multifactorial ANOVA analysis, the *session* variable significantly influenced the incidence of the GAO ($F = 4.98$; $P < 0.034$) and GAO-GA-AO ($F = 4.30$; $P < 0.048$) structures.

As for the narrative microstructure, the SLI children produced significantly shorter utterances ($MLU_{SLI} = 4.17$; $MLU_{TD} = 5.62$; $F = 6.37$; $p \leq 0.040$) and less verbs per utterance than their TD peers ($M_{SLI} = 1.02$; $\sigma = 0.35$; and $M_{TD} = 1.57$; $\sigma = 0.19$; $F = 8.78$; $p \leq 0.025$). Moreover, in the SLI group, the narrative macrostructure (SS) highly interacted with the narrative microstructure (*verb lexical diversity*) (see Table 5).

The SS correlated positively to the verb LTR in the SLI children, while it correlated negatively to the noun LTR in the TD peers. In addition, in the SLI children,

Table 5. Correlation between some macro- and microstructural measures in preschoolers

	SS	Noun LTR	Verb LTR	Noun/verb ratio
	SLI children, $N = 12$			
SS	1			
Noun LTR	0.026	1		
Verb LTR	0.86*	0.26	1	
Noun/verb ratio	0.82*	−0.0446	0.93**	1
	TD children, $N = 12$			
SS	1			
Noun LTR	−0.71*	1		
Verb LTR	−0.07	0.21	1	
Noun/verb ratio	0.23	−0.17	−0.29	1

* – $p \leq 0.05$; ** – $p \leq 0.02$.

the verb LTR correlated negatively to the percentage of verbs among all words ($r = -0.95^{**}$). The *session* variable significantly influenced the rate of grammatical and lexical errors in both groups but in opposite directions. The SLI children produced more grammatical ($F = 6.3$; $P = 0.066$) and lexical ($F = 38.6$; $P = 0.003$) errors per utterance in the second session, while the TD children produced more grammatical errors ($F = 5.8$; $P = 0.043$) in the first session.

Although the total number of linguistic disfluencies was almost equal between the groups, some types of disfluencies (unfilled hesitations and incomplete utterances) were more frequent in the SLI group (consequently, $F = 3.63$; $p \leq 0.07$ and $F = 4.45$; $p \leq 0.05$), whereas other disfluencies (fillers and word repetitions) were more numerous in the TD group (consequently, $F = 9.34$; $p \leq 0.01$ and $F = 3.74$; $p \leq 0.07$).

Results of Study 2

A simple comparative one-way ANOVA analysis has not revealed any significant quantitative macrostructural differences between the groups. However, a detailed estimation of the episode structure has demonstrated some distinctions between the dyslexics and TD peers, similarly to Study 1. The multifactor dispersion ANOVA analysis has shown a significant impact of independent variables such as *group*, *session*, story *complexity*, and *mode* on the distribution of complete and incomplete episode structures. The incidence of the complete (GAO) structure was almost the same in both groups, but the *group* variable significantly influenced the distribution of the GA and the AO (respectively, $F = 4.8$; $P = 0.034$; effect size = 0.11 for the GA; $F = 4.08$; $P = 0.05$; effect size = 0.095 for the AO) structures. The GA structures were more prevalent in the TD children, while the AO structures were more prevalent in the dyslexic group. The *session* variable significantly influenced the distribution of the GA and the GO structures. The GO structures prevailed in the first session, while the GA ones were more frequent in the second session. However, *story complexity* was the most influential variable. It had a significant impact on the incidence of the GAO ($F = 5.33$; $P = 0.028$), the GO ($F = 12.5$; $P = 0.001$), and the AO ($F = 4.26$; $P = 0.047$) structures. For instance, the less informative GO structure, which did not include any description of the protagonists' actions, was much more frequent (3 times in the TD children and 4 times in the dyslexics) in the more complex *Baby-Goats* story than in the less complex *Baby-Birds* one. The TD children produced the GAO structures more often in the *Baby-Birds* than in the *Baby-Goats* story ($F = 4.62$; $P = 0.057$).

The microstructure indices, however, did not discriminate the groups. The dyslexics produced significantly more lexical errors per word than the TD peers

($F = 7.13$; $P = 0.014$). In the dyslexics, storytelling according to the more complex picture sequence, the *Baby-Goats*, contained more lexical errors than the easier one, the *Baby-Birds*; this tendency was not revealed in the TD children. Also, only in the DYS group, the number of GO structures positively correlated with the number of lexical errors per word ($r = 0.628$; $P < 0.029$).

The statistical analysis of disfluencies has revealed only one significant distinction between the dyslexic and the TD children, i.e. a higher percentage of lexical corrections among all corrections in the dyslexics.

Discussion

Narrative production according to a picture sequence is a complex multimodal activity. In the course of this activity, children create a text that expresses both explicit and implicit meaning. The proportion of these two constituents depends on the different children's ability to produce simultaneously a coherent story and create a cohesive discourse. In the majority of scientific publications, the narrative text measures have been discussed as the constant manifestations of language competence (Berman & Slobin, 1987; Gonzalez et al., 2012; Thorne et al., 2007). Our data provide evidence that intrinsic and external circumstances influence this process and the final product, i.e. a narrative text. When evaluating language skills in clinical populations, it seems reasonable to take into account the set of these multiple determinants (Bliss & McCabe, 2006). The narrator, as an actor, and the story-(re)telling process are rather sensitive to multiple psychological circumstances. In this regard, the data about narrative competence in the SLI children are uneven. In different studies, controversial limitations in the narrative language have been revealed. In the present study, the analysis of the narrative production of the participants has proven the influence of independent variables, such as *clinical status*, *story complexity*, *mode*, and *session*; this confirms our hypothesis. The power of these determinants and the most sensitive processes were distinct in different clinical groups. According to our presupposition, in the SLI children, both macro- and microstructure were sensitive to *session* and *mode*. The children produced shorter utterances and less complete episode structures in the telling than the retelling mode, and they produced more complete (GAO) episode structures in the second session than in the first one. On the other hand, in the second session, they produced more lexical errors than in the first one. This relation could be explained by competition for cognitive resources between a construction of the episode structure and a selection of a proper lexical item. Similar evidence of competing between content and form has been obtained in the study by Colozzo et al. (2011). It is interesting to note that the story structure (SS) significantly correlated to lexical diversity. The SS correlated positively to the verb LTR and the noun/verb ratio in the SLI children; however, it correlated negatively to the noun LTR in the TD peers. According to our previous experience, the noun/verb ratio appears to be a valid measure for the so-called narrativity (Ricoeur, 1980). The lower the noun/verb ratio, the higher the narrativity value. Still, in the SLI children, the verb LTR is in concurrent relations with the percentage of verbs among all tokens: the higher the verb LTR, the rarer the verbs production in a narrative. This might be a consequence of competing for limited cognitive resources in the SLI children but not in the TD peers. Taking into account the central role of a verb phrase in the description of events (Berman & Slobin, 1987), the concurrent relations (the number of verbs vs verb diversity) in the SLI children might prevent them from creating productive but still lexically rich narratives.

As for the macrostructure measures in storytelling, the GAO was the most prevalent episode structure in the TD preschoolers, while the AO was the most frequent in the SLI children, who produced a significant number of incomplete event descriptions.

Episode completeness was dependent on external factors in both clinical groups, but this impact was different between the SLI and the dyslexic children. The SLI children were more sensitive to the story *mode*, while the dyslexics were more sensitive to the story *complexity*. When telling the story based on a more complex *Baby-Goats* sequence, the children tended to produce minimally informative GO structures and to omit the description of the protagonists' actions. This should be treated as a trade-off effect, since the children demonstrated sufficient understanding of the stories when answering comprehension questions. In the study of Gonzalez et al. (2012), similar data about the influence of pictorial complexity on the narrative production were obtained. Contrary to this study, the SLI children under the present investigation were less sensitive to the story *complexity* variable. A possible explanation of this dissimilarity is the age range difference between our investigation and the study by Gonzalez et al. (2012). In our study, dyslexics were very sensitive to the story *complexity*, and their age was closer to the subjects of the given publication.

The microstructure of the reading-disabled children was not influenced by any independent variables. This might be explained by the sufficient grammar processing of oral language in the dyslexics.

Conclusions

The results of our two studies have confirmed that the specifically reading-disabled children (dyslexics) have many common features with specifically language-impaired (SLI) children. Nevertheless, this data do not conform with the assumptions that dyslexia and specific language impairments share the same nature (Bishop & Snowling, 2004). On the contrary, the two clinical groups demonstrate many differences clearly revealed in the dynamic assessment.

Despite the promising results of the study, some limitations should be noted. First, the size of the experimental (DYS and SLI) and the control (TD) group was rather small in order to make broader generalizations. Thus, the experimental population will be extended in the future. Second, only two transcribers were involved, and the agreement measure between the first and the second transcriber was not estimated. However, to sum up, the results of the present study have provided us with novel evidence of the advantages of the dynamic approach to the narrative analysis and the assessment of clinical populations.

Acknowledgement

The scientific data analysis and a preparation of the manuscript for publication were supported by a research grant No.18-18-00114 from the Russian Science Foundation.

Our sincere thanks are due to the editors of this volume and two anonymous reviewers, for their helpful suggestions and comments on previous versions of this chapter.

References

Balčiūnienė, I., & Kornev, A. N. 2016. Doing new things with language: Narrative language in SLI preschoolers. *Estonian Papers in Applied Linguistics* 12, 25–42.

Berman, R. A., & Slobin, D. I. 1987. Five ways of learning to talk about events: A crosslinguistic study of children's narratives. *Berkeley Cognitive Science Report* 46. Berkeley, CA: University of California.

Bishop, D. V. M., & Snowling, M. J. 2004. Developmental dyslexia and specific language impairment: Same or different? *Psychological Bulletin* 130, 858–886. https://doi.org/10.1037/0033-2909.130.6.858

Bliss, L. S. & McCabe, A. 2006. Comparison of discourse genres: Clinical implications. *Contemporary Issues in Communication Science and Disorders* 33(2), 126–137.

Catts, H. W., Bridges, M. S., Little, T. D., & Tomblin, J. B. 2008. Reading achievement growth in children with language impairments. *Journal of Speech, Language, and Hearing Research* 51(6), 1569–1579. https://doi.org/10.1044/1092-4388(2008/07-0259)

Catts, H. W., Fey, M. C., Zhang, X., & Tomblin J. B. 2001. Estimating the risk of future reading difficulties in kindergarten children: A research-based model and its clinical implementation. *Language, Speech, and Hearing Services in Schools* 32, 38–50. https://doi.org/10.1044/0161-1461(2001/004)

Coggins, T. E., Friet, T., & Morgan, T. 1998. Analysing narrative productions in olderschool-age children and adolescents with fetal alcohol syndrome: An experimental tool for clinical applications. *Clinical Linguistics & Phonetics* 12(3), 221–236. https://doi.org/10.3109/02699209808985223

Colozzo, P., Gillam, R. B., Wood, M., Schnell, R. D., & Johnston, J. R. 2011. Content and form in the narratives of children with specific language impairment. *Journal of Speech, Language, and Hearing Research* 54(6), 1609–1627. https://doi.org/10.1044/1092-4388(2011/10-0247)

Duinmeijer, I., de Jong, J., & Scheper, A. 2012. Narrative abilities, memory and attention in children with a specific language impairment. *International Journal of Language & Communication Disorders* 47(5), 542–555. https://doi.org/10.1111/j.1460-6984.2012.00164.x

Fey, M. E., Catts, H. W., Proctor-Williams, K., Tomblin, J. B., & Zhang, X. 2004. Oral and written story composition skills of children with language impairment. *Journal of Speech, Language, and Hearing Research* 47(December), 1301–1318. https://doi.org/10.1044/1092-4388(2004/098)

Fiestas, C. E., Bedore, L. M., Peña, E. D., & Nagy, V. J. 2005. Use of mazes in the narrative language samples of bilingual and monolingual 4- to 7-year old children. In J. Cohen, K. T. McAlister, K. Rolstad, & J. MacSwan (Eds.), *Proceedings of the 4th International Symposium on Bilingualism* (pp. 730–740). Somerville, MA: Cascadilla Press.

Gagarina, N., Klop, D., Kunnari, S., Tantele, K., Välimaa, T., Balčiūnienė, I., Bohnacker, U. & Walters, J. 2012. *MAIN: Multilingual Assessment Instrument for Narratives*. Berlin: ZAS.

Gagarina, N., Klop, D., Kunnari, S., Tantele, K., Välimaa, T., Balčiūnienė, I., Bohnacker, U., & Walters, J. 2015. Assessment of narrative abilities in bilingual children. In Armon-Lotemk, S., de Jong, J. , & Meier, N., et al. (Eds.), *Assessing multilingual children: Disentangling bilingualism from language impairment* (pp. 243–276). Bristol: Multilingual Matters. https://doi.org/10.21832/9781783093137-011

Gonzalez, D. O., Cáceres, M. A., Bento-Gaz, A. C. P. & Befi-Lopes, D. M. 2012. The complexity of narrative interferes in the use of conjunctions in children with specific language impairment. *Jornal da Sociedade Brasileira de Fonoaudiologia* 24, 152–156. https://doi.org/10.1590/S2179-64912012000200011

Grigorenko, E. L., Kornev, A. N. & Rakhlin, N. 2011. Reading-related skills, reading achievement, and inattention: A correlational study. *Journal of Cognitive Education and Psychology* 10(2), 140–156. https://doi.org/10.1891/1945-8959.10.2.140

Holm, A., Crosbie, S., & Dodd, B. 2007. Differentiating normal variability from inconsistency in children's speech: Normative data. *International Journal of Language & Communication Disorders* 42(4), 467–486. https://doi.org/10.1080/13682820600988967

Kapa, L. L., Plante, E. & Doubleday, K. 2017. Applying an integrative framework of executive function to preschoolers with specific language impairment. *Journal of Speech, Language, and Hearing Research* 60(8), 2170–2184. https://doi.org/10.1044/2017_JSLHR-L-16-0027

Kornev, A. N. 1995. *Disleksija i disgrafija u detej* [Dyslexia and dysgraphia in children]. St. Petersburg: Gippokra.

Kornev, A. N. & Balčiūnienė, I. 2014. Story (re-)telling and reading in children with dyslexia: Language or cognitive resource deficit? In *LSCD 2014: Workshop on Late Stages in Speech and Communication Development* (pp. 23–26). London: UCL.

Kornev, A. N., & Balčiūnienė, I. 2015. Narrative production weakness in Russian dyslexics: Linguistic or procedural limitations? *Estonian Papers in Applied Linguistic* 11, 141–157.

Kornev, A. N., & Balčiūnienė, I. 2017. Fictional narrative as a window to discourse development: A psycholinguistic approach. In J. Badio (Ed.), *Events and Narratives in Language* (pp. 171–188). Bern: Peter Lang.

Kornev, A. N. & Ishimova O. A. 2010. *Metodika diagnostiki disleksii u detej* [Methodology in diagnosing dyslexia]. St. Petersburg: Izdatel'stvo Politehnicheskogo universiteta.

Leonard, L. R. 2000. *Children with Specific Language Impairment.* Cambridge, MA: The MIT Press.

Lyon, G. R., Shaywitz, S. E., & Shaywitz, B. A. 2003. A definition of dyslexia. *Annals of Dyslexia* 53(1), 1–14. https://doi.org/10.1007/s11881-003-0001-9

Mackie, C., & Dockrell, J. E. 2004. The nature of written language deficits in children with SLI. *Journal of Speech, Language, and Hearing Research* 47(6), 1469–1483. https://doi.org/10.1044/1092-4388(2004/109)

MacWhinney, B. 2017a. *Tools for analyzing talk, Part 1: The CHAT program* <http://talkbank.org/manuals/CHAT.pdf> (19 August, 2017).

MacWhinney, B. 2017b. *Tools for analyzing talk, Part 2: The CLAN program* <http://talkbank.org/manuals/CLAN.pdf> (19 August, 2017).

Nippold, M. A., Mansfield, T. C., Billow, J. L. & Tomblin, J. B. 2008. Expository discourse in adolescents with language impairments: Examining syntactic development. *American Journal of Speech-Language Pathology* 17(4), 356–366. https://doi.org/10.1044/1058-0360(2008/07-0049)

Petersen, D. B., Gillam, S. L., & Gillam, R. B. 2008. Emerging procedures in narrative assessment: The index of narrative complexity. *Topics in Language Disorders* 28(2), 115–130. https://doi.org/10.1097/01.TLD.0000318933.46925.86

Puranik, C. S., Lombardino, L. J., & Altmann, L. J. 2007. Writing through retellings: An exploratory study of language-impaired and dyslexic populations. *Reading and Writing* 20(3), 251–272. https://doi.org/10.1007/s11145-006-9030-1

Ricoeur, P. 1980. Narrative time. *Critical Inquiry* 7(1), *On Narrative*, 169–190. https://doi.org/10.1086/448093

Schneider, P., Dubé, R. V. & Hayward, D. 2005. *The Edmonton narrative norms instrument*. Retrieved from University of Alberta Faculty of Rehabilitation Medicine website <www.rehabresearch.ualberta.ca/enni> (10 October, 2018).

Stein, N. L., & Albro, E. R. 1997. Building complexity and coherence: Children's use of goal-structured knowledge in telling stories. In M. G. W. Bamberg (Ed.), *Narrative development: Six approaches* (pp. 5–44). Mahwah, NJ: Lawrence Erlbaum Associates.

Stein, N. L., & Glenn, C. G. 1975. An analysis of story comprehension in elementary school children: A test of a schema. <http://files.eric.ed.gov/fulltext/ED121474.pdf>

Stein, N. L., & Glenn, C. G. 1979. An analysis of story comprehension in elementary school children. In R. Freedle (Ed.), *Discourse processing: Multidisciplinary perspectives* (pp. 53–120). Norwood, NJ: Ablex.

Thorne, J. C., Coggins, T. E., Olson, H. C., & Astley, S. J. 2007. Exploring the utility of narrative analysis in diagnostic decision making: Picture-bound reference, elaboration, and fetal alcohol spectrum disorders. *Journal of Speech, Language, and Hearing Research* 50(2), 459–474. https://doi.org/10.1044/1092-4388(2007/032)

Ukrainetz, T. A., & Blomquist, C. 2002. The criterion validity of four vocabulary tests compared with a language sample. *Child Language Teaching and Therapy* 18(1), 59–78. https://doi.org/10.1191/0265659002ct227oa

Vygotsky, L. S. 1962. *Thought and language*. Cambridge, MA: The MIT Press. https://doi.org/10.1037/11193-000

Real-time comprehension of sentences in children with SLI

Evidence from eye movements

Llorenç Andreu,[1] Nadia Ahufinger,[1,2] Laura Ferinu,[1,2]
Fernanda Pacheco,[2] Roser Colomé[2] and Mònica Sanz Torrent[2]
[1]Universitat Oberta de Catalunya / [2]Universitat de Barcelona

Verbs play an essential role in enabling sentences to be interpreted rapidly in real time. The objective of this work is to investigate how verb information is used during real-time comprehension of sentences in Spanish. Twenty-five children (aged 5.3–8.2 years) with specific language impairment (SLI), fifty typically developing children (aged 3.3–8.2 years), and thirty-one normal adults participated in three eye-tracking experiments involving spoken language comprehension. Participants listened to simple sentences in the presence of four depicted objects, only one of which satisfied the semantic restrictions of the verb. Eye movements revealed that children with SLI were able to recognize and retrieve the meaning of the verb rapidly enough to anticipate the upcoming semantically appropriate referent.

Keywords: specific language impairment, eye movements, comprehension, sentence processing, verb semantics

Introduction

Real-time sentence comprehension requires the rapid activation of conceptual and linguistic information. In this process, language users' implicit knowledge of lexical semantics, especially their knowledge of verbs, plays an essential role in enabling sentences to be interpreted rapidly in real time (Andreu, Sanz-Torrent, & Trueswell, 2012). Previous studies with adults have shown that the recognition of a verb includes rapid activation of the semantic and syntactic specifications of the verb, including detailed semantic information associated with each argument (e.g. Altmann & Kamide, 1999; Carlson & Tanenhaus, 1988; Mauner & Koenig, 2000;

https://doi.org/10.1075/z.223.09and

MacDonald, Pearlmutter, & Seidenberg, 1994; Trueswell & Tanenhaus, 1994). For example, Altmann and Kamide (1999) found that listeners can anticipate upcoming referents in a sentence based on verb information (e.g. anticipating a reference to edible objects upon hearing *eat* in *The boy will eat…*).

In this work, we study verb-based anticipatory information in the context of sentence comprehension in children with specific language impairment (SLI). SLI is an oral language disorder characterized by developmental delays in verbal abilities that can affect both expressive and receptive language where there is an absence of clear neurological, sensory-motor, non-verbal cognitive or social–emotional deficits (Bishop, 1997; Leonard, 1998). Children with SLI characteristically produce syntactically simpler sentences, show deficits in their use of inflectional morphology such as verb tense and agreement, and show significant delays in lexical acquisition, especially verbs, in comparison to age-matched peers (e.g. Bedore & Leonard, 2001; Bishop, 1997; Grinstead et al., 2009; Leonard, 1998; Leonard & Deevy, 2006; Sanz-Torrent, Serrat, Andreu, & Serra, 2008).

There are relatively few real-time comprehension studies that investigate the ability of children with SLI to recognize words embedded within sentences. For instance, using a word-monitoring paradigm, Montgomery, Scudder, and Moore (1990), Stark and Montgomery (1995) and Montgomery (2000, 2002) found that children with SLI are slower at recognizing words embedded in a sentence than their typically developing age-matched peers. In contrast, Marinis and van de Lely (2007) found that in children with SLI with grammatical deficits (G-SLI), lexical retrieval is not slowed. Using a cross-modal picture priming task, they found that these children, when hearing filler-gap dependencies, reactivated filler-antecedents upon hearing a verb, but failed to do so at the location of the syntactic gap.

The present work is based on the so-called "visual world paradigm" (Tanenhaus, Spivey-Knowlton, Eberhard, & Sedivy, 1995). This paradigm provides a moment-by-moment record of where people are looking as they hear sentences that describe their visual referent world (Trueswell, 2008). Using this methodology, the objective of this work is to investigate how Spanish-speaking children with SLI use sematic verb information during real-time sentence comprehension. Through three experiments we will analyse: (1) if children with SLI are able to recognize and retrieve the meaning of a verb, embedded in a sentence, rapidly enough to anticipate the upcoming semantically appropriate referent, before it is mentioned (Experiment 1), (2) if, in the case of anticipation, it is produced by verb-specific semantic restrictions or instead reflects knowledge of simple lexical co-occurrences (Experiment 2), and (3) if children with SLI are able to access the meaning of verbs rapidly enough so as to anticipate their possible arguments and adjuncts (Experiment 3).

Based on the problems found in previous studies in verb production in children with SLI (e.g. Bedore & Leonard, 2001; Grinstead et al., 2009; Sanz-Torrent, Serrat, Andreu, & Serra, 2008), the assumption is that children with SLI should either display use of verb information to anticipate the upcoming semantically appropriate referent or that this anticipation should take place to a lesser degree than with children with typical development.

Experiment 1

Experiment 1 is an adaptation of the study by Altmann and Kamide (1999). The aim is to replicate their results in adults and to explore the effects in children with typical language development and children with SLI.

Methodology

Participants

Four groups took part in this study. The first one consisted of 31 adults that were students or junior faculty at various universities in the Barcelona area (mean age = 30.76 years; *SD* = 7.01 years; range (19.2–45.7 years). The second group consisted of 25 children (18 boys, 7 girls) with specific language impairment (SLI), ranging from ages 5.3 to 8.2. The third group consisted of 25 children (18 boys, 7 girls) matching the children with SLI in terms of age, sex and mother tongue, ranging from 5.3 to 8.2 years of age. The fourth group consisted of 25 children (18 boys, 7 girls) matched according to mean length of utterance in words (MLU-w), sex and mother tongue with the children with SLI, ranging from ages 3.3 to 7.1. Table 1 presents a summary of descriptive data for the three groups of children.

Materials

Twelve simple sentences were constructed (see Appendix A). All contained the same structure: Noun Phrase (NP) + Verb + Adverb + NP/Prepositional Phrase (PP), which always corresponded to Agent + Verb + Adverb + Theme/Patient. All sentences began with one of four possible agents: *the woman, the man, the girl* or *the boy*. These were assigned randomly to sentences and six were male and six female. Twelve different verbs were used. There were ten adverbs denoting the manner of the action (*quickly (3), slowly (2), strongly* (2), *carefully (3)*) and two denoting the frequency of the action (*sometimes*).

Sentences were recorded by a male native Spanish speaker and sampled at 44,100 Hz. A digital audio editor was used to adjust each sentence so that the

Table 1. Group age, cognitive measures and performance in language

	Group			
	SLI group	Age controls	MLU-w controls	Pairwise
	Mean (S.D.)	Mean (S.D.)	Mean (S.D.)	
Age (years)	6.69 (0.90)	6.72 (0.92)	5.51 (1.05)	SLI = AC, SLI > MLU*, AC > MLU*
NVIQ	96.1 (7.9)	106.3 (6.0)	93.13 (9.32)	SLI = AC, SLI = MLU, AC = MLU
PPVT-III	89.58 (9.56)	112.07 (14.37)	92 (12.87)	SLI = AC, SLI = MLU, AC = MLU
ELI-Phonetics*	6.37 (4.27)	2.12 (2.23)	4.47 (3.87)	SLI > AC**, SLI = MLU, AC = MLU
ELI-Receptive vocabulary*	36.27 (18.84)	73.07 (17.97)	67.85 (26.13)	SLI = AC**, SLI = MLU, AC = MLU
ELI-Expressive vocabulary*	8.62 (1.8)	60.38 (15.06)	52.27 (28.84)	SLI < AC**, SLI < MLU**, AC = MLU
ELI-Pragmatics*	53.64 (25.99)	80.38 (15.60)	62.56 (14.34)	SLI < AC**, SLI = MLU, AC > MLU**
MLU-w	3.95 (1.39)	6.86 (1.76)	3.97 (1.45)	SLI < AC**, SLI = MLU, AC > MLU**

Note. Chronological age in years; NVIQ (Nonverbal Intelligence Quotient) in standard score (mean=100; SD: 15); PPVT-III (Peabody Picture Vocabulary Test III. Spanish version) in standard score (mean=100; SD: 15); ELI (Evaluación del Lenguaje Infantil); ELI-Phonetics in mean number of errors; ELI-Receptive vocabulary, ELI-Expressive vocabulary and ELI-Pragmatics in percentiles; MLU-w (Mean Length of Utterance in words). *Values only calculated for children under age 6. Comparison made by two-tailed Mann–Whitney U-test. **$P < 0.05$.

Agent NP, the Verb and the Adverb each lasted one second (words + silence lasted 1000 ms). This facilitated the subsequent analysis of data without having any effect on auditory stimuli. Utterances sounded natural and unedited to adult native speakers. All the authors had rated the naturalness of the utterances on a scale of 1 to 5. Any stimuli that had been given a rating of less than 4 were reedited until they were rated above 4.

Visual images were constructed and paired with each sentence. Each image consisted of four pictures located in the centre of four quadrants on the screen. For every trial, there was one target picture depicting the target Theme/Patient and three distracter pictures that could not be semantically possible Themes/Patients of the verb (see Figure 1). The position of the target picture in each quadrant was randomized. The audio and the visual image for each item were merged together in a video file lasting 5000 ms, using VirtualDubMod software. In each video, the onset of the spoken sentence coincided with the onset of the visual stimuli.

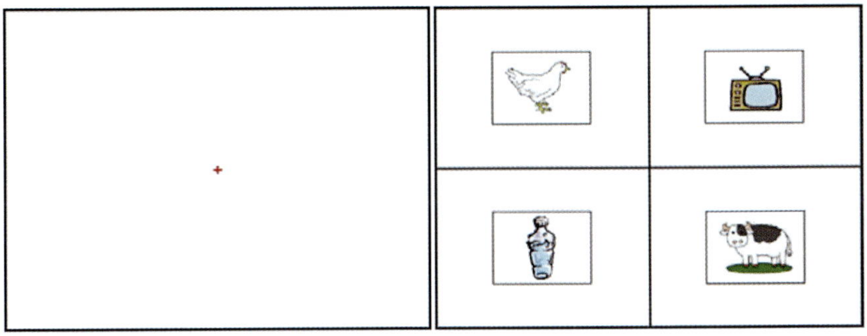

Figure 1. Stimuli example: *El hombre ordeña con cuidado la vaca* [the man carefully milks the cow]. (target: *vaca* [cow]; distracters: *gallina* [chicken] / *botella* [bottle] / *televisión* [television])

Procedure

Participants were seated approximately 22″ in front of a Tobii T120 eye tracker with an integrated 17" TFT monitor. Tobii Studio software was used to present the stimuli and collect the eye-tracking data. Stimuli videos were made using 800 x 600-pixel images presented on a screen set to 1024 x 768 pixels. The sounds of the stimuli were presented to participants via a mono channel split between two loudspeakers positioned on either side of the viewing monitor. Eye position was sampled at 120 Hz (approximately 8-ms intervals).

Participants were instructed to listen to the sentences and inspect the images, trying to understand both sentences and depicted scenes. The test videos were presented randomly in two blocks. All participants were given both blocks. Between each trial, participants were presented with a crosshair (on which they had been instructed to fixate) for approximately 2000 ms, to ensure that the direction of the gaze in each trial would start from the same point (the centre of the four quadrants).

The horizontal and vertical eye position data obtained using Tobii Studio software were used to assess eye position. A value of one was given to every eye-tracking sample that fell within a region of interest (as defined by a rectangle surrounding each image); otherwise it was assigned a zero. From this we calculated the proportion of looks made by the participants to the target picture and the distracters.

Results

Figures 2 through 5 present the proportion of looks, from sentence onset, to the target referent in comparison to the average proportion of looks to the three distracter objects. As we can see in Figure 1, one picture represented the target and the other three served as distracter pictures. For this reason, we divided the proportion of looks to the distracter objects by three. Vertical lines indicate the exact onset of the verb and the adverb. The dotted line indicates the onset of the object NP/Prepositional Phrase (PP).

As a simple estimate of the degree of anticipatory eye movements, each trial for each subject was given a binary code (1 = target look; 0 = otherwise) based on the eye position at the offset of the adverb (3000 ms), just prior to hearing the target NP (marked with the discontinuous vertical line). Consistent with what is graphed at 3000 ms in Figures 2–5, the adult group had the highest proportion of target looks.

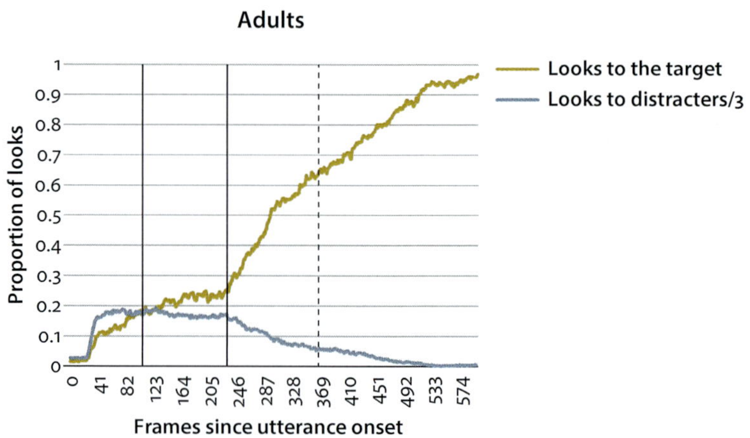

Figure 2. Proportion of looks to the target and distracters from onset of image and sound for the adult group

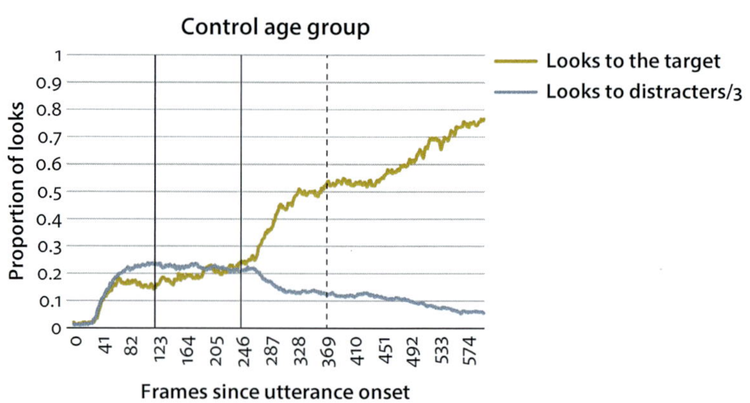

Figure 3. Proportion of looks to the target and distracters from onset of image and sound for the control age group

In order to determine if the SLI group differed from each of the comparison groups in terms of target looks, separate analyses of variance (ANOVAs) were conducted on E-Logit transformations of subject and item means of the proportional data (see Barr, 2008) with group (SLI vs. comparison group) as a factor. As can be seen in Table 1, anticipatory target looks for children with SLI were indeed reliably different from adults and from age-matched controls, but they were not different from MLU controls, indicating that children with SLI were undertaking slightly less anticipatory processing than children of similar ages.

Crucially, however, there is ample evidence that all four groups, including children with SLI, were capable of anticipatory referential processing. It means that all the groups looked more at the target than the distracters.

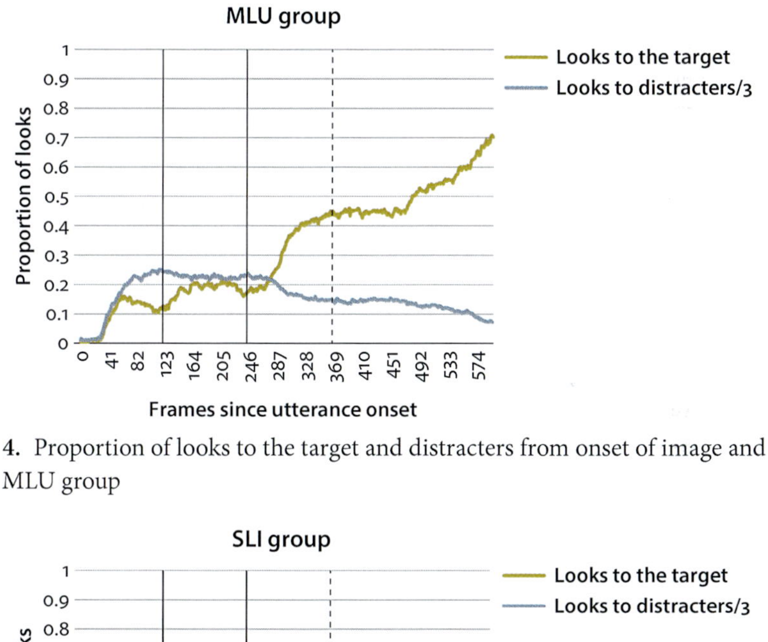

Figure 4. Proportion of looks to the target and distracters from onset of image and sound for the MLU group

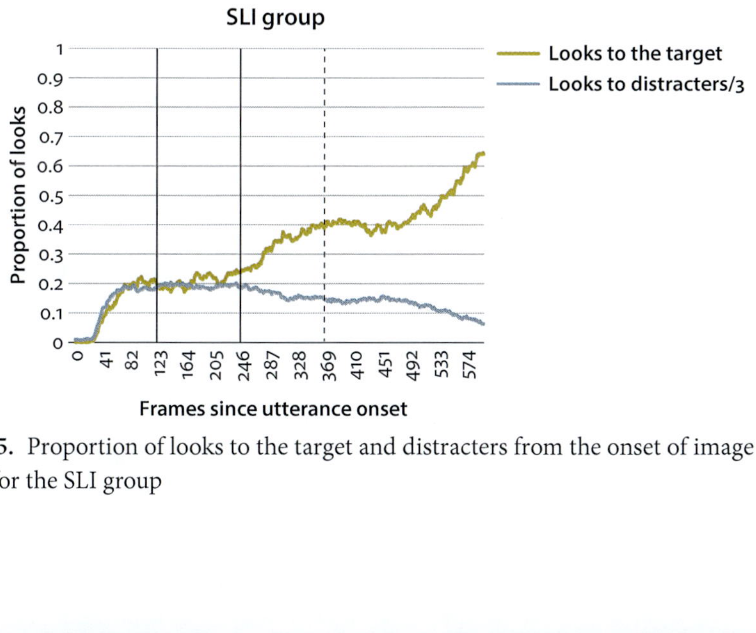

Figure 5. Proportion of looks to the target and distracters from the onset of image and sound for the SLI group

Table 2. Analyses of variances (ANOVAs) comparing SLI children to each participant group

Comparison	Effect	Subject means			Item means		
		F	d.f.	*p*	*F*	d.f.	*p*
SLI vs. Adults	Group	10.63	1.53	0.002	23.65	1.11	0.0005
SLI vs. Age	Group	4.39	1.47	0.042	5.55	1.11	0.038
SLI vs. MLU	Group	0.54	1.47	n.s.	2.11	1. 11	n.s.

Note. SLI=Children with specific language impairment; MLU=Children matched by mean length of utterance; Age=Children matched by age; n.s.=not significant.

Discussion

All groups, including the children with SLI, showed anticipatory processing of the target while hearing the adverb but not while hearing the verb. This was probably due to the fact that the participants needed to listen to most of the verb to process the meaning and then needed a minimum latency time of between 150 and 180 ms to plan and launch a saccade (Fischer, 1992; Martin, Shao, & Boff, 1993; Saslow, 1967).

On the other hand, while hearing the adverb that followed the verb, all groups showed a rise in the number of looks to the target referent as compared to looks to the distracter objects. This rise occurred prior to hearing the target NP. Adults showed the sharpest rise, but all three groups of children, including children with SLI, performed similarly.

Children with SLI were able to use verb-specific semantic information rapidly enough during spoken sentence comprehension to anticipate upcoming referents, just like the other groups of subjects. Although anticipatory looks to the target were significantly lower for the SLI group when compared to the age-matched controls and adults, the looking pattern for children with SLI was indistinguishable from that of MLU-matched controls.

Experiment 2

It is possible that the child groups' successful performance in launching anticipatory eye movements towards typical Patients/Themes in Experiment 1 may not reflect quick use of verb-specific semantic restrictions but rather reflect knowledge of simple lexical co-occurrences (*milk-cow*). To address this issue, the present experiment compared anticipatory eye movements for both typical and atypical Patient/Theme relationships. In some trials, participants heard a typical Patient/Theme relationship such as *The man quickly closes the door* while viewing a door among a set of "unclosable" objects (e.g. a cloud, a tree, a stamp). In other trials, they heard an atypical Patient/Theme relationship such as *The man suddenly pushes the flower pot* while viewing a flower pot among "unpushable" objects (e.g. a house, a street lamp, a road). Here, "push" and "flower pot" tend not to co-occur in the language, and are clearly not word associates, yet the flower pot is the most likely thing to be pushed in this visual context. Past studies with adults have shown that anticipatory eye movements occur with both atypical and typical arguments (Boland, 2005; Kamide, Altmann, & Haywood, 2003).

Methodology

Participants

The same participants took part in this experiment as in Experiment 1.

Materials

Twenty simple sentences were constructed (see Appendix B). All of these sentences contained the same structure as in Experiment 1 (*NP* + Verb + Adverb + NP/PP). Ten sentences ended with a typical Theme/Patient for the verb and ten sentences ended with an atypical Theme/Patient for the verb. The sentences were recorded and the visual images were constructed as in Experiment 1.

Procedure

The same procedure was used in the present experiment as for Experiment 1.

Results

Figures 6 through 9 present the proportion of looks over time to the target referent compared to the average proportion of looks to the three distracter objects, as split by condition (typical vs. atypical target). As in Experiment 1, the most remarkable aspect of the results is the similarity across all groups of subjects. Children with SLI and all other groups showed significant anticipatory processing for both typical and atypical referents, although the anticipatory effects were greater for typical referents. While hearing the adverb and prior to hearing the target NP, there was a rise in looks to the target referent as compared to looks at distracter objects for all groups, with sharper rises for typical targets. Children with SLI demonstrated slightly less anticipatory processing than other children, but overall the results from all groups of children were quite similar, in that they all showed signs of anticipatory processing for both typical and atypical targets.

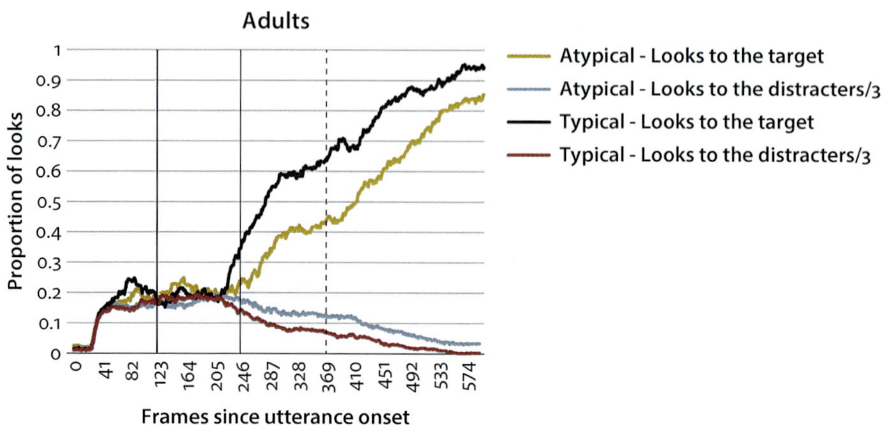

Figure 6. Proportion of looks to the target and distracters from image and sound onset under both typical and atypical conditions for the adult group

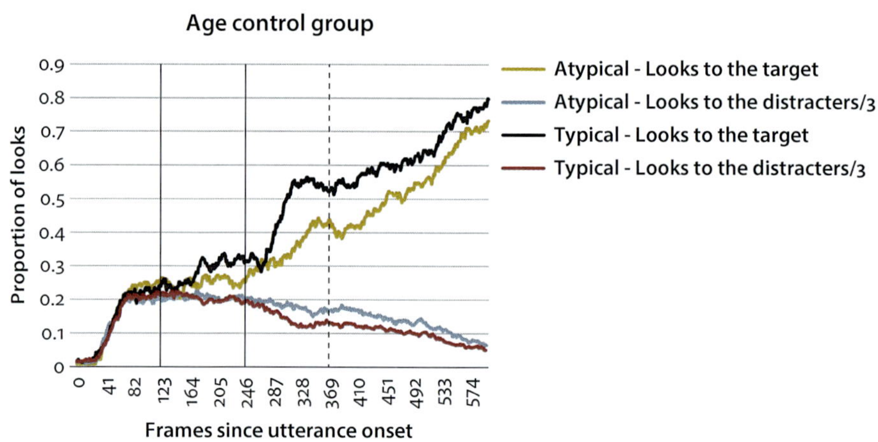

Figure 7. Proportion of looks to the target and distracters from image and sound onset under both typical and atypical conditions for the control age group

In order to determine if the SLI group differed from each of the comparison groups in terms of anticipatory processing, separate analyses of variance (ANOVAs) were conducted on E-Logit transformations of subject and item means of the proportional data (see Barr, 2008) with group (SLI vs. comparison group) and target type (atypical vs. typical) as factors. As can be seen in Table 3, anticipatory target looks for children with SLI were indeed reliably different from adults and from age-matched controls, as shown by the reliable group effect in each of these comparisons. However, as in Experiment 1, children with SLI were no different from the MLU controls, indicating that children with SLI were undertaking less anticipatory processing than children of similar ages. A group by

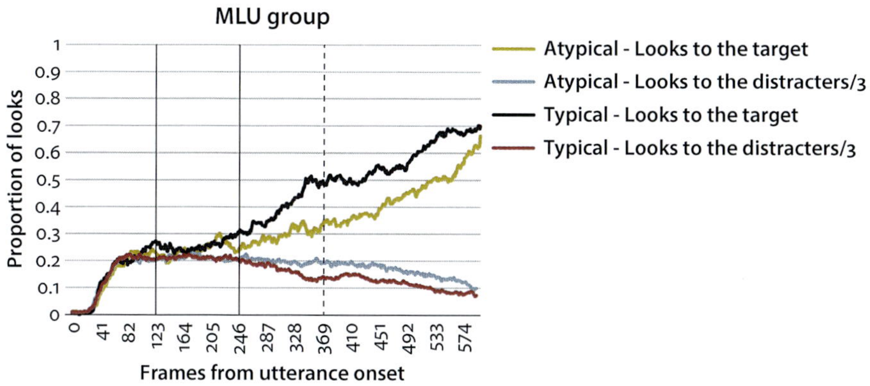

Figure 8. Proportion of looks to the target and distracters from image and sound onset under both typical and atypical conditions for the MLU group

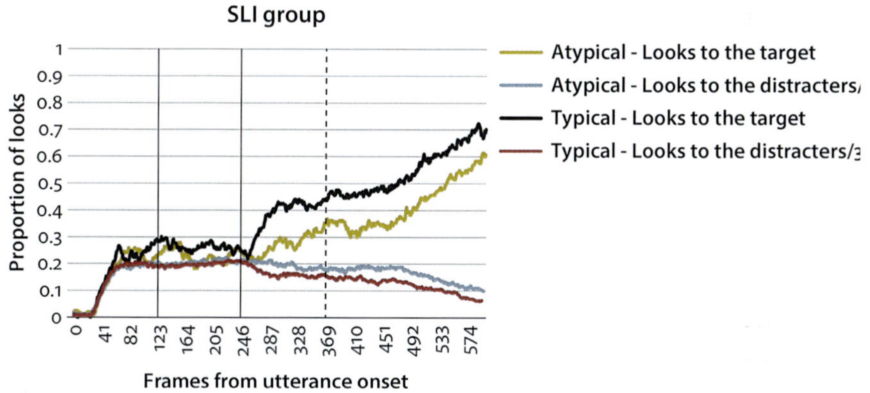

Figure 9. Proportion of looks to the target and distracters from image and sound onset under both typical and atypical conditions for the SLI group

target type interaction was only significant when comparing the SLI and adult groups, suggesting that the effect of typicality was slightly greater in adults than in children with SLI.

Crucially, however, as in Experiment 1, there is ample evidence that all four groups, including children with SLI, were capable of anticipatory referential processing. In addition, this anticipatory processing occurred for both typical and atypical targets.

Table 3. Analyses of variances (ANOVAs) comparing SLI to each participant group

Comparison	Effect		Subject means			Item means	
		F	d.f.	*p*	*F*	d.f.	*p*
	Group	7.70	1.54	0.008	9.11	1.9	0.015
SLI vs. Adults	Target type	43.42	1.54	<0.001	1.96	1.9	n.s.
	Group x target type	6.59	1.54	0.013	1.86	1.9	n.s.
	Group	5.66	1.47	0.022	7.23	0.19	n.s.
SLI vs. Age	Target type	4.94	1.47	<0.001	0.750	0.19	n.s.
	Group x target type	0.06	1.47	n.s.	0.19	0.19	n.s.
	Group	0.47	1.48	n.s.	0.39	0.19	n.s.
SLI vs. MLU	Target type	23.04	1.48	<0.001	1.77	0.19	n.s.
	Group x target type	1.27	1.48	n.s.	1.61	0.19	n.s.

Note. SLI=Children with specific language impairment; MLU=Children matched by mean length of utterance; Age=Children matched by age; n.s.=not significant.

Discussion

All groups of participants showed reliable signs of anticipatory processing for both typical and atypical targets. This pattern suggests that more than simple lexical association is behind the performance of children with SLI (and the other groups of participants). Even with items for which the upcoming NP was not lexically predictable but was likely given the scenario's alternatives (i.e. an atypical target referent in the presence of objects that were not possible Patients/Themes), children with SLI behaved like the other children and generated anticipatory eye movements towards the atypical target. Moreover, all groups of children as well as the adults directed more looks at the typical Patients/Themes than the atypical ones. This latter pattern replicates the adult findings of Kamide et al. (2003, Experiment 1 & 2) and Boland (2005, Experiment 2), where effects of typicality on anticipatory processing were observed.

Experiment 3

The previous experiments suggest that children with SLI are able to use verb-specific semantic information rapidly enough during spoken sentence comprehension to anticipate upcoming Patient/Theme referents. In Experiment 3 we investigated another aspect of the use of verb information during real-time sentence comprehension. Specifically, we examined if children use verbs to predict arguments and adjuncts in sentence comprehension. Some psycholinguistic theories of parsing (e.g. Boland & Boehm-Jernigan, 1998; Frazier & Clifton, 1996; Stevenson, 1998) have distinguished between arguments and adjuncts. The thematic roles of theme, patient and source–goal are arguments because they are essential participants that must be specified in the sentence. Adjuncts, on the other hand, are considered to be supplements that are not selected by the verb although they can complete its meaning and their deletion does not cause ungrammaticality. In general, instruments, locatives and comitatives, among others, are considered adjuncts (Bosque & del Monte, 1999).

Methodology

Participants

The same participants took part in this experiment as in Experiment 1.

Materials

We selected different sentences in which arguments (themes, sources–goals, instruments) and adjuncts (comitatives and locatives) played different thematic roles with respect to the predicate (see Appendix C). We categorized the sentences according to four conditions:

- Transitive verb/Theme: *La niña come despacio la tarta con la cuchara* [The girl slowly eats cake with a spoon]. Pictures – Target: *tarta* [cake]; Competitor: *cuchara* [spoon]; Distracters: *sombrero* [hat], *dinosaurio* [dinosaur].
- Verb of motion/Source-Goal: *El hombre entra despacio en casa con la maleta* [The man slowly enters the house with the suitcase]. Pictures – Target: *casa* [house]; Competitor: *maleta*; Distracter: *luna* [moon], *tractor* [tractor].
- Verb of action/Instrument: *La mujer esquia deprisa con el trineo por la montaña* [The woman skis down the mountain fast with the sled]. Pictures – Target: *trineo* [sled]; Competitor: *montaña* [mountain]; Distractor: *vaso* [glass], *playa* [beach].
- Intransitive verb/Locative: *La niña duerme siempre en la cama con el osito* [The girl always sleeps in bed with a teddy bear]. Pictures – Target: *cama* [bed]; Competitor: *osito* [teddy bear]; Distracter: *arbol* [tree], *bombilla* [light bulb].

Twenty-four simple sentences were constructed. All contained the same structure: Noun Phrase (NP) + Verb + Adverb + Target Phrase (NP or Prepositional Phrase, PP) + PP, which always corresponded to Agent + Verb + Adverb + Theme/Instrument/Locative/Source–Goal + Instrument/Locative/Comitative. The distribution of the 24 target phrases was as follows: six themes, six instruments, six locatives, and six locations that had the thematic roles of goal (four of them) and source (two of them). In order to minimize the restrictive effect the verb has on subsequent elements, all the sentences began with one of four possible agents: *the woman, the man, the girl* or *the boy*. These were randomly assigned to sentences and for every condition there were three male and three female. Twenty-four different verbs were used. An adverb or adverbial phrase was placed after the verb to establish a temporary space for processing verb information. The adverbs used denoted the manner of the action (attentively, quickly, slowly, suddenly, carefully, sadly and cheerfully) or the temporal properties of the action (always and every day). The target phrases followed three locatives and three instruments in the "theme" condition, six comitatives in the "source–goal" condition, six locatives in the "instrument" condition and three comitatives and three instruments in the "locative" condition.

The sentences were recorded and the visual images were constructed as in Experiment 1.

Procedure

The same procedure was used in the present experiment as for Experiment 1.

Results

Figures 10 through 13 present the proportion of looks at the referent targets over time for adult, control age, MLU and SLI groups. The black vertical line in the graphs divides the two temporal windows selected to analyse anticipatory eye movements towards the target. The first was from verb onset to offset (which included 1000–2000 ms from video onset) and the second was between adverb onset and offset (which included 2000–3000 ms from video onset). Analyses of variance (ANOVAs) by participant and by item were conducted over the means of the proportional data for each window of analysis with group (SLI, control age, MLU, adults) and argument type (theme, source–goal, instrument, locative) as independent variables.

In the verb window (1000–2000 ms), results showed that neither argument type [$F1(3.306) = 2.497$, $p = 0.060$; $F2(3.80) = 0.746$, $p = 0.528$] nor group [$F1(3.102) = 0.147$, $p = 0.93$; $F2(3.80) = 0.072$, $p = 0.975$], nor the interaction between these two variables [$F1(9.306) = 0.502$, $p = 0.873$; $F2(9.80) = 0.167$, $p = 0.997$], had any effect. Figure 4 shows the differences in the mean of the proportion of looks with respect to the argument type in each group of the sample.

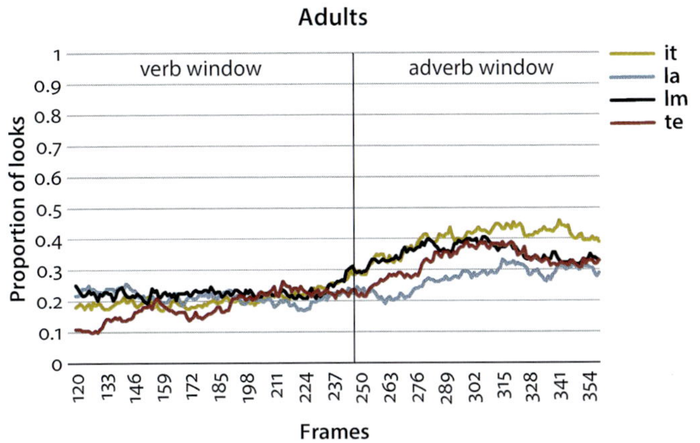

Figure 10. Proportion of looks at instrument (it), locative (la), source–goal (lm) and theme (te) referents in verb and adverb windows for the adult group

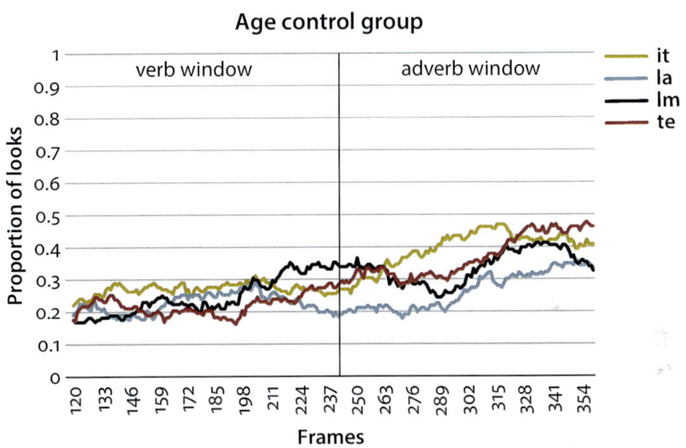

Figure 11. Proportion of looks at instrument (it), locative (la), source–goal (lm) and theme (te) referents in verb and adverb windows for the age control group

In the adverb window (2000–3000 ms), results showed significant differences by argument type [$F1(3.306) = 10.821$, $p < 0.001$; $\varepsilon 2 = 0.096$; $F2(3.80) = 2.891$, $p = 0.04$; $\varepsilon 2 = 0.098$] but not between groups [$F1(3.102) = 1.044$, $p = 0.377$; $F2(3.80) = 0.725$, $p = 0.54$]. The interaction between these two variables was also not significant [$F1(9.306) = 0.802$, $p = 0.615$; $F1(9.80) = 0.222$, $p = 0.99$]. Post-hoc comparison revealed that the differences related to argument type were restricted to the comparison between locatives and the rest of the arguments. Figure 15 shows the differences in the mean of the proportion of looks with respect to the argument type in each group of the sample.

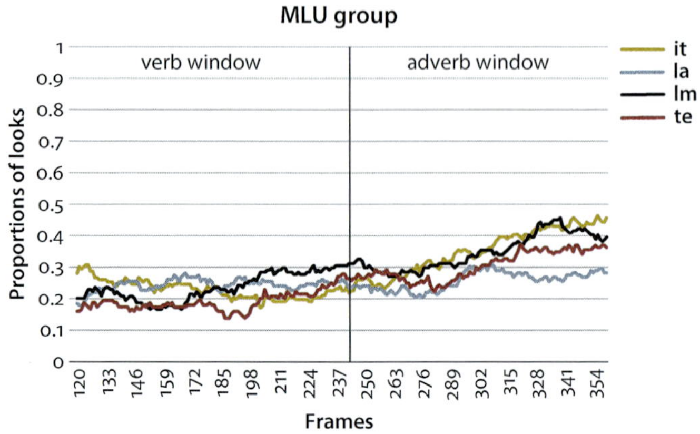

Figure 12. Proportion of looks at instrument (it), locative (la), source–goal (lm) and theme (te) referents in verb and adverb windows for the MLU group

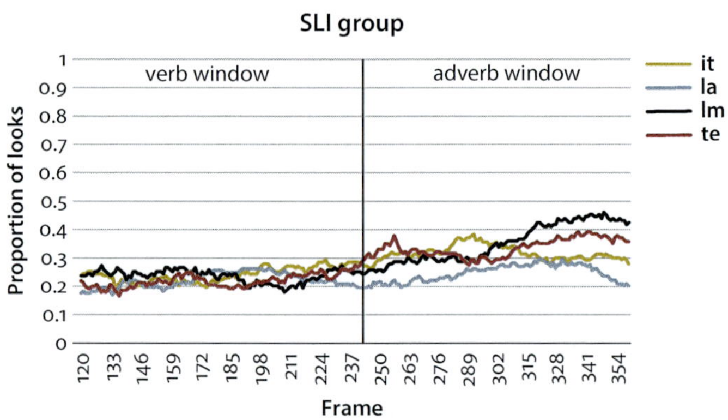

Figure 13. Proportion of looks at instrument (it), locative (la), source–goal (lm) and theme (te) referents in verb and adverb windows for the SLI group

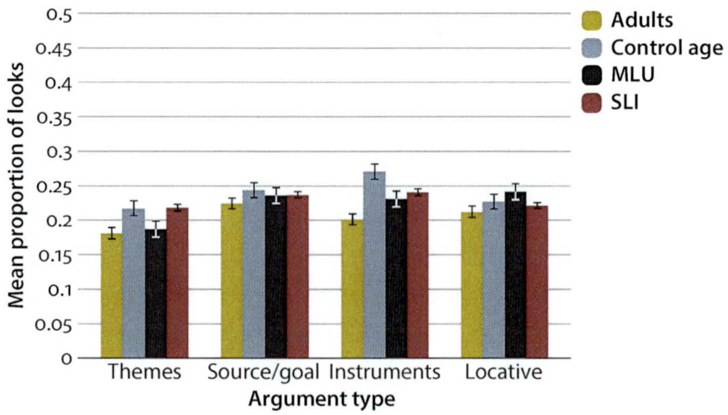

Figure 14. Proportion of looks at theme, instrument, locative and source–goal referents binned into the verb window by group

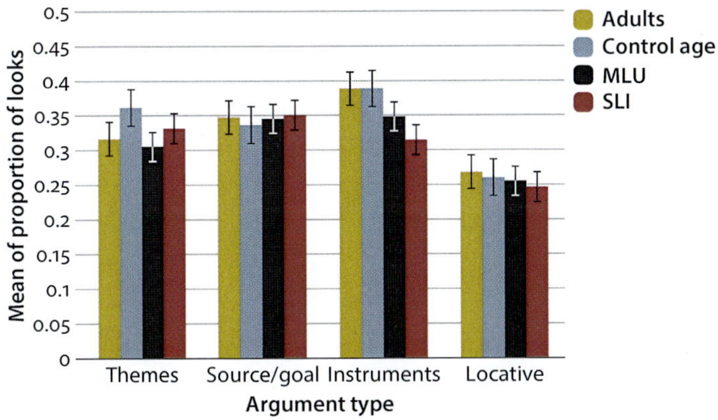

Figure 15. Proportion of looks at theme (te), instrument (it), locative (la) and source–goal (lm) referents binned into the adverb window by group

Discussion

In this experiment, we compared anticipatory looks at the themes, sources–goals, instruments (arguments) and locatives (adjuncts). Contrary to our expectations, all groups of participants showed that the proportion of looks at the theme, source–goal and instrument referents was significantly higher than for looks at locatives. This pattern was found for adults and children with and without SLI. These results suggest that children with SLI do not suffer impairment in retrieving the verb's semantic information in order to anticipate arguments and adjuncts in sentence comprehension: like adults and age-matched children, children with SLI can anticipate upcoming referents based on verb information.

General discussion

The purpose of this study was to investigate if children with SLI use verb information during real-time sentence comprehension in Spanish. For this purpose, in three eye-tracking studies we used the visual world paradigm to analyse anticipatory looks at a visual referent of arguments and adjuncts in the context of simple sentences in children with SLI.

Based on the problems found in verb production in children with SLI in previous studies (e.g. Bedore & Leonard, 2001; Grinstead et al., 2009; Sanz-Torrent, Serrat, Andreu, & Serra, 2008), the assumption was that children with SLI would show no use of verb information to anticipate the upcoming semantically appropriate referent or that this anticipation would be to a lesser degree than in children with typical development.

However, children with SLI used verb-specific semantic information rapidly enough during spoken sentence comprehension to anticipate upcoming referents of arguments and adjuncts. Moreover, all groups of children and adults appeared to be sensitive to typicality. In summary, this work shows that children with SLI use selectional information conveyed by a verb to anticipate upcoming information in sentence comprehension.

The results of this work suggest that children with SLI present less atypical comprehension than would be expected due their problems with language production. Further studies should analyse the causes of these differences and the influence of verb semantics on sentence comprehension and production.

Appendix A. Sentences used in Experiment 1

1. La mujer abre de prisa la puerta (TARGET: puerta, DISTRACTERES: lápiz, gato, elefante).
1. *The woman opens quickly the door (TARGET: door, DISTRACTERS: pencil, cat, elephant).*
2. El niño recorta con cuidado el papel (T: papel, D: despertador, zorro, dinosaurio).
2. *The boy trims carefully the paper (T: paper, D: clock, fox, dinosaur).*
3. El hombre parte con fuerza la barra de pan (T: pan, D: luna, pato, hipopótamo).
3. *The man breaks forcefully the loaf of bread (T: bread, D: moon, duck, hippo).*
4. El hombre construye despacio un castillo (T: castillo, D: libro, león, cabra).
4. *The man builds slowly a castle (T: castle, D: book, lion, goat).*
5. El hombre ordeña con cuidado a la vaca (T: vaca, D: gallina, botella, televisión).
5. *The man milks carefully the cow (T: cow, D: chicken, bottle, television).*
6. La mujer abraza a veces a su padre (T: marido, D: serpiente, radio, clip).
6. *The woman hugs sometimes her father (T: husband, D: snake, radio, paperclip).*
7. La mujer conduce deprisa la ambulancia (T: ambulancia, D: espada, arena, mantequilla).
7. *The woman drives fast the ambulance (T: ambulance, D: sword, sand, butter).*
8. El niño cierra con cuidado los cajones (T: cajones, D: goma, sal, gente).
8. *The boy closes carefully the drawers (T: drawers, D: eraser, salt, people).*
9. La niña ordena a veces los libros (T: libros, D: balcones, azúcar, agua).
9. *The girl organizes sometimes the books (T: books, D: balconies, sugar, water).*
10. La niña derrama con fuerza la sal (T: sal, D: viento, gafas, mochila).
10. *The girl spills forcefully the salt (T: salt, D: wind, glasses, backpack).*
11. La niña lee despacio un cuento (T: cuento, D: coche, bandada de pájaros, flota).
11. *The girl reads slowly a children's story (T: story, D: car, flock of birds, floats).*
12. El hombre reúne deprisa al ejército (T: ejército, D: bosque, guitarra, pan).
12. *The man gathers quickly the army (T: Army, D: forest, guitar, pan).*

Appendix B. Experimental sentences of Experiment 2

Typical target

Block 1

1. El niño rompe de repente un vaso (TARGET: vaso, DISTRACTERES: cohete, moneda, casa).
1. *The boy breaks suddenly a glass (T: glass, D: rocket, coin, house).*
2. El hombre cierra deprisa la puerta (T: puerta, D: nube, árbol, sello).
2. *The man closes quickly the door (T: door, D: cloud, tree, stamp).*
3. El niño quiere siempre un regalo (T: regalo, D: sol, tejado, calle).
3. *The boy wants always a gift (T: gift, D: sun, roof, street).*
4. La niña cuida cada día al perro (T: perro, D: ojo, antena, chimenea).
4. *The girl cares each day for the dog (T: dog, D: eye, antenna, chimney).*
5. La mujer cura con cuidado la herida (T: herida, D: nube, plancha, reloj).
5. *The woman disinfects carefully the wound (T: wound, D: cloud, iron, clock).*

Block 2

6. El niño encuentra de repente una moneda (T: moneda, D: relámpago, planeta, desierto).
6. *The boy finds suddenly a coin (T: coin, D: lightning, planet, desert).*
7. La mujer escucha siempre la radio (T: radio, D: mesa, manzana, zapatos).
7. *The woman listens always to the radio (T: radio, D: table, apple, shoes).*
8. La niña abre a veces la ventana (T: ventana, D: escoba, planta, percha).
8. *The girl opens sometimes the window (T: window, D: broom, plant, hanger).*
9. El hombre conduce deprisa el coche (T: coche, D: calcetín, silla, puerta).
9. *The man drives fast the car (T: car, D: sock, chair, door).*
10. La mujer compra a veces patatas (T: patatas, D: iglú, helicóptero, cocodrilo).
10. *The woman buys sometimes potatoes (T: potatoes, D: igloo, helicopter, crocodile).*

Atypical target

Block 1

1. La mujer lava con cuidado la corbata (T: corbata, D: flor, estrella, enchufe).
1. *The woman washes carefully the tie (T: tie, D: flower, star, plug).*
2. La niña peina siempre al gato (T: gato, D: corazón, lápiz, sofá).
2. *The girl combs always the cat (T: cat, D: heart, pencil, sofa).*
3. El niño empuja de repente la maceta (T: maceta, D: casa, farola, carretera).
3. *The boy pushes suddenly the flower pot (T: flower pot, D: house, street lamp, road).*
4. La niña grita siempre a la tortuga (T: tortuga, D: árbol, tejado, sofá).
4. *The girl yells always at the turtle (T: turtle, D: tree, roof, sofa).*
5. El hombre mastica despacio la hierba (T: hierva, D: rueda, guitarra, banco).
5. *The man chews slowly grass (T: grass, D: wheel, guitar, bank).*

Block 2

6. El hombre pesca de repente la bota (T: bota, D: espejo, bombilla, luna).
6. *The man fishes out suddenly the boot (T: boot, D: mirror, lamp, moon).*
7. El niño pela cada día la piña (T: piña, D: teléfono, zapato, escoba).
7. *The boy peels each day the pineapple (T: pineapple, D: phone, shoe, broom).*
8. El hombre escribe a veces la partitura (T: partitura, D: cámara de fotos, nariz, ratón).
8. *The man writes sometimes the music score (T: music score, D: camera, nose, mouse).*
9. La mujer come despacio el jabalí (T: jabalí, D: maleta, ordenador, carpeta).
9. *The woman eats slowly the boar (T: boar, D: bag, computer, folder).*
10. La niña sopla a veces el saxo (T: el saxo, D: bolígrafo, fresas, pie).
10. *The girl blows sometimes the sax (T: sax, D: pen, strawberry, foot).*

Appendix C. Sentences used in the Experiment 2

Themes

La mujer compra cada día el pan en la panadería.
(TARGET: pan; COMPETIDOR: panadería; DISTRACTORS: playa, sol)
[The woman buys everyday bread in the bakery.
(TARGET: bread; COMPETITOR: bakery; DISTRACTORS: beach, sun)].
El hombre lee con atención un cuento en la cama.
(T: cuento; C: cama; D: armario, uvas)
[The man reads carefully a story on the bed.
(T: story book; C: bed, D: wardrobe, grapes)].
La niña come despacio la tarta con la cuchara.
(T: tarta, C: cuchara; D: sombrero, dinosaurio)
[The girl eat slowly the cake with the spoon.
(T: cake t, C: spoon; D: hat, dinosaur)].
El niño lanza deprisa la pelota en la canasta.
(T: pelota; C: canasta; D: palmera, nariz)
[The boy throws quickly the ball in the basket.
(T: ball; C: basket; D: palm, nose)].
El niño recorta con cuidado una hoja con las tijeras.
(T: hoja; C: tijeras; D: caramelo, martillo)
[The boy cuts carefully a sheet with the scissors.
(T: sheet; C: scissors; D: caramel, hammer)].
La niña pinta con cuidado el dibujo con los colores.
(T: dibujo; C: colores; D: cuchillo, sombrilla.
[The girl paints carefully the drawing with the colors.
(T: drawing; C: color; D: knife, umbrella)].

Sorces and goals (locations with verbs of motion)

El niño va deprisa a la escuela con la mochila.
(T: escuela; C: mochila; D: planeta, fuego)
[The boy goes quickly to school with the backpack.
(T: school; C: backpack; D: planet, fire].
La niña viene con alegría de la feria con un muñeco.
(T: feria; C: muñeco; D: sol, elefante)
[The girl comes with joy from the fair with a doll.
(T: fair, C: doll, D: Sun, elephant)].
El hombre cae de repente al pozo con el coche.
(T: pozo; C: coche; D: camiseta, imán)
[The man suddenly falls into the well with the car].
(T: well, C: car; D: shirt, magnet)
El hombre entra despacio en casa con la maleta.
(T: casa; C: maleta; D: luna, tractor)
[The man comes slowly home with the suitcase.
(T: house; C: suitcase; D: Moon, tractor)].
La mujer se sienta con cuidado en el sofá con el cojín.
(T: sofá C: cojín; D: cactus, león)
[The woman sits carefully on the sofa with a cushion.
(T: C sofa: cushion; D: cactus, lion)].
La mujer sale con tristeza del hospital con muletas.
(T: hospital; C: muletas; D: nevera, Tierra)
[The woman leaves with sadness the hospital with crutches.
(T: hospital; C: crutches; D: fridge, Earth].

Locatives

La niña camina cada día por el parque con los zapatos.
(T: parque; C: zapatos; D: tobogán, televisión)
[The girl walks every day through the park with shoes.
(T: park, C: shoes; D: slide, television].
La mujer pasea despacio por la montaña con el bastón.
(T: montaña, C: bastón; D: sol, lápiz)
[The woman walks slowly through the mountain with his cane.
(T: mountain, C: cane; D: Sun, pencil)].
El hombre vuela deprisa por el cielo con el avión.
(T: cielo, C: avión; D: casa, silla)
[The man flies fast across the sky with the plane.
(T: sky, C: plane; D: home, chair)].
La niña duerme siempre en la cama con el osito.
(T: cama; C: osito; D: árbol, bombilla)
[The girl always sleeps in the bed with the teddy bear.
(T: bed; C: teddy bear; D: tree, bulb)].

El niño canta con alegría en el escenario con la guitarra.
(T: escenario, C: guitarra; D: Luna, olla)
[The boy sings with joy on stage with the guitar.
(T: stage C: guitar, D: Moon, pot)].
El niño corre deprisa por el bosque con la radio.
(T: bosque, C: radio; D: avión, ordenador)
[The boy quickly runs through the forest with the radio.
(T: forest, C: radio; D: aircraft, computer)].

Instruments

El niño nada deprisa con el flotador en la piscina.
(T: flotador; C: piscina; D: botas, castillo)
[The boy quickly swims to float in the pool.
(T: float; C: pool; D: boots, castle)].
La niña resbala de repente con el plátano en la acera.
(T: plátano; C: acera; D: globo, parque)
[The girl suddenly slips with the banana on the sidewalk.
(T: banana; C: sidewalk; D: balloon, park)].
El hombre navega despacio con el barco por el lago.
(T: barco; C: lago; D: libro, camino)
[The man slowly navigates with the boat on the lake.
(T: boat; C: lake; D: book, road)].
La mujer patina con cuidado con el patinete por las escaleras.
(T: patinete; C: escaleras; reloj, jardín)
[The women carefully skating with the scooter down the stairs.
(T: scooter; C: stairs; D: clock, garden)].
El hombre bucea despacio con el tubo en el mar.
(T: tubo; C: mar; D: estrella, cama)
[The man slowly dives with the pipe into the sea.
(T: tube; C: sea; D: star, bed)].
La mujer esquía deprisa con el trineo por la montaña.
(T: trineo; C: montaña; D: vaso, playa)
[The Woman skies fast with the sled up the mountain.
(T: sled; C: mountain; D cup, beach)].

References

Andreu, L., Sanz-Torrent, M., Trueswell, J. 2012. Anticipatory sentence processing in children with SLI: Evidence from eye movements during listening. *Applied Psycholinguistics* 34, 5–44. https://doi.org/10.1017/S0142716411000592

Altmann, G. T. M., & Kamide, Y. 1999. Incremental interpretation at verbs: Restricting the domain of subsequent reference. *Cognition* 73, 247–264. https://doi.org/10.1016/S0010-0277(99)00059-1

Barr, D. 2008. Analyzing 'visual world' eyetracking data using multilevel logistic regression. *Journal of Memory and Language* 59, 457–474. https://doi.org/10.1016/j.jml.2007.09.002

Bedore L., & Leonard L. (1998) Specific language impairment and grammatical morphology: A discriminant function analysis. *Journal of Speech, Language, and Hearing Research*, 41, 965–1220.

Bedore, L. M., & Leonard, L. B. (2001). Grammatical Morphology Deficits in Spanish-Speaking Children With Specific Language Impairment. *Journal of Speech, Language, and Hearing Research*, 44(4), 905–924. https://doi.org/10.1044/1092-4388(2001/072)

Bishop, D. 1997. *Uncommon understanding*. London: Psychology Press.

Boland, J. E. 2005. Visual arguments. *Cognition* 95, 237–274. https://doi.org/10.1016/j.cognition.2004.01.008

Boland, J. E., and Boehm-Jernigan, H. (1998). Lexical constraints and prepositional phrase attachment. *Journal of Memory and Language*, 394, 684–719.

Bosque, I., and Demonte, V. (eds.) (1999). *Gramática descriptiva de la lengua española*. Madrid: Espasa-Calpe.

Carlson, G., & Tanenhaus, M. 1988. Thematic roles and language comprehension. In W. Wilkins (Ed.), *Thematic relations*. New York, NY: Academic Press.

Fischer, B. (1992). Saccadic reaction time: Implications for reading,dyslexia and visual cognition. In K. Rayner (Ed.),*Eye movementsand visual cognition: Scene perception and reading*(pp. 31–45).New York: Springer Verlag.

Frazier, L., and Clifton, C. (1996). *Construal*. Cambridge, MA: MIT Press.

Grinstead, J., De la Mora, J., Pratt, A. & Flores, B. 2009. Temporal interface delay and root nonfinite verbs in Spanish-speaking children with Speciic Language Impairment: Evidence from the grammaticality choice task. In *Hispanic Child Languages: Typical and Impaired Development* [Language Acquisition and Language Disorders 50], J. Grinstead (ed.), 239–264. Amsterdam: John Benjamins.

Kamide, Y., Altmann, G. T. M., & Haywood, S. 2003. Prediction and thematic information in incremental sentence processing: Evidence from anticipatory eye-movements. *Journal of Memory and Language* 49, 133–156. https://doi.org/10.1016/S0749-596X(03)00023-8

Leonard, L. 1998. *Specific Language Impairment*. Cambridge, MA: The MIT Press.

Leonard, L. B., & Deevy, P. 2006. Cognitive and linguistic issues in the study of children with specific language disorders. In M. Traxler & M. Gernsbacher (Eds.), *Handbook of psycholinguistics* (2nd ed.). Boston, MA: Elsevier. https://doi.org/10.1016/B978-012369374-7/50031-6

MacDonald, M. C., Pearlmutter, N. J., & Seidenberg, M. S. 1994. The lexical nature of syntactic ambiguity resolution. *Psychological Review* 101, 676–703. https://doi.org/10.1037/0033-295X.101.4.676

Marinis, T., & van der Lely, H. K. J. 2007. On-line processing of wh-questions in children with G-SLI and typically developing children. *International Journal of Language & Communication Disorders* 42(5), 557–582. https://doi.org/10.1080/13682820601058190

Martin, E., Shao, K. C., & Boff, K. R. (1993). Saccadic overhead: Infor-mation processing time with and without saccades. *Perception & Psychophysics*, 53, 372–380.

Mauner, G., & Koenig, J. P. 2000. Linguistic vs. conceptual sources of implicit agents in sentence comprehension. *Journal of Memory and Language* 43, 110–134. https://doi.org/10.1006/jmla.1999.2703

Montgomery J. 2000. Verbal working memory and sentence comprehension in children with specific language impairment. *Journal of Speech, Language, and Hearing Research* 43(2), 293–308. https://doi.org/10.1044/jslhr.4302.293

Montgomery, J. W. 2002. Examining the nature of lexical processing in children with specific language impairment: Temporal processing or processing capacity deficit? *Applied Psycholinguistics* 23, 447–470. https://doi.org/10.1017/S0142716402003077

Montgomery, J. W., Scudder, R. R., & Moore, C. 1990. Language-impaired children's real time comprehension of spoken language. *Applied Psycholinguistics* 11, 273–290. https://doi.org/10.1017/S0142716400008894

Saslow, M. G. (1967). Effects of components of displacement-step stimuli upon latency for saccadic eye movement. *Journal of the Optical Society of America*, 57, 1024–1029.

Stark, R. E., & Montgomery, J. W. 1995. Sentence processing in language impaired children under conditions of filtering and time compression. *Applied Psycholinguistics* 16, 137–154. https://doi.org/10.1017/S0142716400007050

Stevenson, S. (1998). Parsing as incremental restructuring. In *Reanalysis in Sentence Processing*, eds J. D. Fodor and F. Ferreira (Dordrecht: Kluwer Academic Publishers), 327–363.

Tanenhaus, M. K., Spivey-Knowlton, M. J. Eberhard, K. M., & Sedivy, J. C. 1995. Integration of visual and linguistic information in spoken language comprehension. *Science* 268, 1632–1634. https://doi.org/10.1126/science.7777863

Trueswell, J. C. 2008. Using eye movements as a developmental measure within psycholinguistics. In I. A. Sekerina, E. M. Fernández, & H. Clahsen (Eds.), *Language processing in children* (pp. 73–96). Amsterdam: John Benjamins.

Trueswell, J. C., & Tanenhaus, M. K. 1994. Toward a lexicalist framework for constraint-based syntactic ambiguity resolution. In Clifton, C., Frazier, L., & Rayner, K. (Eds.) *Perspectives in sentence processing* (pp. 155–179). Hillsdale, NJ: Lawrence Erlbaum Associates.

PART III

Deafness

Emotion recognition skills in children with hearing loss

What is the role of language?

Francesc Sidera,[1] Elisabet Serrat,[1] Anna Amadó[1] and Gary Morgan[2]
[1]Universitat de Girona / [2]City, University of London

Previous studies have found a deficit in emotion recognition skills in children with hearing loss linked to their linguistic development. Our aim is to explore how different linguistic-communicative skills influence the capacity to recognise emotions from faces, at different developmental points, in children with and without hearing loss. We administered language measures and a task of emotion recognition (ER) to 166 children (75 with hearing loss). Results show that ER was linked to various linguistic-communicative skills in children with hearing loss, whereas fewer connections existed in hearing children. As these relations varied with age, we discuss how the importance of the different linguistic and communicative skills for ER varies throughout development and as a function of hearing status.

Keywords: emotion recognition, vocabulary, linguistic-communicative skills, hearing loss, children

Introduction

Several studies have shown that language is important for the development of sociocognitive skills, and particularly, for emotion understanding (e.g. Astington & Jenkins 1999; Rieffe & Wiefferink, 2017). It follows that hearing-impaired (from now on, HI) children with linguistic difficulties might have social understanding delays (see, for example, Peterson, Wellman, & Slaughter, 2012). Such social understanding delays might be explained by difficulties in formal aspects of language (Dyck, Farrugia, Shochet, & Holmes-Brown, 2004) like vocabulary or grammar development, but also by deficits in early communication abilities that

https://doi.org/10.1075/z.223.10sid

emerge out of social interactions and conversations (Meristo, Strid, & Hjelmquist, 2016; Morgan et al., 2014). In this regard, the objectives of this study are: a) to understand better how different aspects of language are related to the capacity to recognise emotions at different developmental points; and b) to study whether this relationship evolves similarly in children with or without linguistic difficulties.

Deficits in emotion recognition in children with hearing loss

Controversy exists in relation to whether HI children have a deficit in their capacity to recognise emotions. On the one hand, various studies have found difficulties in recognising facial emotions (for example Dyck et al., 2004; Gray, Hosie, Russell, Banks, & Ormel, 2001; Wang et al., 2011), even in non-verbal tasks (Wang, Su & Yan, 2016; Wiefferink et al., 2013). The age of the child at assessment and type of emotion evaluated are very relevant for determining these difficulties. In the study by Sidera et al., (2017) the specific emotions that HI children had difficulty with in comparison to hearing children varied with age. In that study, the young HI group (3- and 4-year-olds) were significantly delayed in the recognition of fear, the medium aged HI group (5- and 6-year-olds) had difficulty in the recognition of disgust and surprise, and the oldest HI group (7- and 8-year-olds) found recognition of surprise and fear complicated. However, the HI group followed the same developmental order in the recognition of emotions as the hearing comparison group (see also Ziv, Most, & Cohen, 2013). Wang et al., (2016) report evidence that young HI children (aged 4 years) who have had relatively little experience with aided hearing (because of their age) even struggle to label basic emotions (e.g. happy, sad, fear). According to the developmental model of Widen, and Russel (2013) these basic emotions are the first labels to be acquired in typically developing children. In summary, HI children have been shown to have delays in labeling, emotions.

On the other hand, there are studies that have not found evidence of this delay. This can be attributed to various factors: a) these studies did not include late-acquired labels for emotion faces, such as disgust or surprise (see: Laugen, Jacobsen, Rieffe, & Wichstrøm, 2017; Mancini et al., 2016); b) these studies involved older study participants (see: Hopyan-Misakyan, Gordon, Dennis, & Papsin, 2009; Most and Aviner, 2009), who might have caught-up with their peers; or c) these studies compared a group of HI children with a group of hearing children of a younger age (see: Hosie et al., 1998 in their young group; Ziv et al., 2013).

Another important aspect to be considered is the child's level of hearing loss. Some authors have found emotion recognition (ER) difficulties in children with profound hearing loss but not with severe to moderate hearing losses (see for example, Most & Michaelis, 2012). Methodological aspects also matter, e.g. Jones,

Gutierrez, and Ludlow (2017) found that HI children (including users of sign language) labelled facial emotional expressions better when they were dynamic (from a video) rather than in static pictures (without movement).

Language and emotion recognition in children with hearing loss

In wider research, it is thought that the development of language and emotion concepts is interdependent, and language is a powerful tool for developing an understanding of emotion (Mancini et al., 2016). It is possible that different aspects of emotion understanding may be more or less dependent on language (see Dyck et al., 2004). Thus, research on how the linguistic delays of HI children affect their understanding of emotions may help us understand the role that language has in constructing emotional concepts more generally.

However, some researchers have failed to find a relationship between language and ER, even in verbal tasks (Jones et al., 2017), but this study only used one linguistic measure, and did not compare whether HI children were actually linguistically delayed. Other studies have found such a relationship (for example, Dyck et al., 2004). Sidera et al., (2017) found language-related difficulties (in vocabulary and linguistic-communicative skills) in HI children when they were labelling facial emotions depicted in drawings. If language is a likely reason for ER delays in HI children, there may be other important contributors. Sidera et al., (2017) found that even after matching vocabulary, non-verbal reasoning and chronological age, the HI group was still delayed in ER compared to the hearing group. More research is needed to better understand how HI children develop language and ER.

The ability to label and understand emotions at an age appropriate level is important for wider mental health and social development. For example, several studies have linked delays in emotion understanding to risks in the development of cognitive regulation (Carlson & Wang, 2007; Botting et al., 2016).

In the present study, we extend Sidera et al., (2017) by considering how the relationship between linguistic and ER skills changes across different developmental points in HI and hearing children. This will allow us to better understand which aspects of language are most connected to HI and ER at different ages. As language and ER skills develop with age, we expect that diverse linguistic components will be linked to ER at different ages. The existent literature does not allow us to make predictions about how these relationships evolve, so in this sense this study is exploratory.

Methodology

Participants

For this study, we used the same sample as in Sidera et al.'s (2017) study, which we briefly detail next (see this study for more details). It consisted of 166 children (91 hearing and 75 with hearing loss) aged between 39 and 107 months (Mean = 71.96 months; *SD* = 18.39). The groups with and without hearing loss were very similar in terms of age (children with hearing loss: Mean = 71.01 months; *SD* = 17.87; hearing children: Mean = 72.84 months, *SD* = 18.86; Mann Whitney's $U = 3226.5$, $p = .546$) and cognitive ability (children with hearing loss: Mean = 131.31; *SD* = 44.54; hearing children: Mean = 135.31, *SD* = 40.67; Mann Whitney's $U = 3088.5$, $p = .293$). The percentage of boys and girls was also similar in both groups (45.3% of girls in the HI group, and 50.5% in the hearing group), and the Chi-Square test showed that there were no significant group differences ($\chi^2 = .448$; $p = .503$). Children with reported learning difficulties or other pathologies apart from HI were not included in the sample.

Regarding the characteristics of the HI group, all children had prelocutive (onset before the age of 12 months) bilateral hearing loss and attended mainstream oral schools, which is the most common educational option in Catalonia, the region where data were collected. The mean age of detection of the hearing loss was 19.24 months (*SD* = 19.43; range = 0 to 75), and the mean age of hearing devices fitting was 26.91 months (*SD* = 18.39; range = 4 to 81). From the 75 HI children, 36 had a cochlear implant (with or without additional hearing aids) while 38 had only hearing amplification devices (including here a child with a bone-attached hearing implant); one had never had sensory aids. Speech therapists and teachers reported that none of the children used sign language. As far as the level of hearing loss (in the better ear) is concerned, one child had mild hearing loss (from 21 to 40 dB of loss), 25 moderate (from 41 to 70 dB), 12 severe (from 71 to 90 dB) and 37 profound (from 91 dB). Level of hearing was reported by the speech therapist of each child through a questionnaire (see materials section).

It is noteworthy that when we compared the sample with and without hearing loss in the linguistic tasks (in expressive vocabulary and linguistic-communicative-skills) we found that the mean scores of HI children in both tasks were located between the percentile 17 and 18 of the scores from our sample of hearing children.

Materials

Children were evaluated on the following tasks:

1. *Naming vocabulary* subtest of the British Ability Scales–2 (BAS–2). In this expressive vocabulary task children have to label pictures (Elliot et al., 1996; Spanish adaptation by Arribas & Corral, 2011). Depending on the age of the child, children are shown a different set of pictures. We used the aptitude score of the test which transforms the raw score by considering the particular level of difficulty administered to each child.
2. Cognitive ability.
   The pattern construction subtest of the BAS-2 (Elliot et al., 1996; Spanish adaptation Arribas & Corral, 2011) was used to control for the non-verbal reasoning skills of the child. The test is a good proxy of general cognitive ability. In this task, children have to reproduce visual patterns by using squares and/or cubes. Again, as different children may be administered different items according to their age and performance, the aptitude score was used.
3. Facial emotion recognition task.
   We administered a facial ER task that required children to identify emotion labels and match them to facial emotional expressions, which may be more dependent on language skills than emotion-matching or emotion discrimination tasks (see: Wang et al., 2016; Rieffe & Wiefferink, 2017). It consisted of six coloured cartoons of a girl depicting happiness, sadness, fear, anger, surprise and disgust (published in Sidera et al., 2017). All drawings were placed in front of the child (in two lines of three drawings, in random order) and they were asked: *"Could you point to the girl looking…* and then: *happy, sad, scared, angry, surprised or disgusted"* (in Catalan language, which corresponds to the labels of "contenta", "trista", "espantada", "enfadada", "sorpresa" and "fàstic"). After children gave an answer, the experimenter only said "Ok" before moving to the next emotion. The order of presentation of the questions was counterbalanced using a Latin-square design. The researcher took notes of children's responses, and awarded 1 point for each correct answer. Their scores in this task varied from 0 to 6 (ER score), corresponding to the number of drawings they correctly pointed to.
4. Questionnaire with sociodemographic and audiological data.
   This questionnaire included the following sociodemographic information: date of birth, number of siblings, mother tongue of the mother and father, language used by the mother and father with the child, educational level of the parents, communicative systems (oral language, written language, sign languages, cued speech, lip-reading, or others) used at home and school, preferred communicative system of the child and age of the first word. For the children with hearing loss, the questionnaire also included a part on audiological information, where we asked about the cause of the hearing loss, the level of hearing loss in each ear, the use of hearing devices, the existence

of relatives with hearing loss and the knowledge of different communication systems. Speech therapists for the HI and teachers for the typically hearing children filled out this information. Take note that not all the information are provided in this paper because it is not needed to our aim.

5. Linguistic Proficiency Profile – 2 (LPP–2).
   The same professionals responded to the LPP–2, a tool designed to assess the linguistic-communicative skills of HI children but which is also suitable for hearing children (Bebko & McKinnon, 1993).

LPP–2 is a measure of general language development (see Bebko, Calderon & Treder, 2003). The original author gave permission to translate the scale from the Spanish version into the Catalan language. The tool assesses five areas of expressive language and communication skills: Form, Content, Reference, Cohesion, and Use (each subscale has 9, 12, 11, 11 and 13 items, respectively). A person who is familiar with the child's speech has to evaluate their level of mastery for each item, which can be described as: a) not acquired (0 points); b) emerging (1 point); c) or acquired/past (2 points). In the original scale the total score of the scale is 112. However, since 87 from the 166 participants had, at least, one item not answered (the LPP–2 contemplates that respondents may be insecure about the level of the child), we decided to score the scale with percentages (from these 87 children, the mean number of unanswered items was 2.12, apart from a child whose LPP–2 could not be obtained). Hence, we calculated the percentage of the Total LPP–2 score, as the number of points obtained by the child divided by the maximum number of points they could obtain without considering the unanswered items. So, for example, if a child had one blank item, his percentage of points would be calculated by dividing his total score per 110, instead of per 112 (as each item has a maximum score of 2). The same procedure was followed in each of the 5 LPP–2 subscales. This also permitted us to compare the percentage of points from one subscale to another, as not all subscales have the same number of items.

Procedure

Parental informed consent was obtained for each child before conducting the study, and permission by the school centers and Catalan Department of Education were also obtained. Children were individually interviewed at their own schools, in a quiet room. Tasks were administered by a researcher in one session lasting from 35 to 55 minutes. Children with hearing loss were administered the tasks with the presence of their speech therapist.

For purposes of data analysis the sample was split into three age groups (young group: 3- and 4-year-olds, medium group: 5- and 6- year olds and old group: 7- and

8-year-olds) based on the following rationale. The first age group is still developing their core language and ER. From the medium age group onwards, based on previous data (Widen & Rusell, 2013), we would typically expect to observe the onset of ER and emotion language development. We expect this phenomenon to continue in the old group. At 8 years of age, we would expect hearing children to have a firm understanding of emotion labels and social-cognitive reasons for expressing different (including false) emotions.

The young group had 20 HI children and 23 hearing children; the medium group 33 HI children and 37 hearing children, and the old group 22 HI children and 31 hearing children. As described in Table 1, Mann–Whitney's U test revealed that in all groups there were no differences between the children with and without hearing loss in cognitive ability scores or age.

Table 1. Mean age in months (and SD), and mean cognitive ability score (and SD) as a function of age group and hearing status

	Cognitive ability			Age		
	HI children	Hearing children	Comparison	HI children	Hearing children	Comparison
Young group $N = 43$	85.00 (28.71)	82.57 (30.47)	$U = 207.5$ $p = .582$	48.8 (5.45)	47.96 (5.49)	$U = 211.5$ $p = .651$
Medium group $N = 70$	138.42 (33.81)	144.30 (25.57)	$U = 548.5$ $p = .464$	70.15 (8.13)	70.73 (7.56)	$U = 579$ $p = .710$
Old Group $N = 53$	162.73 (36.69)	163.71 (20.76)	$U = 301$ $p = .469$	92.5 (6.60)	93.52 (7.4)	$U = 320$ $p = .704$

Data were analysed using IBM SPSS version 23.

Results

Descriptive statistics

First of all, we compared ER score between the groups with and without hearing loss (see Figure 1). Mann–Whitney's U test showed that while there were no significant differences between HI and hearing children in the young group ($U = 192.5$, $p = .351$), differences in ER appeared in both the medium group ($U = 368.5, p = .003$) and the old group ($U = 193, p = .002$). Following Field (2009), we calculated the effect size of these comparisons (and of all Mann–Whitney comparisons in the study) with the formula $r = Z/\sqrt{N}$. Effect sizes in the medium group were $r = 0.36$, and $r = 0.42$ in the old group. According to Cohen (1988,

1992), when $r = 0.1$, the effect size is small, when $r = 0.3$ the effect is medium, and when $r = 0.5$, the effect is large (see Field, 2009). Therefore, the abovementioned effects were medium.

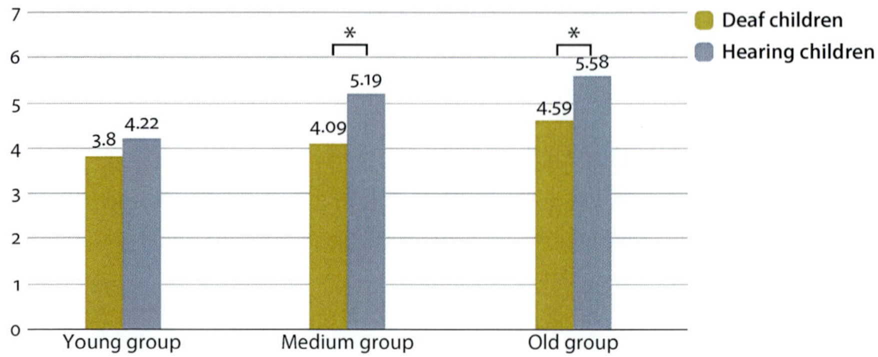

Figure 1. ER score (means) as a function of hearing status and age group

Note: Asterisks represent significant differences ($p < .005$).

In relation to the linguistic variables, Mann–Whitney's U test was used to compare the scores in vocabulary and LPP–2 (Total and subscales) between HI and hearing children in the three age groups (see Table 2). Results showed that: a) in the young group, HI children only showed lower scores than hearing children in the LPP–2 Form (medium effect size); b) in the medium group, HI children showed lower scores than hearing children in all the LPP–2 subscales, in the Total LPP–2 score, and in the vocabulary score (medium and large effect sizes); c) in the old group, HI children obtained lower scores in the LPP–2 subscales of Content, Reference and Cohesion (medium and large effect sizes), but not in the subscales of Form and Use. Significant differences were also found in this age group in the vocabulary score and in the total LPP–2 score.

Regarding audiological variables, HI children with cochlear implants obtained higher scores on ER ($N = 36$; $M = 4.25$; $SD = 1.48$) than children without cochlear implant ($N = 39$; $M = 4.08$; $SD = 1.46$), but these differences were not statistically significant ($U = 655$, $p = .606$). Regarding the level of hearing loss, we compared the score on ER between children with profound hearing loss ($N = 37$; $M = 4.16$; $SD = 1.59$) and children with lower levels of hearing loss (mild, moderate and severe grouped together: $N = 38$; $M = 4.16$; $SD = 1.35$). Mann–Whitney's U test showed no significant differences between the two groups. The combined effect of the variables *cochlear implant* and *level of hearing loss* could not be analyzed, as only 4 children with profound hearing loss did not have cochlear implant (while 33 had a CI), and only 3 children with lower levels of hearing loss had a cochlear implant (while 35 did not).

Table 2. Means (and SD) of linguistic skills as a function of hearing status and age group

		Vocabulary	Form	Content	Reference	Cohesion	Use	LPP-2 Total	Summary
Young	HI	99.45	72.08	67.34	65.79	45.21	61.23	63.44	Form: HI < H
Group	*N* = 20	(20.67)	(21.97)	(20.59)	(20.13)	(23.56)	(22.45)	(20.28)	
	Hearing	103.22	86.83	72.61	70.30	52.58	60.24	67.51	
	N = 23	(16.12)	(11.88)	(25.11)	(17.58)	(29.20)	(19.81)	(19.60)	
	U	193	132*	180	206	202.5	226	203.5	
			r = .37						
Medium	HI	101.18	77.95	77.44	70.34	57.89	71.21	71.37	In all variables:
group	*N* = 32	(18.38)	(20.67)	(18.37)	(20.91)	(24.03)	(23.13)	(20.44)	HI < H
	Hearing	122.19	96.79	95.00	93.28	83.30	86.23	89.72	
	N = 37	(11.50)	(7.72)	(93.28)	(9.33)	(16.17)	(10.47)	(11.26)	
	U	207.5***	257.5***	151***	188.5***	238***	363.5**	227***	
		r = .56	*r* = .53	*r* = .66	*r* = .59	*r* = .52	*r* = .33	*r* = .46	
Old group	HI	112.36	82.59	86.74	79.73	67.57	83.21	79.65	Vocab. Content
	N = 22	(16.76)	(18.29)	(12.24)	(14.38)	(26.59)	(16.88)	(15.86)	Ref. Coh. Total
	Hearing	129.48	90.28	94.86	93.28	87.82	84.07	89.77	LPP-2 HI < H
	N = 31	(10.68)	(12.47)	(6.70)	(9.72)	(19.47)	(15.68)	(10.42)	
	U	133.5***	258	204.5*	141***	167.5**	327.5	202.5*	
		r = .52		*r* = .35	*r* = .50	*r* = .44		*r* = .34	

Note: "U" refers to Mann–Whitney's U scores. Asterisks represent: ****p*. <. 001; ***p* < .01; **p* < .05 *. HI stands for hearing-impaired children and H for hearing. Effect sizes of significant comparisons were calculated using "*r*".

Correlations between emotion recognition and language

As it can be observed in Table 3, significant correlations (aged controlled) were found between ER and linguistic variables only in the HI group. Specifically, vocabulary and the LPP-2 subscales of Form, Reference and Use correlated with the ER score.

Table 3. Spearman partial correlations (age controlled) between emotion recognition, linguistic variables and cognitive ability

	Vocab.	Form	Cont.	Ref.	Coh.	Use	LPP-2 Total	Cog. ability
ER HI children *N* = 72	.356**	.254*	.227	.254*	.206	.296*	.254*	.203
ER hearing children *N* = 88	.053	.089	.133	.036	.057	.124	.105	.145

Note: Numbers correspond to "r" values. Asterisks represent: ***p <. 001; **p < .01; * p < .05.

Spearman partial correlations (aged controlled) between linguistic variables and ER were also carried out in each of the three age groups and separating the HI and hearing groups (see Table 4). In the group of HI children, significant correlations between linguistic variables and ER were found only in the medium age group. As far as the hearing group is concerned, we found two significant correlations with ER: a negative one with vocabulary in the young group, and a positive one with the Use subscale in the old group.

Table 4. Spearman partial correlations (age controlled) between emotion recognition, linguistic variables and cognitive ability as a function of age group

		Vocab	Form	Content	Ref.	Coh.	Use	LPP-2 Total	Cognitive ability
Young Group	HI *N* = 17	.321	−.069	.057	.009	.047	.247	−.005	.043
	Hearing *N* = 20	−.521*	.175	.214	−.002	.093	.144	.181	.060
Medium group	HI *N* = 30	.481**	.447*	.363*	.393*	.314	.391*	.398*	.160
	Hearing *N* = 34	.073	.166	−.047	−.093	.119	−.112	−.027	.034
Old group	HI *N* = 19	.258	.075	−.074	.135	.121	.209	.168	.429
	Hearing *N* = 28	.119	.004	.174	−.170	.060	.414*	.264	.065

Note: Numbers correspond to "r" values. Asterisks represent: ***p <. 001; **p < .01; * p < .05.

Predictors of emotion recognition

A linear regression analysis was conducted in order to find the predictors of ER using the forward method (see Table 5). Results showed that in hearing children the best predictor of ER was cognitive ability, while in HI children the best predictor of ER was vocabulary.

Table 5. Linear regression (forward method) with emotion recognition as a dependent variable, and linguistic variables (vocabulary, form, content, reference, cohesion, use and LPP-2 Total), cognitive ability, and age (in months) as predictors

Coefficients							**Summary of the model**	
	Predictors	***B***	**Stand. error**	**Standarised coefficients-Beta**	***t***	**Sig.**	**R squared**	**Adjusted R Squared**
HI children *N* = 74	Constant	.639	.925		.691	.492	.170	.158
	Vocabulary	.034	.009	.412	3.833	.000		
Hearing children *N* = 90	Constant	2.983	.419		7.119	.000	.238	.230
	Cognitive ability	0.16	.003	.488	5.247	.000		

Discussion

There is great theoretical interest in the interaction between language and cognition (e.g. Gooch, Thompson, Nash, Snowling, & Hulme 2016). While many aspects of language and cognition develop in parallel, it is not clear what the mutual influence is of one on the other. One way of looking at this is to explore contexts where one of these two factors is delayed significantly and to explore the effects of these delays on the other system. In previous work, language variables were found to predict ER score in HI but not hearing children (Sidera et al. 2017). The current study extends previous work by delineating how the diverse linguistic variables are related to ER at different developmental points. Our findings (see Table 3) support the view that different linguistic and communicative skills (especially the Form, Reference and Use of language, as well as vocabulary) are important for the development of ER (see Dyck et al. 2004). Correlations between language and ER were not found in hearing children when the whole group was considered, and when we divided it into 3 age groups, fewer correlations were found than in HI children. Nevertheless, this does not imply that language is less important for learning to recognise emotions in hearing children than in HI children. It could also be the case that the recognition of basic emotions is easily attained for children with a certain level of linguistic and communicative abilities. In the case of HI children, if these tools are not properly developed, the recognition of basic emotions might be affected too (Wang et al., 2016).

A criticism of our study could be that children's capacity to recognise emotions was measured using linguistic labels, thus it is possible that a non-verbal assessment of ER capacities might have led to different results. However, studies like Wang et al., (2016) or Wiefferink et al., (2013) have found differences between HI and hearing children even in non-verbal ER tasks, which also support the idea that a deficit in HI children in recognizing emotions is not just a linguistic problem related to labeling emotions in specific tasks, but a conceptual one. In this regard, Jones et al., (2017) reported that HI children are better with dynamic than with static faces. This suggests that increasing the saliency of the stimuli would lower their difficulties in ER. However, Jones et al. (2017) did not confirm that the HI children in their study had a linguistic delay. Furthermore if the moving face helped it was not for all emotions as HI children struggled with the dynamic expression of disgust. Many of the participants in Jones et al. (2017) were sign users, and it is not clear if results can be extended to non-signers. In any case, as these authors argue, children can learn about emotions in both formats (static and dynamic), so difficulties with ER in any format might be relevant. Future research should investigate differences in even more ecological situations, like videos of people expressing real emotions in specific contexts, rather than emotions from actors.

Our results that considered the different age groups separately showed that for the group of HI children different linguistic and communicative skills were important for ER, but only in the group of 5- and 6-year-olds. On the other hand, it is possible that correlations between language and ER were not observed in the young HI group because linguistic differences with the hearing group were minimal. In relation to the oldest group, despite linguistic differences between HI and hearing children, no correlations between language and ER were observed in this group. One possible interpretation is that most HI children at this age have already acquired the necessary linguistic tools for ER, so individual differences do not depend so much on language but on their emotion-related social experiences. In the case of hearing children, we found a negative correlation between vocabulary and ER in the young group and a correlation between Use of language and ER in the old group. Therefore, in the group of hearing children, the linguistic-communicative skill from the LPP-2 most linked to ER was language Use. In this sense, the pragmatic aspect of language could be an important linguistic aspect used to learn to recognize emotions.

There are a couple of reasons why language use and ER are linked, which we propose here. The first is related to the developmental experience of hearing impairment which is generally very different to that of hearing children. In the first two years of life, typically developing children cultivate an understanding of other's intentions to communicate via joint attention and triadic interactions (Ninio & Bruner, 1978; Tomasello & Todd, 1983). The outcome of this early period of social-communicative routines is not only vocabulary development, but also emotion regulation. Consequently, a disruption to this early period of establishing meaningful interactions will have an impact on both language and emotion recognition (Carlson & Wang, 2007; Botting et al., 2016). The second possibility (and not mutually exclusive) is that during the ER task itself children are mediating performance by self-directed speech. Previous work in hearing children with language delays has demonstrated that self-directed speech was less optimal and was a factor involved in reduced performance on similar tasks (Lidstone, Meins, & Fernyhough, 2012).

More research concerning early experience of emotion talk in HI children is needed to explore these issues further. This could also help us to interpret the negative correlation found between vocabulary and ER in the youngest hearing group, while in the whole sample of HI children, vocabulary was found to be the best predictor of ER. In this respect, results might have been different if our vocabulary task had included vocabulary on emotions or mental states, as they have been found to correlate with ER tasks that involve labeling (Rieffe & Wiefferink, 2017). According to Widen (2013), children's development of concepts referring to facial expressions of emotion (e.g. surprised, happy) does not only depend on vocabulary by connecting a label to a face but also on establishing relationships between different components of emotion understanding (e.g. understanding the causes and consequences of emotions). Finally, the small sample in the young HI group may also be a reason for such a correlation. Indeed, when a regression was carried out with the whole sample of hearing children, the best predictor of ER was not a linguistic variable, but cognitive ability.

As already mentioned, one limitation of our study is that, despite having a fairly large sample of HI children, this might not have been large enough to study the effects of different age groups. This was especially relevant when trying to study the effects of cochlear implant (CI) on ER skills. We did not find differences between CI and non CI children, but this result might have been obscured by the fact that the majority of children with CI had a profound hearing loss, while the majority of children without CI had better hearing. Another limitation of the present study may have been that the young HI children had a minimal linguistic delay. Future research could focus attention on this young group of children in order to detect which are the linguistic variables most intertwined with ER. Another interesting line of research refers to the origins of the difficulties in ER and emotion understanding in early communicative experiences. What are the conditions that promote this important social-cognitive development in the early parent–child interactions that happen daily in the first 12 months and how does hearing loss disrupt these early interactions leading to both language and social-cognitive delays?

In sum, we have observed that both formal language and different linguistic-communicative skills (especially the use of language) play an important role in the development of ER. Due to the central role of this crucial aspect of social cognition in daily life, it is important that any delays are detected as soon as possible and remediation offered in order to improve the inclusion of HI children in wider society.

Acknowledgements

We thank the resource centres for children with hearing loss (CREDA) in Catalonia for their help, as well as speech therapists, teachers, schools and children who participated in the study.

This work was supported by the Spanish Ministerio de Economía y Competitividad and the Fondo Europeo de Desarrollo Regional (PSI2015-69419-R; MINECO-FEDER). Morgan's work was supported by the Economic and Social Research Council of Great Britain [grant number RES-620-28-0002], Deafness, Cognition and Language Research Centre (DCAL).

References

Arribas, D., & Corral, S. 2011. *BAS2, Escalas de aptitudes intelectuales. Madrid: TEA Ediciones.*

Astington, J., & Jenkins, J. 1999. A longitudinal study of the relation between language and Theory of Mind development. *Developmental Psychology* 35, 1311–1320. https://doi.org/10.1037/0012-1649.35.5.1311

Bebko, J. M., Calderon, R., & Treder, R. 2003. The language proficiency profile-2: Assessment of the global communication skills of deaf children across languages and modalities of expression. *Journal of Deaf Studies and Deaf Education* 8, 438–451. https://doi.org/10.1093/deafed/eng034

Bebko, J. M., & McKinnon, E. E. 1993. *The Language Proficiency Profile-2* (Unpublished assessment tool). York University, Toronto, Canada.

Botting, N., Jones, A., Marshall, C., Denmark, T., Atkinson, J., & Morgan, G. 2016. Non-verbal executive function is mediated by language: A study of deaf and hearing children. *Child Development* 88(5), 1689–1700. https://doi.org/10.1111/cdev.12659

Carlson, S. M., & Wang, T. S. 2007. Inhibitory control and emotion regulation in preschool children. *Cognitive Development* 22, 489–510. https://doi.org/10.1016/j.cogdev.2007.08.002

Cohen, J. (1988). Statistical power analysis for the behavioural sciences (2nd ed.). New York: Academic Press

Cohen, J. (1992). A power primer. *Psychological Bulletin*, 112(1), 155–159.

Dyck, M. J., Farrugia, C., Shochet, I. M. & Holmes-Brown, M. 2004. Emotion recognition/understanding ability in hearing or vision-impaired children: Do sounds, sights, or words make the difference? *Journal of Child Psychology and Psychiatry* 45, 789–800. https://doi.org/10.1111/j.1469-7610.2004.00272.x

Elliot, C. D., Smith, P., & McCulloch, K. (1996) British ability scales (2nd ed.). Slough, UK: National Foundation of Educational Research.

Field, A. P. 2009. *Discovering statistics using SPSS: And sex and drugs and rock 'n' roll* (3rd ed.). London: Sage.

Gooch, D., Thompson, P., Nash, H. M., Snowling, M. J., & Hulme, C. 2016. The development of executive function and language skills in the early school years. *Journal of Child Psychology and Psychiatry* 57, 180–187. https://doi.org/10.1111/jcpp.12458

Gray, C., Hosie, J., Russell, P., Banks, J., & Ormel, E. 2001. Emotional development in deaf children: Understanding facial expressions, display rules, and theory of mind. In M. Marschark, D. Clark, & M. Karchmer (Eds.), *Context, cognition, and deafness*. Washington, DC: Gallaudet University Press.

Hopyan-Misakyan, T. M., Gordon, K. A., Dennis, M., & Papsin, B. 2009. Recognition of affective speech prosody and facial affect in deaf children with unilateral right cochlear implants. *Child Neuropsychology* 15, 136–146. https://doi.org/10.1080/09297040802403682

Hosie, J., Gray, C., Russell, P., Scott, C., & Hunter, N. 1998. The matching of facial expressions by deaf and hearing children and their production and comprehension of emotion labels. *Motivation and Emotion* 22, 293–313. https://doi.org/10.1023/A:1021352323157

Jones, A. C., Gutierrez, R., & Ludlow, A. K. 2017. The role of motion and intensity in deaf children's recognition of real human facial expressions of emotion. *Cognition and Emotion*, 1–14. https://doi.org/10.1080/02699931.2017.1289894

Laugen, N. J., Jacobsen, K. H., Rieffe, C., & Wichstrøm, L. 2017. Emotion understanding in preschool children with mild-to-severe hearing loss. *The Journal of Deaf Studies and Deaf Education* 22(2), 155–163. https://doi.org/10.1093/deafed/enw069

Lidstone, J. S. M., Meins, E., & Fernyhough, C. 2012. Verbal mediation of cognition in children with specific language impairment *Development and Psychopathology* 24, 651–660. https://doi.org/10.1017/S0954579412000223

Mancini, P., Giallini, I., Prosperini, L., D'alessandro, H. D., Guerzoni, L., Murri, A., … Nicastri, M. 2016. Level of emotion comprehension in children with mid to long-term cochlear implant use: How basic and more complex emotion recognition relates to language and age at implantation. *International Journal of Pediatric Otorhinolaryngology* 87, 219–232. https://doi.org/10.1016/j.ijporl.2016.06.033

Meristo, M., Strid, K., & Hjelmquist, E. 2016. Early conversational environment enables spontaneous belief attribution in deaf children. *Cognition* 157, 139–145. https://doi.org/10.1016/j.cognition.2016.08.023

Morgan, G., Meristo, M., Mann, W., Hjelmquist, E., Surian, L., & Siegal, M. 2014. Mental state language and quality of conversational experience in deaf and hearing children. *Cognitive Development* 29, 41–49. https://doi.org/10.1016/j.cogdev.2013.10.002

Most, T., & Aviner, C. 2009. Auditory, visual, and auditory–visual perception of emotions by individuals with cochlear implants, hearing aids, and normal hearing. *Journal of Deaf Studies and Deaf Education* 14, 449–464. https://doi.org/10.1093/deafed/enp007

Most, T., & Michaelis, H. 2012. Auditory, visual, and auditory-visual perception of emotions by young children with hearing loss versus children with normal hearing. *Journal of Speech, Language, and Hearing Research* 55, 1148–1162. https://doi.org/10.1044/1092-4388(2011/11-0060)

Ninio, A., & Bruner, J. 1978. The achievement and antecedents of labeling. *Journal of Child Language* 5(1), 1–15. https://doi.org/10.1017/S0305000900001896

Peterson, C. C., Wellman, H. M., & Slaughter, V. 2012. The mind behind the message: Advancing theory of mind scales for typically developing children, and those with deafness, autism, or Asperger syndrome. *Child Development* 83(2), 469–485.

Rieffe, C., & Wiefferink, C. H. 2017. Happy faces, sad faces: Emotion understanding in toddlers and preschoolers with language impairments. *Research in Developmental Disabilities* 62, 40–49.

Sidera, F., Amadó, A. & Martínez, L. 2017. Influences on facial emotion recognition in deaf children. *The Journal of Deaf Studies and Deaf Education* 22(2), 164–177. https://doi.org/10.1093/deafed/enw072

Tomasello, M., & Todd, J. 1983. Joint attention and lexical acquisition style. *First Language* 4, 197–212. https://doi.org/10.1177/014272378300401202

Wang, Y., Su, Y., Fang, P., & Zhou, Q. 2011. Facial expression recognition: Can preschoolers with cochlear implants and hearing aids catch it? *Research in Developmental Disabilities* 32, 2583–2588. https://doi.org/10.1016/j.ridd.2011.06.019

Wang, Y., Su, Y., & Yan, S. 2016. Facial expression recognition in children with cochlear implants and hearing aids. *Frontiers in Psychology* 7, 1989. https://doi.org/10.3389/fpsyg.2016.01989

Widen, S. C. 2013. Children's interpretation of facial expressions: The long path from valence-based to specific discrete categories. *Emotion Review* 5(1), 72–77. https://doi.org/10.1177/1754073912451492

Widen, S. C., & Russell, J. A. 2013. Children's recognition of disgust in others. *Psychological Bulletin* 139, 271–299. https://doi.org/10.1037/a0031640

Wiefferink, C. H., Rieffe, C., Ketelaar, L., De Raeve, L., & Frijns, J. H. 2013. Emotion understanding in deaf children with a cochlear implant. *Journal of Deaf Studies and Deaf Education* 18, 175–186. https://doi.org/10.1093/deafed/ens042

Ziv, M., Most, T., & Cohen, S. 2013. Understanding of emotions and false beliefs among hearing children versus deaf children. *Journal of Deaf Studies and Deaf Education* 18, 161–174. https://doi.org/10.1093/deafed/ens073

Executive functions and eye fixations in children with Cochlear Implant

María Fernanda Lara Díaz, Carolina Rivera and Silvia Raquel Rodriguez
Universidad Nacional de Colombia

This study is meant to describe the executive functions (EFs) and eye fixation in a group of 13 children with Cochlear Implants (CI) and their controls with the purpose to establish the relationship between the mentioned skills and language. Children with CI showed a significantly lower performance and need more time in tasks of inhibition, mental flexibility, and working memory. Children with CI have different visual fixation patterns in which they tend to stare longer in peripheral areas, which might explain a less effective executive functioning. These findings coincide with the general domain of hearing theory, which states that hearing loss can affect other cognitive domains that are not related with auditory input and has implications for different sensorial systems.

Keywords: Cochlear Implant, ocular fixation, executive functions, language, deafness

Introduction

Deafness has been considered the fifth cause of disability (Kral et al., 2016). According to the World Health Organization, five percent of the world's population presents some degree of hearing loss, and 0.4% of them are children (Surowiecki et al., 2002). After its development, the Cochlear Implant (CI) has become an alternative for the treatment of sensorineural profound hearing loss. Despite the significant evolution of technology, surgical techniques, and intervention approaches, there is a strong heterogeneity in rehabilitation results in terms of speech perception, word recognition, and linguistic abilities (Beer et al., 2011). These variables account for the cause of deafness, age of onset, age of implantation, anatomic conditions, family, and rehabilitation procedures. In the same way, other variables related to cognitive functions have been observed such as attention,

https://doi.org/10.1075/z.223.11dia

memory, and EFs that may influence the acquisition and development of language after the implantation. These cognitive functions directly account for the heterogeneity mentioned above (Kronenberger et al., 2014). Similarly, those factors can be affected because of hearing loss and are related with poor linguistic, social, and educational development (Blair & Razza, 2007).

Executive functions refers to attention shifting, working memory, and inhibitory control cognitive processes that are utilized in planning, problem solving, and goal-directed activities (Miyake, Fridman, Emerson, Witzki, & Howerter, 2000). An atypical development of EFs can be observed in children who use CI (Beer et al., 2011). The children perform less efficiently than hearing children in short-term memory (auditory and verbal), working memory, fluency, and inhibitory control (Pisoni et al., 2011). On the other hand, strong development in visuospatial cognitive tasks, visual memory, and organization are identified (Kronenberger et al., 2013).

This could be explained due to an interruption in neural development caused by deafness, which affects cerebral regions responsible for auditory processing and affects the frontal lobe – the main site for the functioning of EFs (Neville et al., 1998). Children with hearing loss who develop language using CI are two to five times more likely to have clinically significant difficulties with the domain of EFs than the children with normal audition (Kronenberger et al., 2014).

According to Oberg and Lukomski (2011), visual attention could play a major role in the equipping of skills related with EFs. However, there are many perspectives explaining the way visual attention affects those with CI. Figueras et al. (2008) does not find differences in visual attention of children with hearing loss using a CI, to children who do not use a CI, and children with normal hearing. In contrast, other studies observed differences (Mitchell & Maslin, 2007; Khan et al., 2005). A possible explanation is related to the impulsivity in the resolution of these kinds of tasks that can be associated with executive functioning or with the use of visual codification strategies to obtain information from the environment, which results in a higher assignation on fixations and attention to central and peripheral visual fields (Parasnis et al., 2003).

Bavelier et al. (2000) state that deaf people need to use a larger visual field to obtain more information while their hearing peers only trust in their central visual field and process additional information through hearing. Furthermore, the answer latency of the population with hearing loss when facing some tasks could be slower as well, due to the need to handle the visual field more efficiently and the desire to be able to answer in a more accurate way (Sladen et al., 2005). The reason for that could be that hearing is the sense that can provide a more precise spatial location when processing a non-visible stimulus. Individuals with severe to profound hearing loss do not dispose of enough aural information to monitor events that are not in the centre of the visual window. In such a way, it might be speculated that deaf people differ from individuals with normal hearing in terms of their answer capacity to events in the visual periphery (Rothpletz et al., 2003).

To test visual attention, researchers use Eye Trackers to register ocular movements during the execution of cognitive tasks. An Eye Tracker is a fundamental tool for studying visual perception and its relationship with the performance of EFs in a population with CI. This tool allows researchers to expand on the knowledge about attentional mechanisms underlying hearing loss, and the way they play a role in cognitive tasks of a superior order. This present study has two main objectives: (1) To examine the EFs of inhibition, mental flexibility, and working memory in children with CI and hearing children (2) To examine the relationship of visual fixation patterns on language development and executive functions in children with CI and hearing children. Based on previous studies, we hypothesize that the executive functioning in children with CI will be less effective than in hearing children. Secondly, we hypothesize that the children with CI will demonstrate distinct visual fixation patterns, particularly looking at peripheral areas of a stimulus, than hearing children, since hearing loss imposes limitations on daily life, it is possible that children with CI use differential visual strategies to obtain more information from the environment.

Methodology

Participants

There were 26 children who participated, including 13 who use cochlear implants and 13 who do not use them. The CI group consisted of 7 boys and 6 girls, and the normal-hearing listener group also consisted of 7 boys and 6 girls. All the participants with CI were attending Auditory-Verbal Therapy focused on aural-verbal aspects.

For the selection of participants with CI, the following criteria were considered: profound bilateral sensorineural deafness, an age of onset under the age of three, implantation before seven years old with a minimum use of three years, and constant attendance to a rehabilitation program focused on the development of oral language. Children with normal hearing needed to have normal peripheral bilateral hearing, based on an audiometry of average pure tones of 20 dB or less. Members of both groups have a normal level of reading, normal or corrected vision, have not been diagnosed with any neurological or cognitive condition or any other syndrome associated with deafness.

Materials

Non-verbal Cognition: Kaufman's Brief Intelligence Test (K-BIT) (Kaufman & Kaufman, 1983). This study used the Matrices subtest, in which the participant observes one picture and then has to select from a series of possible answers. Next, he or she has to select the picture amongst the possible answers that he or she considers that best match for the first picture.

Language: Clinical Evaluation of Language Fundamentals®-Preschool-2 Spanish (CELF®-Preschool-2 Spanish) (Wiig et al., 2004): this test evaluates expressive and comprehensive language in children from 3 years to 6 years 11 months. Core Language is a measure of general language ability that quantifies children's overall language performance. The score was derived by summing the scores from the subtests that discriminate best typical language from disordered language. Even though the participants with and without CI were older than 6 years 11 months years, they were assessed with this instrument considering the aural age of participants with CI.

Executive Functions: Battery of frontal lobes and executive functions (BANFE*)* (Flórez Lazaro, Ostrosky-Solis & Lozano Gutierrez, 2012) this instrument includes most of the neuropsychological tests that are supported by scientific literature and have been internationally applied. All the sections have been adapted for a Spanish speaking population. The conceptual paradigm that guided its design is based upon the proposals of Stuss & Levine (2002) and Zelazo & Muller (2002).

Additionally, 6 subtests were administered: Mazes, Semantic classification, Hannoi Tower, Visuospatial memory, Stroop, and Self-ordered pointing. First, Mazes is a task that evaluates participant's capacity to respect limits (impulsivity control), follow rules, and plan motor execution to reach a specific goal (planning). It requires the individual to trace a maze without touching the walls or going through them (Levin, Song, Swing-Cobbs & Roberson, 2001). Secondly, Semantic classification evaluates the capacity to analyse and to group animal figures in the highest possible number of semantic categories. The development of this test requires the abilities of abstraction, initiative, and mental flexibility (Delis, Squire, Birhle & Massman, 1992). Thirdly, Hannoi Tower evaluates the capacity to plan a series of actions in a specific order allowing one to reach a goal. It estimates the ability to anticipate actions (sequential planning) (Borys, Spitz & Dorans, 1982).

Fourthly, visuospatial memory estimates the capacity to retain and actively reproduce the sequential order of a series of objects that are situated in a space. It is based on the test of Corsi Cubes (Corsi, 1972), introducing the variable proposed by Goldman-Rakic (1998) and Petrides (2000), which includes figures that represent real objects. Fifthly, Stroop evaluates participants' capacity to inhibit an automatic response and to select an answer considering arbitrary criteria (MacLeod, 1991). And sixthly, self-ordered pointing evaluates the capacity to use the visuospatial working memory to autonomously point out a series of figures without repeating or omitting any of them. This task implies visuospatial memory and the development of effective strategies (Flores Lázaro, Ostrosky-Solis, & Lozano Gutiérrez, 2012). It is important to clarify that the first three subtests are assessed with a pen and paper method, whereas the last three subtests were completed on a computer screen. The Eye Tracker was set up and recorded at the beginning of these last three subtests.

The Eye Tracker Tobii TX 300 recorded participants' ocular movement, and the Tobii Studio 3.2.1. Software was used to register and analyse the data. The movements were later analysed and used to explore executive functioning. To obtain the measures, the software requires the establishment of Areas of Interest (AoI). For this study, two areas (the centre of the image and the periphery) were selected in agreement with the background presented in relation to the performance of children with CI in EFs. The measurement used for the analysis of visual fixation patterns was the total time that it took to look at the (AoI), known as the length of the visits.

Procedure

For the evaluation through the *Eye Tracker,* the BANFE sheets were scanned and presented in a 23" screen with a resolution of 1920 x 1080 pixels. The same indications suggested in the test battery were followed for the administration of each one of the subtests and the presentation of the stimulus was developed with the *Tobii* Studio 3.2.1. software. Because children were evaluated, only the data with a reliability average above 70% were considered.

Participants sat in the test chair ensuring a necessary distance of 60 cm between their eyes and the computer screen creating a 90° angle. A calibration system was automatically programmed for a total of 9 points. Because the tests required that participants point to the screen, pointing, a small laser pointer of 25 centimetres was used to avoid sudden movements from the participant and the consequent absence of ocular register. Table 1 presents a summary of the implemented tests and the evaluated skills.

Table 1. Summary of the implemented tests and the evaluated skills

Test	Sub test	Measures	Evaluated skill
K- BIT	Matrices	Non-Verbal IQ	Cognition
Language	Remembering sentences	Core language Expressive language	Comprehensive and expressive language
	Words structure	Comprehensive language Content of language	
	Concepts and following directions	Structure of language	
	Expressive vocabulary		
	Sentences structure		
	Types of words (expressive and comprehensive		
Executive Functions	Mazes	Dead-end	Motor planning
		Go through	Limits respect
		Time	Impulsivity
	Semantic classification	Total punctuation	Mental flexibility
		Number of abstract categories	Abstraction
		Total number of categories	Lexical recursion
		Total average of animals	
	Hanoi Tower	Time	Anticipation
		Number of movements	
	Visuospatial memory(eye tracker)	Maximum sequence	Working memory
		Perseverations	
		Order errors	
	Stroop(eye tracker)	Stroop errors	Inhibitory/Impulsivity Control
		Time	
		Number of hits	
	Self-ordered pointing(eye tracker)	Omissions	Working memory Visuospatial and Organization
		Time	
		Hits	

Data Analysis

Data management and analysis were performed using the SPSS 22 software. U Mann Whitney non-parametric tests were used to compare the results obtained in both groups. Multiple linear regression models with stepwise backward elimination were constructed to analyse independent factors (EFs and visual fixation patterns) with the dependent variable as Core Language. Non-significant variables associated with language (at the $p < .05$ level) were excluded from the models. Significant variables associated with language were analysed in terms of the amount of added variance they accounted for (R^2).

Results

Before the tests, participants were compared in terms of their sociodemographic characteristics. Findings suggest significant differences in terms of hearing age between the CI group and the control group (Table 2).

Table 2. Participants' characteristics

Variables	CI group $n = 13$	Control group $n = 13$	Mann-Whitney U	p	Z
Non-verbal cognition (K-BIT)	88.23 (11.46)	93.46 (13.02)	59	.190	−1.309
Chronological Age	8.61 (1.55)	8.61 (1.60)	84	.979	−0.026
Hearing Age	5.43 (1.43)	8.61 (1.60)	13	.000	−3.698

*Data expresses the average of the group. Standard deviation in parentheses.

Language

Language performance in both groups confirmed a low development in the group with CI in the evaluated components except for the content, as it can be observed in Table 3.

Table 3. Results in the language test

Sub test	CI group	Control group	Mann-Whitney U	p	Z
Core Language	75.23 (17.76)	144.07 (6.15)	4.5	.000	−4.108
Receptive Language	84.16 (12.39)	111.75 (15.74)	6	.001	−3.134
Expressive Language	71.75 (22.90)	111.50 (11.60)	14	.003	−2.499
Content	87.83 (22.24)	119.00 (11.41)	13	.007	−2.577
Structure	70.16 (17.34)	117.62 (14.48)	4	.001	−2.900

*Data expresses the average of the group. Standard deviation in parentheses.

Executive Functions

As seen in Table 4, there are differences in some of the areas that were evaluated for executive functioning. For the subtests that evaluated planning (mazes), anticipation (Tower of Hannoi), and visual memory, there are no differences between groups. However, in the tasks that evaluated cognitive flexibility, abstraction, inhibition, and working memory, children with CI had significantly lower performances.

Table 4. Comparison of averages in EFs

Test	CI group	Control group	Mann-Whitney U	*p*	Z
Mazes (Planning)					
Go through	2.15 (2.85)	2.30 (3.61)	79	.766	−0.297
Dead-end	3.92 (2.78)	5.61 (3.77)	60	.206	−1.264
Time	219.53 (88.94)	223.69 (80.02)	81	.858	−0.179
Semantic classification (Cognitive Flexibility)					
Total Categories	3.00 (1.35)	6.07 (2.43)	10	.000	−3.421
Total Abstract	0.30 (0.63)	2.15 (1.46)	19	.001	−3.396
Categories	65.90 (170.2)	67.26 (141.25)	83	.938	−0.643
Total animals	4.76 (2.68)	13.23 (4.96)	10.5	.000	0.077
Total score					
Hannoi Tower (Anticipation)					
Movements	18.92 (12.76)	14.07 (8.46)	64	.289	−3.914
Time	94.15 (57.64)	61.92 (50.08)	52.50	.101	−1.059
Visuospatial Working Memory (MT visual)					
Maximum sequence	2.07 (1.11)	2.69 (1.18)	59.5	.185	−1.804
Perseverations	0.07 (0.27	0.38 (0.65)	52.5	.101	−1.326
Order Errors	2.30 (1.65)	2.76 (1.42)	69	.412	−1.642
Stroop (inhibitory control)					
Stroop Error	8.07 (5.78)	3.38 (3.64)	44	.036	−1.496
Time	141.84 (54.96)	117 (40.53)	54	.118	−0.820
Hits	75.92 (5.78)	80.61 (3.64)	44	.036	−2.095
Self-ordered pointing (working/organization memory)					
Time	121.07 (72.38)	73.38 (31.60)	60	.038	−1.564
Hits	13.00 (4.28)	16.84 (3.76)	42	.029	−2.095
Perseverations	3.30 (2.17)	6.46 (4.61)	52	.101	−1.668
Omissions	7.38 (3.5)	5.53 (3.01)	58.5	.179	−2.188

*Data expresses the average of the group. Standard deviation in parentheses.

Visual Fixation Patterns

In order to analyse visual fixations in EFs subtests (Visuospatial memory, Stroop, and Self-ordered pointing), we selected two Areas of Interest, (AoI): one completely surrounding the stimulus denominated in the centre and one outside the stimulus denominated in the periphery. It is possible to affirm that children with CI visit peripheral areas of an image for longer amounts of time than children in the control group (Table 5).

Table 5. Comparison of visual patterns (total of visits in AoI)

Subtest	AoI	CI group	Control group	Mann-Whitney *U*	*p*	*Z*
Visuospatial memory	Centre	74.04 (36.75)	60.36 (30.84)	72	.521	−0.641
	Periphery	57.40 (44.60)	48.10 (25.72)	83	.939	−0.077
Stroop	Centre	34.93 (13.12)	24.90 (10.96)	48	.061	−1.872
	Periphery	6.59 (5.82)	1.89 (1.98)	40	.022	−2.228
Self-ordered pointing	Centre	1.96 (2.10)	2.89 (3.74)	60	.209	−1.256
	Periphery	2.48 (1.66)	1.69 (1.24)	38	.017	−2.386

*Data expresses the average of the group. Standard deviation in parentheses.

A multiple linear regression model was used to examine the independent variables of EFs and eye fixations while core language was the dependant variable (Table 6). There are significant differences between the two groups. In the CI group, 65% of the variance is explained by Semantic classifications in the first model, which is related to the linguistic nature of the task. A second model includes fixation in the periphery area in the same task, in which semantic classification helps to explain 81% of the variance. In the control group, fixation in the centre area in the Stroop task explains 27% of the variance.

Table 6. Summary of stepwise multiple regression model

	Variables entered	R^2	Adjusted R^2	*F*	*β*	*p*
	CI group					
Model 1	Semantic classification	.68	.65	22.08	0.30	.001
Model 2	Semantic classification				0.98	.000
	Fixation in a periphery area Semantic classification	.84	.81	25.14	−0.43	.013
	Control group					
Model 1	Fixation in a centre area in *Stroop*	.34	.27	5.2	0.58	.045

Discussion

The present study hypothesized that (1) the executive functioning in children with CI will be less effective than in normal hearing children (2) the children with CI will demonstrate distinct visual fixation patterns, particularly looking more at peripheral areas of a stimulus, than hearing children. Our hypotheses were supported by the language, executive functioning, and visual attention tests. In terms of language, the component of content does not show any significant difference, which indicates that children with CI have the resources to complete tasks, such as, following simple instructions, expressing vocabulary in the level of a word, and comprehending simple associations related to functionality. These children have participated in therapeutic processes of Auditory-Verbal Therapy for an average of 5.4 years. Because one of the main objectives of this kind of therapy is to strengthen aural skills, it establishes a strong connection with the content of language. Another plausible explanation is the difference between the comprehensive and expressive components of language amongst these individuals; in other words, children with CI comprehend more than what they can express (Ulanet et al., 2014).

As some authors state (Beer et al., 2014; Beer et al., 2011; Figueras et al., 2008; Greiner, 2010), it is not possible to perform consistently on EFs tests. This lack of consistency is a limitation that deserves careful consideration for future research. Theoretical conceptualizations related with EFs suggest that rather than being unitary functions, they encompass a wide range of dissociable skills; in that way, it is possible for an individual to fail in some EF tasks while he or she succeeds in the others (Garavan et al., 2002). This could mean that some skills related with the EFs can follow independent developments; some of them are strongly related with language and could be more affected by deafness. The variability in the results can also be associated to the differential nature of the EF task, as it is evident that those skills with less effective performances are directly related with tasks that are verbal or have a linguistic component in contrast with the performances obtained in more procedural tasks (Oberg & Lukomski, 2011; Daza & Phillips-Silver, 2013). The results are consistent with Ullman's (2001) explanation about the procedural declarative model in relation with language.

Through the use of technology, visual tracking patterns during the tasks were identified and compared in order to further our understanding of EFs. In agreement with Rothpletz et al. (2003), it was observed that the significant differences between the fixation patterns of the groups were condensed in the peripheral in comparison with hearing children who focused their attention on central visual areas. Sladen et al. (2005) affirmed that these behaviours would be related with the tendency of individuals with hearing loss to use strategies of visual codification to obtain additional visual information from the environment that they can't obtain through hearing. Recent studies indicate that deaf individuals tend to codify a strategy to obtain information from the environment in a holistic way, in which they direct their attention to central and peripheral visual fields in different proportions (Proksch & Bavelier, 2002; Tharpe et al., 2008; Codina et al., 2011). This conclusion would imply that people with deafness need to use a wider visual field to obtain environmental information while individuals with normal hearing can rely on their central visual field and process the required additional information by hearing.

In this regard, it is interesting to understand the level of influence that a larger attention to peripheral visual fields has on the results of standardised tests related with EFs, the impact of these fixation patterns in deaf children's daily lives, and its effect in variables such as vocabulary and language acquisition. Brooks and Meltzoff (2008) recognise an important relationship between the length of time a visual stimulus is presented and the location of visual fixation for infants with an adequate lexical development. Likewise, the fact that children with CI focus their attention in peripheral visual fields could explain the low performance of this group in attention abilities, inhibitory control, and working memory (Kronenberger et al., 2014; Figueras et al., 2008; Dye & Hauser, 2014). This understanding could positively impact the search for strategies to enhance social, academic, and therapeutic performance in this population.

Findings in this present study indicate that visual fixation may have an impact on executive performance of children with CI. The fact that this population experiences a tendency to stare at peripheral visual fields in a higher proportion than hearing individuals impacts the development of language. This could be a positive aspect to be considered within the variability observed for children with CI regarding their linguistic and cognitive development. In the same way, these findings coincide with the general domain of hearing theory proposed by Houston et al. (2012), which states that hearing privation can affect other cognitive domains that are not related with auditory input and have implications for different sensorial systems. Undoubtedly, this would become an important aspect to consider when designing future strategies for auditory rehabilitation.

References

Bavelier, D., Tomann, A., Hutton, C., Mitchell, T., Corina, D., Liu, G., & Neville, H. 2000. Visual attention to the periphery is enhanced in congenitally deaf individuals. *Journal of Neuroscience* 20(17), RC93–RC93. https://doi.org/10.1523/JNEUROSCI.20-17-j0001.2000

Beer, J., Kronenberger, W. G., Castellanos, I., Colson, B. G., Henning, S. C. & Pisoni, D. B. 2014. Executive functioning skills in preschool-age children with Cochlear Implants. *Journal of Speech, Language, and Hearing Research* 57(4), 1521–1534. https://doi.org/10.1044/2014_JSLHR-H-13-0054

Beer, J., Kronenberger, W. G. & Pisoni, D. B. 2011. Executive function in everyday life: implications for young Cochlear Implant users. *Cochlear Implants International* 12(Suppl 1), S89–S91. https://doi.org/10.1179/146701011X13001035752570

Blair, C., & Razza, R. P. 2007. Relating effortful control, executive function, and false belief understanding to emerging math and literacy ability in kindergarten. *Child Development* 78(2): 647–663. https://doi.org/10.1111/j.1467-8624.2007.01019.x

Borys, S. V., Spitz, H. H., & Dorans, B. A. 1982. Tower of Hanoi performance of retarded young adults and nonretarded children as a function of solution length and goal state. *Journal of Experimental Child Psychology* 33(1): 87–110. https://doi.org/10.1016/0022-0965(82)90008-X

Brooks, R., & Meltzoff, A. N. 2008. Infant gaze following and pointing predict accelerated vocabulary growth through two years of age: A longitudinal, growth curve modelling study. *Journal of Child Language* 35(1), 207–220. https://doi.org/10.1017/S030500090700829X

Corsi, P. M. 1972. Human memory and the medial temporal region of the brain (Unpublished doctoral dissertation). McGill University, Montreal.

Codina, C., Buckley, D., Port, M., & Pascalis, O. 2011. Deaf and hearing children: A comparison of peripheral vision development. *Developmental Science* 14(4), 725–737. https://doi.org/10.1111/j.1467-7687.2010.01017.x

Curtis, C. E., Zaid, D. H., & Pardo, J. V. 2000. Organization of working memory in the human prefrontal cortex: A PET study of self-ordered object working memory. *Neuropsychologia* 38(11), 1503–1510. https://doi.org/10.1016/S0028-3932(00)00062-2

Daza, M. T., & Phillips-Silver, J. 2013. Development of attention networks in deaf children: Support for the integrative hypothesis. *Research in Developmental Disabilities* 34(9), 2661–2668. https://doi.org/10.1016/j.ridd.2013.05.012

Delis, D. C., Squire, L. R., Bihrle, A., & Massman, P. 1992. Componential analysis of problem-solving ability: Performance of patients with frontal lobe damage and amnesic patients on a new sorting test. *Neuropsychologia* 30(8), 683–697. https://doi.org/10.1016/0028-3932(92)90039-O

Dye, M. W. G., & Hauser, P. C. 2014. Sustained attention, selective attention and cognitive control in deaf and hearing children. *Hearing Research* 309, 94–102. https://doi.org/10.1016/j.heares.2013.12.001

Figueras, B., Edwards, L., & Langdon, D. 2008. Executive function and language in deaf children. *Journal of Deaf Studies and Deaf Education* 13(3), 1–16. https://doi.org/10.1093/deafed/enm067

Flores Lázaro, J. C., Ostrosky-Solis, F., & Lozano Gutiérrez, A. 2012. Batería de funciones ejecutivas y lóbulos frontales (BANFE). México: Manual Moderno.

Garavan, H., Ross, T., Murphy, K., Roche, R., & Stein, E. 2002. Dissociable executive functions in the dynamic control of behavior: Inhibition, error detection, and correction. *Neuroimage* 17(4), 1820–1829. https://doi.org/10.1006/nimg.2002.1326

Goldman-Rakic, P. S., 1998. The prefrontal landscape: implications of functional architecture for understanding human mentation and the central executive. In *The Prefrontal Cortex: Executive and Cognitive Functions*, A. C. Roberts, T. W. Robbins, & L. Weiskrantz (eds), 87–102. Oxford: Oxford University Press, Oxford.

Greiner, L. A. 2010. Measures of executive function in children with Cochlear Implants (Unpublished MA thesis). The University of Iowa.

Houston, D. M., Beer, J., Bergeson, T. R., Chin, S. B., Pisoni, D. B., & Miyamoto, R. T. 2012. The ear is connected to the brain: Some new directions in the study of children with Cochlear Implants at Indiana University. *Journal of the American Academy of Audiology* 23(6), 446–463.

Kaufman, A. S., & Kaufman, N. L. 1983. *K-ABC--Kaufman assessment battery for children: Administration and scoring manual.* Circle Pines, MN: American Guidance Service.

Khan, S., Edwards, L., & Langdon, D. 2005. The cognition and behaviour of children with Cochlear Implants, children with hearing aids and their hearing peers: A comparison. *Audiology and Neurotology* 10(2), 117–126. https://doi.org/10.1159/000083367

Kral, A., Kronenberger, W. G., Pisoni, D. B., & O'Donoghue, G. M. 2016. Neurocognitive factors in sensory restoration of early deafness: A connectome model. *The Lancet Neurology* 15(6), 610–621. https://doi.org/10.1016/S1474-4422(16)00034-X

Kronenberger, W., Beer, J., Castellanos, I., Pisoni, D., & Miyamoto, R. 2014. Neurocognitive risk in children with Cochlear Implants. *JAMA Otolaryngology Head Neck Surgery* 140(7), 608–615. https://doi.org/10.1001/jamaoto.2014.757

Kronenberger, W., Pisoni, D., Henning, S., & Colson, B. 2013. Executive functioning skills in long-term users of Cochlear Implants: A case control study. *Journal of Pediatric Psychology* 38(8), 902–914. https://doi.org/10.1093/jpepsy/jst034

Levin, H. S., Song, J., Swing-Cobbs, L. & Roberson, G. 2001. Porteus maze performance following traumatic brain injury in children. *Neuropsychology* 15(4), 557-567. https://doi.org/10.1037/0894-4105.15.4.557.

Lezak, M. D., Howieson, D. B., & Loring, D. W. 1995. *Neurological assessment.* New York, NY: Oxford University Press.

MacLeod, C. M. 1991. Half a century of research on the Stroop effect: An integrative review. *Psychological Bulletin* 109(2), 163–203. https://doi.org/10.1037/0033-2909.109.2.163

Mitchell, T. V., & Maslin, M. T. 2007. How vision matters for individuals with hearing loss. *International Journal of Audiology* 46(9), 500–511. https://doi.org/10.1080/14992020701383050

Miyake, A., Friedman, N. P., Emerson, M. J., Witzki, A. H., Howerter, A., & Wager, T. D. 2000. The unity and diversity of executive functions and their contributions to complex "frontal lobe" tasks: A latent variable analysis. *Cognitive Psychology* 41(1), 49–100. https://doi.org/10.1006/cogp.1999.0734

Neville, H. J., Bavelier, D., Corina, D., Rauschecker, J., Karni, A., Lalwani, A., Braun, A., Clark, V., Jezzard, P., & Turner, R. 1998. Cerebral organization for language in deaf and hearing subjects: Biological constraints and effects of experience. *Proceedings of the National Academy of Sciences* 95(3), 922–929. https://doi.org/10.1073/pnas.95.3.922

Oberg, E., & Lukomski, J. 2011. Executive functioning and the impact of a hearing loss: performance-based measures and the Behavior Rating Inventory of Executive Function (BRIEF). *Child Neuropsychology: A Journal on Normal and Abnormal Development in Childhood and Adolescence* 17(6), 521–545. https://doi.org/10.1080/09297049.2011.555760

Parasnis, I., Samar, V. J., & Berent, G. P. 2003. Deaf adults without attention deficit hyperactivity disorder display reduced perceptual sensitivity and elevated impulsivity on the Test of Variables of Attention (T.O.V.A.). *Journal of Speech, Language, and Hearing Research* 46(5), 1166–1183. https://doi.org/10.1044/1092-4388(2003/091)

Petrides, M. 2000. Dissociable Roles of Mid-Dorsolateral Prefrontal and Anterior Inferotemporal Cortex in Visual Working Memory. *The Journal of Neuroscience* 20(19):7496-7503. https://doi.org/10.1523/jneurosci.20-19-07496.2000.

Pisoni, D., Kronenberger, W., Roman, A., & Geers, A. 2011. Measures of digit span and verbal rehearsal speed in deaf children following more than 10 years of Cochlear Implantation. *Ear and Hearing* 32(Suppl), 60S–74S. https://doi.org/10.1097/AUD.0b013e3181ffd58e

Proksch, J., & Bavelier, D. 2002. Changes in the spatial distribution of visual attention after early deafness. *Journal of Cognitive Neuroscience* 14(5), 687–701. https://doi.org/10.1162/089892902760138591

Rothpletz, A. M., Ashmead, D. H., & Thorpe, A. M. 2003. Responses to targets in the visual periphery in deaf and normal-hearing adults. *Journal of Speech, Language, and Hearing Research* 46(6), 1378–1386. https://doi.org/10.1044/1092-4388(2003/107)

Sladen, D. P., Tharpe, A. M., Ashmead, D. H., Grantham, D. W., & Chun, M. M. 2005. Visual attention in deaf and normal hearing adults: Effects of stimulus compatibility. *Journal of Speech, Language, and Hearing Research* 48(6), 1529–1537. https://doi.org/10.1044/1092-4388(2005/106)

Stuss, D. T., & Levine, B. 2002. Adult clinical neuropsychology: Lessons from studies of the frontal lobes. *Annual Review of Psychology* 53(1), 401–433. https://doi.org/10.1146/annurev.psych.53.100901.135220

Surowiecki, V. N., Maruff, P., Busby, P. A., Sarant, J., Blamey, P. J., & Clark, G. M. 2002. Cognitive processing in children using Cochlear Implants: The relationship between visual memory, attention, and executive functions and developing language skills. *Annals of Otology, Rhinology & Laryngology* 189(suppl), 119–126. https://doi.org/10.1177/00034894021110S524

Tharpe, A., Ashmead, D., Sladen, D., Ryan, H., & Rothpletz, A. M. 2008. Visual attention and hearing loss: Past and current perspectives. *Journal of the American Academy of Audiology* 19(10), 741–747. https://doi.org/10.3766/jaaa.19.10.2

Ulanet, P. G., Carson, C. M., Mellon, N. K., Niparko, J. K., & Ouellette, M. 2014. Correlation of neurocognitive processing subtypes with language performance in young children with Cochlear Implants. *Cochlear Implants International* 15(4), 230–240. https://doi.org/10.1179/1754762814Y.0000000077

Ullman, M. T. 2001. A neurocognitive perspective on language: The declarative/procedural model. *Nature Reviews Neuroscience* 2(10), 717–726. https://doi.org/10.1038/35094573

Wiig, E. H., Secord, W. & Semel, E. M. 2004. *CELF preschool 2: Clinical evaluation of language fundamentals preschool.* San Antonio, TX: Pearson/PsychCorp.

Zelazo, P. D., & Müller, U. 2002. Executive function in typical and atypical development. In U. Goswami (Ed.), *Handbook of childhood cognitive development* (pp. 445–469). Oxford: Blackwell. https://doi.org/10.1002/9780470996652.ch20

PART IV

Genetic syndromes with intellectual disabilities

The relationship between the lexicon and grammar in Spanish-speaking children with Down syndrome

Donna Jackson-Maldonado,[1] Miguel Galeote[2] and María Fernanda Flores Guerrero[2]
[1]Universidad Autónoma de Querétaro, México / [2]Universidad de Málaga, España

A strong association between early vocabulary comprehension and production has been shown in typically developing children (TD), and there is robust evidence for a lexicon-grammar association. These relations have been inconsistent in children with Down Syndrome (DS). In this study, ten Spanish-speaking children with DS were observed for vocabulary comprehension, production and initial morphosyntax using a parental report, the Down-CDI. Results showed high individual differences and developmental patterns were not similar to the literature of children with TD. The relation between vocabulary size, composition, sentence length and complexity was inconsistent. Thus, some developmental patterns of TD children are similar in children with DS. There is an association between grammar and vocabulary at the general level, but not within specific components.

Keywords: lexicon, grammar, Down Syndrome, Spanish

Introduction

The relationship between the lexicon and grammar in child language has been the topic of discussion between modular and functional models of language acquisition (Bates & Goodman, 1997, 1999). Whereas modular models (Chomsky, 1988) would propose separate modules, "that our capacity for grammar is innate, and that this capacity comprises a dedicated, special-purpose learning device that has evolved for grammar alone" (Bates & Goodman, 1999:p. 30), functional models have consistently shown, across typical (monolingual and bilingual) and atypical language development, that there is an association between the lexicon and

https://doi.org/10.1075/z.223.12jac

grammar when lexical development has reached a critical mass (Marchman & Bates, 1994). This relationship changes over time (Bates & Goodman, 1997, 1999). This paper adopts a functional perspective to propose lexical-grammatical associations in a population of Spanish-speaking children with Down Syndrome.

A component of this relationship is vocabulary composition. Most studies have followed a model in which words are divided into three categories: open class (nouns and verbs, adjectives and adverbs that are not time words or places to go), closed class (prepositions, determiners, pronouns) and social words, that include routines and sound effects (Bates et al., 1994; Caselli, Casadio, & Bates to Caselli et al, 1995; Caselli et al., 1999; Conboy & Thal, 2006; Devescovi et al., 2005). Open class words, in turn, can be subdivided into concrete nouns and predicates (referring to relational terms rather than sentence predicates: verbs, adjectives and some adverbs). This division is based on the initial Caselli et al (1995) classification in which adjectives are a form of nominal predication. It has been shown, for monolingual and bilingual populations in multiple languages, including Spanish, that open class words emerge before closed class words and are directly related to the size of the lexicon (see Figure 1; Bates & Goodman, 1997; Bates et al., 1988, 1994; Conboy & Thal, 2006; Goldfield & Reznick, 1990). The initial Caselli et al. proposal included two terms for similar categories: closed class words (pronominals, prepositions, determiners, auxiliaries and conjunctions) and function words (that included space and time adverbials). Caselli, Casadio, & Bates (1999) have suggested a sequence of acquisition in which social expressions are of early acquisition and become less frequent when more referential forms emerge. This, in turn, is related to vocabulary size. The early social expressions may be formulaic, "frozen forms" in which the morphology is not yet analysed. Closed class word

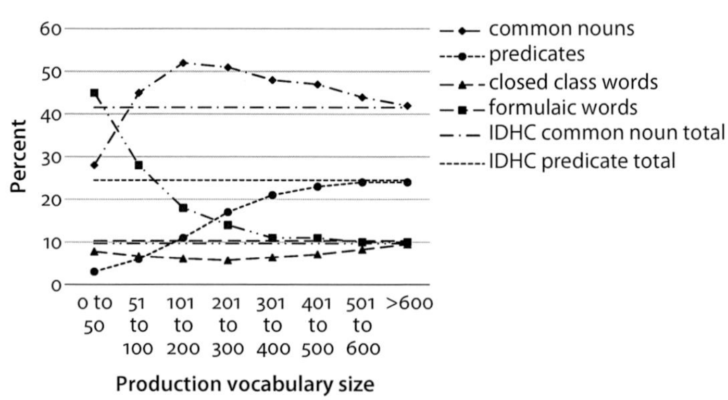

* SMBCDI = Spanish MacArthur Bates Communicative Development Inventories (Jackson-Maldonado et al., 2003)

Figure 1. Vocabulary composition in typically developing children. Norms SMBCDI I & II*

acquisition is highly dependent on the structure of the language, most particularly pronouns, prepositions and determiners (Gentner, 1982). Further, verbs may be acquired before nouns in languages such as Mandarin, Korean, and Tzotzil (Gentner, 1982; de León, 1999).

Several models have shown a strong lexicon-grammar relationship for the emergence of grammar. Early grammar has been studied based on inflectional morphology, mean length of utterance and early sentence complexity. Tomasello (2001) proposes an item-based explanation for the emergence of specific inflectional morphology. Bates and Goodman (1997) and Marchman and Bates (1994) give strong evidence, across different populations, of a regular nonlinear function that illustrates the dependence of grammar on early vocabulary size or a critical mass. It has also been suggested that vocabulary size is a stronger predictor of grammar development than age and gender (Devescovi et al. 2005; Marchman & Bates, 1994; Bates & Goodman, 1997; Dale, Dionne, Eley, & Plomin, 2000). Nevertheless, the directionality of the relationship is still uncertain (Kohnert, Kahn, & Conboy, 2010). Thus, the question emerges whether the lexicon determines the emergence of grammar or whether the emergence of grammar affects the increase in lexical items.

A few studies have addressed the association between the lexicon and grammar in Spanish-speaking children, particularly bilingual English-Spanish or Spanish-Catalan. Conboy & Thal (2006) as well as by Marchman, Martínez-Sussman, & Dale (2004), with English-Spanish bilinguals, proposed that within-language relationships were stronger than across languages. A study by Serrat et al. (2010) evaluated the relationship of verb morphology and verbal lexicon in Spanish-Catalan speakers. They also found a morphological "explosion" along with a critical mass of a verb lexicon that supports a strong relationship between the lexicon and grammar.

Lexical-grammatical relationships in children with Down Syndrome (DS)

Although consistent relationships have been shown across multiple monolingual-bilingual and atypical populations, Bates, Dale, and Thal (1995) had proposed dissociations between vocabulary and grammar in children with DS. Bates and Goodman have suggested that, "In fact there are good reasons to believe that the selective impairment of grammatical morphemes in this group is the by-product of their limitations in auditory perception and/or auditory memory" (1997:p. 17). Fowler (1990) and Miller (1988, 1992) have gone as far as to state that the lexical and grammatical systems were different in this population.

Studies that are more recent have questioned the dissociation or proposed more specific relationships. For instance, for Italian and Spanish children with

DS it has been shown that there is a delay in the transition from vocabulary to grammar when children were matched for vocabulary size (Iverson, Longobardi, & Casselli, 2003; Vicari, Caselli, & Tonucci, 2000; Galeote, Sebastián, Checa, & Sánchez-Palacios, 2014). Further evidence has shown that despite increases in vocabulary size, grammar does not emerge as it does for children who are typically developing (Iverson, Longobardi, & Casselli, 2003). In general, shorter MLU and less sentence complexity have also been found (Caselli, Monaco, Trasciani & Vicari, 2008; Chapman, Seung, Schwartz, & Kay-Raining Bird, 1998; Zampini & D'Odorico, 2011). Yet, there is contradictory evidence (Chapman et al., 2002; Galeote et al., 2014; Rondal, 1978, 1993). In other studies, acquisition of inflectional morphology has been shown to be affected (Caselli et al., 2008; Chapman et al., 1998; Eadie, Fay, Douglas, & Parsons., 2002; Galeote et al., 2014; Roberts, Price, Barnes, et al., 2007; Zampini & D'Odorico, 2011). Despite the contradictions in specific relationships, most studies have found consistent correlations between grammar and the lexicon (Caselli et al., 2008; Galeote et al., 2014; Zampini & D'Odorico, 2011). Thus, it seems that this relationship is more complex in children with DS and data from vocabulary composition and its relation to grammar may aid in the understanding of this problem.

Much of the research with typically developing children to date has been based on data from parent report instruments. Galeote et al. (2014) developed a parent report instrument specifically for children with DS that was based on English and Spanish versions of the MacArthur Bates Communicative Development Instruments (Fenson et al., 2007; Jackson-Maldonado et al., 2003; López Ornat et al., 2005). Galeote and colleagues have published several studies in which they compare children with DS, who were matched for equivalent mental age (EMA), lexical level, gender, and mother's educational level, with typically developing children (TD). When they contrast for EMA in the Galeote et al. (2014) study, children with DS produced shorter sentences that were also less complex. Nevertheless, when contrasting by lexical level (at approximately 200–300 words), there were no differences in mean length of utterances, but there were for complexity and morphological suffixes.

In another study, Checa, Soto and Galeote (2016) analysed the production of nouns, predicates, closed class and social words in 216 children with DS and EMA matched peers. The results showed a high production of social class words at lower vocabulary levels with a decrease as vocabulary levels increased; nouns were highly productive across all levels, but stabilised at larger vocabulary sizes; predicates had a slow increase and then became similar to closed class words, which also increased slowly. These results coincided with findings in an Italian study by Zampini & D'Odorico (2012).

Questions remain to explore further the relationship between the lexicon and grammar in children with DS. Is there an association between vocabulary size and grammar that is similar to what is known for typically developing children? Are patterns of vocabulary composition also similar to typically developing children? To answer these questions, this paper addresses vocabulary and grammar relationships in a Spanish-speaking Mexican group of children with DS. Data were obtained using a parent report instrument, developed specifically for children with DS. The goals of this study are first, to determine associations between the lexicon and early grammatical structures in children with Down syndrome. Specifically, we describe the relationship between vocabulary and two grammar measures: mean length of the three longest utterances in words (M3Lw) and sentence complexity. Secondly, we analyse the relationship between vocabulary size and composition. These contrasts are compared to data of typically developing children and are based on individual cases. We hypothesised, first, that vocabulary and grammar would be associated at early levels of language development. We also propose that vocabulary size will be a strong predictor of types of grammatical words (verbs and closed class words). Further, we predicted that children with DS would have higher percentages of social words than of other word classes.

Method

Participants in this study were part of a larger research project analysing the effects of hippotherapy on the language development of children with DS (Jackson-Maldonado, in process). Data from Wave 1 of the general project were analysed for this study. At the intake, the baseline for the sample of children was obtained. Children were assessed with multiple language and cognition measures, one of which was a parent report instrument of communicative abilities (see below). Only data from this parent report measure will be reported on in this study.

Participants

The initial sample consisted of ten monolingual Spanish-speaking children with DS who were between 4 and 7 years of age and whose equivalent mental age (EMA) was below 3;2 (except for one with an EMA of 3: 5). Language levels (determined by the CDI-Down, see below) and socio-economic status (determined by mother's education) varied across the sample, as did gender. One of these participants only participated in the initial correlational analysis and is not included in the detailed vocabulary study. Table 1 presents descriptive information for each participant, excluding participant 12DS. The remaining nine children were separated by language levels based on the number of words reported to be produced: 0–50, 100–300, 300–500 and, further, into two groups based on vocabulary level and word combinations. Group 1, with 4 children, had low vocabulary levels and no word combinations. Group 2, with 5 children, had higher vocabulary levels and were beginning to combine words (see Table 1). For Group 2 detailed vocabulary composition information is included.

Table 1. Participants by demographic, group, vocabulary and grammatical structures

ID	Age	EMA	Sex	Med	PROD	M3L	VB	CLO	COMP
DS GP1									
02DS	4;2	-3;2	fem	−HS	6	na	na	na	na
07DS	4;3	-3;2	male	+HS	9	na	na	na	na
10SD	4;4	-3;2	male	+HS	10	na	na	na	na
11DS	4;7	3.5	male	+HS	0	na	na	na	na
DS GP2									
01DS	6;8	-3;2	fem	+HS	523	3	3	39	17
03DS	4;5	-3;2	fem	−HS	475	1	0	36	0
04DS	4;9	-3;2	fem	+HS	135	1	0	8	0
06DS	5;10	-3;2	male	+HS	233	4.33	1	11	5
8DS	6;4	-3;2	male	+HS	560	3.3	12	36	9
LC									
01LC	2;4	na	fem	+HS	491	4.33			25
03LC	1;6	na	fem	+HS	446	3			3
04LC	1;6	na	fem	+HS	117	2			0
06LC	1;6	na	male	+HS	203	3			2
08LC	2;4	na	male	*HS	523	3.3			9

DS = Down Syndrome, LC = Language Control, EMA = mental age equivalent, GP = language level group, Med = mother's education, less or more than High School (HS), PROD = total word production, VB = total verbs, CLO = total closed class words, COMP = sentence complexity; na = not available; fem = female.

Vocabulary levels for the participants were quite varied and, it can be observed that despite their advanced age, several children were practically non-verbal, in both comprehension and production, at the beginning of the study. Others were producing very few words, and another group had a low level of word production for their age but was beginning to combine words or already produced full sentences. Although it may seem surprising, these low language levels are, unfortunately, quite common for children with DS in Mexico (see Jackson-Maldonado, de Santiago, & Sánchez, 2010).

For a comparative analysis of Group 2 for vocabulary and grammar, data from five typically developing language (TD) controls was obtained. Participants were paired based on their vocabulary levels and were equivalent in gender and mother's educational level. Because language levels were so low, even in Group 2, language controls were much younger in age than children in DS group. They ranged between 20 and 36 months of age (see Table 1).

Instruments

Although several measures were used in the major study, only those relevant to this paper are presented here. The cognitive scores or mental age equivalents were measured by means of the Reynolds Intellectual Screening Test- Spanish (RIST) (Reynolds & Kamphaus, 2013). Most children scored at or below baseline, that is 3;2, despite their advanced ages. As the baseline for the RIST is 3;2, mental age equivalence is only approximate and could be much lower than the 3;2 level.

Language abilities for this study were observed by a parental report, the Communicative Development Inventory-Down version (CDI-Down; Galeote et al. 2010), adapted to Mexican Spanish by the first author of this paper. The CDI-Down is a parent report that follows the basic format of the English and two Spanish CDI's (Fenson et al., 2007; Jackson-Maldonado et al., 2003; López Ornat et al., 2005). It was developed by Galeote et al. (2010) to be used on children with DS so that it includes more gesture information than the other forms. Also, comprehension and gesture information is extended for all ages. The Mexican-Spanish version of the CDI-Down was modified based on dialectal variations but maintained the rest of the format (for instance, "*catarina*" for "*mariquita*" 'ladybug',

Table 2. CDI-Down categories and items

Category	Number of items
Early Comprehension	11
Comprehension First Phrases	11
Beginning Production	2
Vocabulary List	21 categories, 649 words
Gestures	6 categories
Word Endings	12 questions
Irregular Verbs	20
Word Combinations	Yes/no
3 Longest Utterances (M3L)	3 phrases are written by parent
Sentence Complexity	34 pairs

"*panza*" for "*tripa*"-'belly'). The CDI-Down, Mexican version, consists of 649 words in 21 semantic categories. As in the Spanish MacArthur Communicative Development Inventory-II (SMBCDI-II; "Palabras y Enunciados" or Words and Sentences by Jackson-Maldonado et al., 2003), parents wrote in the child's 3 longest utterances (M3L) and selected the most complex phrases out of 34 sentences in which there were 3 options for each structure: a simpler form, a more complex sentence or the possibility of "my child does not produce anything similar to these sentences" (see Table 2). Only the first two counts were included in this study.

Procedure

Participants were recruited through language clinics and a community centre dedicated to children with Down syndrome for recreational and intervention purposes (Gigi's Playhouse). They were asked to participate in a larger project to test the effects of hippotherapy on the child's language development (Jackson-Maldonado, in process). This study is the first stage of the project in which all language and cognitive instruments were applied before beginning both their traditional language therapy (Wave 2) and the hippotherapy (Wave 3). All parents signed consent forms after an explanation of the full project and the study complied with the Ethical Standards of the university. Children were assessed in the clinic. In particular, the parent report forms were filled out while their children participated in the full assessment protocol. The method for filling out the forms was explained to the parents. Specific examples of comprehension were given, and it was emphasized that children should not repeat the words, but rather say them spontaneously. Further, all styles of phonological productions were accepted. As most parents were not with their children at the moment of filling out the forms, the possibility of the child only repeating the words was easily controlled for.

Data analysis

For the vocabulary composition analysis, the categories were based, mostly, on Conboy & Thal (2006), and the studies cited above. They were divided into semantic categories on the CDI-Down itself. Categories were: nouns (animal names, foods and drinks, vehicles, toys, clothing, body parts, small household items, rooms, and furniture), predicates (main verbs and adjectives), social words and routines (sound effects, games and routines, names of people), and closed-class words (auxiliary verbs, prepositions, pronouns, delimiters and connectors).

Utterance length (M3L) counts and utterance criteria were based on the rules established in Jackson-Maldonado et al. (2003). First, words rather than morphemes were considered (Jackson-Maldonado & Conboy, 2007). Some important considerations in the counts were: the separation of enclitics: content word + clitic ("*damelo-da+me+lo*"-'give it to me' had a count of 3 words), routines were considered as one word, "*uno-dos-tres*"- 'one two three' or coordinate sentences were counted as two separate utterances, "*se fue y trajo pastel*"-'(he) went and brought cake', would be two utterances.

The complexity count, a maximum of 34, also followed general CDI guidelines. The most complex of the two forms was given a count of 1, whereas the simple phrase and the last, "he/she doesn't produce anything similar" were not counted.

Results

The correlations of total vocabulary to grammar as well as the analysis of word types to total vocabulary analysis were carried out with all of the participants, divided by vocabulary level (see above). For specific relationships between word types to M3L and complexity, for obvious reasons, only children reported having word combinations (Group 2) were included in the analysis.

Associations between vocabulary and grammar

Associations were analysed for the children with DS, as it has been done previously for children with TD (see above). To compare vocabulary to grammar measures, Spearman bivariate correlations were carried out because the sample was not normally distributed and was small. Correlations between vocabulary production and grammar (both M3L and Complexity) were high and significant among all variables. Vocabulary and M3L were correlated at $r = .767$, $p = .016$ and as it was to complexity at $r = .753$, $p = .019$. Thus, general associations between vocabulary and grammar were established.

Vocabulary composition and vocabulary levels

The relationship between vocabulary size and vocabulary composition was analysed with the full sample of children with DS. Particularly, we were interested in whether vocabulary size predicted the production of more grammatical words, such as predicates (verbs and adjectives) and closed class words. Figure 2 depicts percent occurrence of each word category. If this figure is compared to Figure 1, based on in typically developing (TD) Spanish-speaking children, there is one large difference: children with DS use more words that are social across all vocabulary levels, while they decrease significantly in TD children. Further, predicates have similar growth curves across vocabulary levels, and both begin to peak at the

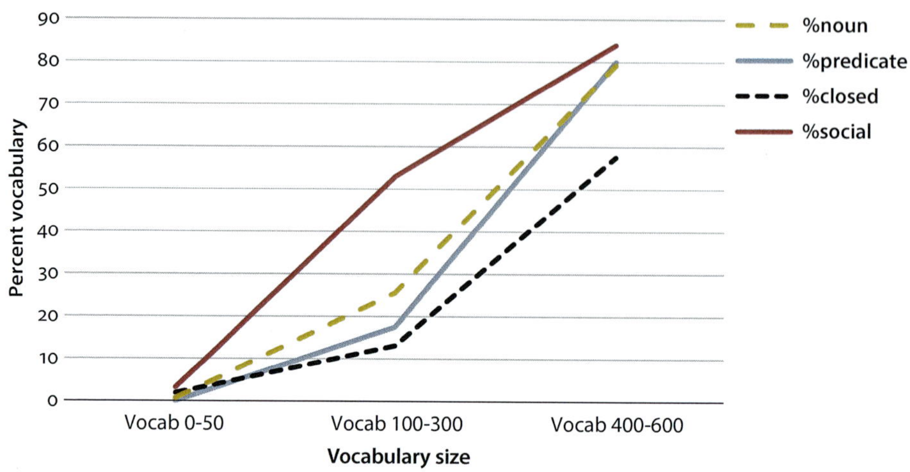

Figure 2. Percent words by vocabulary composition in DS sample by vocabulary level

100–300-word mark. Nouns have a steady increase in children with DS, and have a quick initial increase that is later stabilised in the TD population, but in both groups, nouns are produced more. Closed class words have similar developmental patterns in both populations.

Grammatical word types relationships to grammatical structures in Group 2

To observe the relationship of total vocabulary to closed class words, verbs and grammatical constructions in more detail, a sub-sample of the participants, whose parents reported that they were combining words, was selected. The sub-group consisted of five out of the nine remaining children (see Table 1 for participants and scores). For parts of this analysis, data was also compared to a sample of typically developing children (TD) as shown in Table 1.

The first analysis contrasted grammatical constructions to verbs and closed-class words (see Table 1). It could be predicted that as verbs and closed class words increase so would grammatical constructions. Relationships were not consistent. Whereas some participants with a higher number of verbs also had higher M3Ls, others had a very low verb count and higher M3L and complexity scores. For instance, participant 1DS had the highest complexity score but a low verb and M3L counts. Neither verb nor closed class words were associated with levels of grammatical constructions in higher vocabulary children, but, as would be expected, participants with low vocabulary levels did have fewer verbs, closed class words and low M3L and sentence complexity levels.

The second analysis determined the relationship of total vocabulary scores to M3L and complexity in both the participants with DS and TD, as it can be seen in

Figures 3, and 4 and Table 1. Whereas in children with TD there is a steady relationship between vocabulary size and M3L, this is not observed for children with DS as not all children with higher vocabulary levels have higher M3L scores. This contrast for complexity is slightly different as it is not quite as consistent across both populations. Curiously, there are two participants, one with DS and the other TD with high vocabulary and low complexity scores. This could be a product of the participants rather than a developmental tendency. Looking at the other four

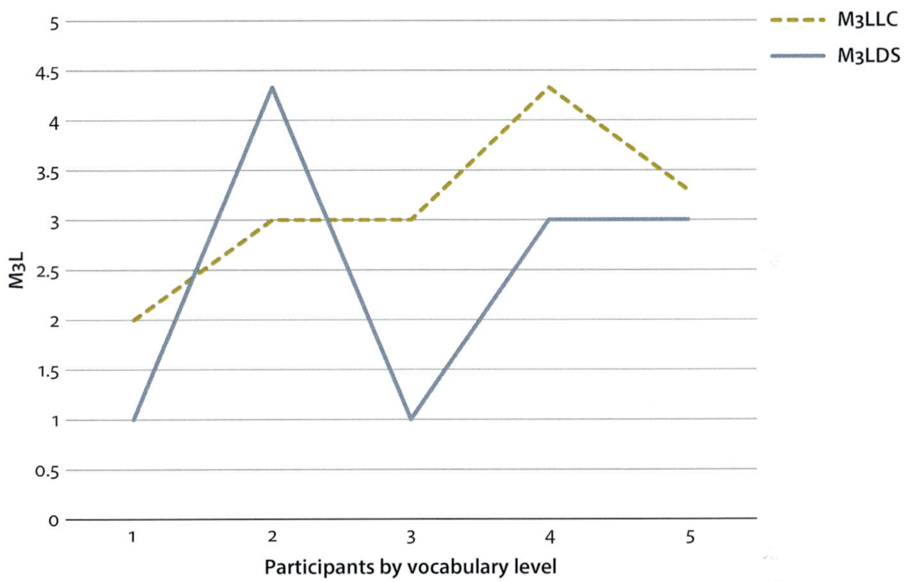

Figure 3. M3L comparisons of Group 2 DS and language control (LC)

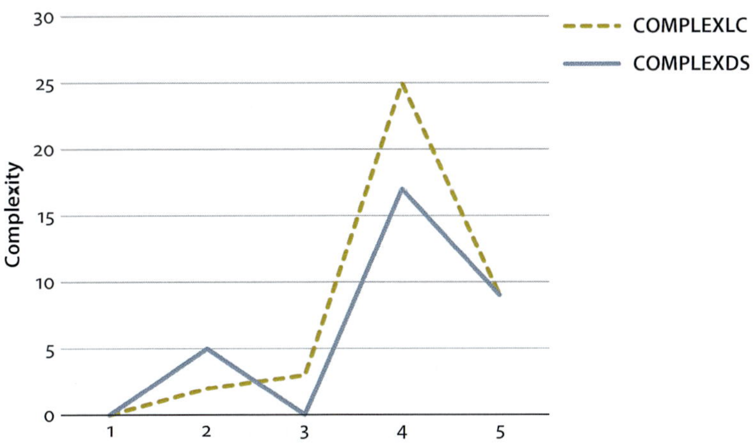

Figure 4. Sentence complexity comparisons of Group 2 DS and language control (LC)

participants, there does seem to be a pattern in which complexity increases with vocabulary levels above 400 words. Part of these inconsistencies could be because, in M3L, parents write in rather than recognise sentences and the complexity section is less straight-forward as parents have to identify types of sentences rather than specific words. In general, there is a less consistent relationship between M3L and vocabulary size.

Discussion

The first prediction of this study was that there would be an association between the lexicon and grammar in children with DS. At the general level, this prediction is supported. High correlations between word production, M3L and sentence complexity were found for the full sample.

The next level of analysis contrasted vocabulary composition to vocabulary size and to grammatical measures. Predictions were, first, that there would be a relationship between vocabulary size and types of words produced as well as to M3L and complexity. These predictions were partially sustained.

There was a general relationship of total vocabulary production to vocabulary composition in children with DS that only coincided with data reported for children with TD relative to nouns and closed class words. Nouns were the strongest category, and closed class words increased after a vocabulary of 400 words in children with DS. Predicates increased after 300 words. If only verbs were considered within predicates, they increased after a vocabulary of 500 words. A distinct finding, which was not consistent with the TD literature, was a high percent use of social words in children with DS. Whereas Checa, Soto, and Galeote (2016) also showed a high percentage of social words in children with DS, they decreased as vocabulary size increased. In this study, this type of words did not decrease. These differences may be because our sample size was small, but the high percentage of social words is quite different if compared to that found in TD literature.

Consistent relationships between vocabulary and grammar have been established for typically developing monolingual and bilingual children at early stages of development (Bates & Goodman, 1997, 1999; Devescovi et al., 2005; Caselli et al., 1995). The evidence for children with DS is slightly different Vicari et al., (2000) suggest that there is a selective disadvantage and grammar, as it "comes apart" and is not dissociated from other linguistic components. In line with this, Zampini and D'Odorico (2011), as well as Checa, Galeote and Soto (2016), find a lexical advantage compared to syntax. These proposals were tested by comparing data for vocabulary size to M3L and complexity scores to children with TD. Whereas the comparison of vocabulary with the complexity was more consistent,

M3L did not seem to be related to vocabulary size. Again, the sample was small, and these sections of the parent report are somewhat less straightforward than the vocabulary parts. Therefore, the data support a "selective disadvantage" with length utterance being more affected than sentence complexity.

When individual cases are analysed, the relationship is more diverse. The participant with the lowest vocabulary levels (below 150 words) did, indeed, have the lowest grammatical measures and used fewer grammatical words. Also, children with lowest vocabulary levels used less closed class words and had lower M3L and complexity scores than those with higher levels of vocabulary production. It has been previously stated that vocabulary size is a sufficient condition for the emergence of function words (that would include closed class words) and word combinations (Bates, Dale, & Thal, 1995; Bates & Goodman, 1997, 1999; Caselli et al., 1995). Data from individual cases in this study does not support this proposal. Some children with high vocabulary scores were not combining words or had low complexity scores, and others with low vocabulary levels had high M3L scores.

This study, based on a small sample of children with DS, has tested and supported the prediction that the lexicon and grammar are associated at the general level. Again, consistent with the DS literature, there seems to be a general delay. Moreover, individual cases do not show such consistent findings and, thus, we would support Vicari et al. (2000) in that there is large variability, and other factors may affect this association. Vocabulary size alone does not predict grammatical maturity. Further studies would require larger samples with more children who are combining words into early syntax and observational data to compare to parent report.

Acknowledgments

This project was funded by *Fondos para el Fortalecimiento de la Investigación*, Universidad Autónoma de Querétaro (FOFIUAQ) No. FLL201604. Special thanks to Gigi's Playhouse and both hippotherapy centres: Pasos Gigantes (Lauren Evans and Fernanda Ruiz) and Rancho Gran Chaparral (Georgina 'Gina' Pérez), as well participating families and volunteers. Particular thanks to, María Guadalupe Solís and Tania Inclán for their generous work on this project.

References

Bates, E., Bretherton, I., & Snyder, L. 1988. *From first words to grammar: Individual differences and dissociable mechanisms*. New York, NY: Cambridge University Press

Bates, E., Dale, P. S., & Thal, D. 1995. Individual differences and their implications for theories of language development. In P. Fletcher & B. MacWhinney (Eds.), *The handbook of child language* (pp. 96–151). Oxford: Blackwell.

Bates, E., & Goodman, J. 1997. On the inseparability of grammar and the lexicon: Evidence from acquisition, aphasia and real-time processing. *Language and Cognitive Processes* 12, 507–586. https://doi.org/10.1080/016909697386628

Bates, E., & Goodman, J. 1999. On the emergence of grammar from the lexicon. In B. MacWhinney (Ed.), *The emergence of language* (pp. 29–79). Mahwah, NJ: Lawrence Erlbaum Associates.

Bates, E., Marchman, V., Thal, D., Fenson, L., Dale, P., Reznick, S., Reilly, J., & Hartung, J. 1994. Developmental and stylistic variation in the composition of early vocabulary. *Journal of Child Language* 21(1), 85–124. https://doi.org/10.1017/S0305000900008680

Caselli, M. C., Casadio, P., & Bates, E. 1999. A comparison of the transition from first words to grammar in English and Italian. *Journal of Child Language* 26, 69–111. https://doi.org/10.1017/S0305000998003687

Caselli, M. C., Bates, E., Casadio, P., Fenson, J., Fenson, L., Sanderl, L., & Weir, J. 1995. A cross-linguistic study of early lexical development. *Cognitive Development* 10(2):159-199. https://doi.org/10.1016/0885-2014(95)90008-X

Caselli, M. C., Monaco, L., Trasciani, M., & Vicari, S. 2008. Language in Italian children with Down Syndrome and with specific language impairment. *Neuropsychology* 22(1), 27–35. https://doi.org/10.1037/0894-4105.22.1.27

Chapman, R. S., Seung, H.-K., Schwartz, S. E., & Kay-Raining Bird, E. 1998. Language skills of children and adolescents with Down Syndrome: II. Production deficits. *Journal of Speech, Language, and Hearing Research* 41, 861–873. https://doi.org/10.1044/jslhr.4104.861

Chapman, R. S., Hesketh, L. J. & Kistler, D. J. 2002. Predicting longitudinal change in language production and comprehension in individuals with Down syndrome: Hierarchical linear modelling. *Journal of Speech, Language, and Hearing Research* 45, 902–915. https://doi.org/10.1044/1092-4388(2002/073)

Checa, E., Galeote, M., & Soto, P. 2016. The composition of early vocabulary in Spanish children with Down Syndrome and their peers with typical development. *American Journal of Speech-Language Pathology* 25(4), 605–619. https://doi.org/10.1044/2016_AJSLP-15-0095

Chomsky, N. 1988. *Language and problems of knowledge: The Managua lectures*. Cambridge, MA: The MIT Press.

Conboy, B. T., & Thal, D. J. 2006. Ties between the lexicon and grammar: Cross-sectional and longitudinal studies of bilingual toddlers. *Child Development* 77(3), 712–735. https://doi.org/10.1111/j.1467-8624.2006.00899.x

Dale, P. S., Dionne, G., Eley, T. C., & Plomin, R. 2000. Lexical and grammatical development: A behavioural genetic perspective. *Journal of Child Language* 27(3), 619–642. https://doi.org/10.1017/S0305000900004281

Devescovi, A., Caselli, M. C., Marchione, D., Pasqualetti, P., Reilly, J., & Bates, E. 2005. A cross-linguistic study of the relationship between grammar and lexical development. *Journal of Child Language* 32(4), 759–786. https://doi.org/10.1017/S0305000905007105

De León, L. 1999. Verbs in Tzotzil (Mayan) early syntactic development. *International Journal of Bilingualism* 3(2–3), 219–239. https://doi.org/10.1177/13670069990030020601

Dixon, J. A., & Marchman, V. A. 2007. Grammar and the lexicon: Developmental ordering in language acquisition. *Child Development* 78(1), 190–212. https://doi.org/10.1111/j.1467-8624.2007.00992.x

Eadie, P. A., Fey, M. E., Douglas, J. M., & Parsons, C. L. 2002. Profiles of grammatical morphology and sentence imitation in children with specific language impairment and Down syndrome. *Journal of Speech, Language, and Hearing Research* 45, 720–732. https://doi.org/10.1044/1092-4388(2002/058)

Fenson, L., Dale, P. S., Reznick, J. S., Thal, D., Bates, E., Hartung, J. P., et al. 2007. *The MacArthur Communicative Development Inventories: User's guide and technical manual*. San Diego, CA: Singular.

Fenson, L., Marchman, V. A., Thal, D. J., Dale, P. S., Reznick, J. S., Bates, & E., et al. 2007. *MacArthur-Bates Communicative Development Inventories: User's guide and technical manual* (2nd ed.). Baltimore, MD: Brookes.

Fowler, A. E. 1990. Language abilities in children with Down Syndrome: Evidence for specific syntactic delay. In D. Cicchetti & M. Beeghly (Eds.), *Children with Down Syndrome: A developmental perspective*, (pp. 302–328). Cambridge: Cambridge University. https://doi.org/10.1017/CBO9780511581786.010

Galeote, M., Soto, P., Sebastián, E., Checa, E., & Sánchez-Palacios, C. 2014. Early grammatical development in Spanish children with Down Syndrome. *Journal of Child Language* 41(1), 111–131. https://doi.org/10.1017/S0305000912000591

Galeote, M., Rey, R., Checa, E., & Sebastián, E. 2010. El desarrollo de la morfosintaxis en niños con síndrome de Down: Primeros datos normativos. *Revista Síndrome de Down* 27(4), 107.

Galeote, M., Soto, P., Sebastián, E., Rey, R., & Checa, E. 2012. La adquisición del vocabulario en niños con síndrome de Down: Datos normativos y tendencias de desarrollo. *Infancia y Aprendizaje* 35(1), 111–122. https://doi.org/10.1174/021037012798977502

Galeote, M., Checa, E., Sánchez-Palacios, C., Sebastián, E., & Soto, P. 2016. Adaptation of the MacArthur-Bates Communicative Development Inventories for Spanish children with Down Syndrome: Validity and reliability data for vocabulary. *American Journal of Speech-Language Pathology* 25(3), 371–380. https://doi.org/10.1044/2015_AJSLP-15-0007

Galeote, M., Soto, P., Checa, E., Gómez, A., & Lamela, E. 2008. The acquisition of productive vocabulary in Spanish children with Down Syndrome. *Journal of Intellectual & Developmental Disability* 33, 292–302. https://doi.org/10.1080/13668250802441870

Galeote, M., Soto, P., Lamela, E., Checa, E., Pulido, L., & Rey, R. 2006. Adaptación de los Inventarios de Desarrollo Comunicativo MacArthur-Bates para el estudio del desarrollo del lenguaje en niños con síndrome de Down [Adaptation of the MacArthur-Bates Communicative Development Inventories for the study of language development of children with Down syndrome]. *Revista de Atención Temprana* 9, 4–16.

Gentner, D. 1982. Why nouns are learned before verbs: Linguistic relativity vs natural partitioning. In S. Kuczaj (Ed.), *Language development, Vol. 2: Language, cognition and culture*, (pp. 301 – 334). Hillsdale, NJ: Lawrence Erlbaum Associates.

Goldfield, B., & Reznick, J. 1990. Early lexical acquisition: Rate, content, and the vocabulary spurt. *Journal of Child Language* 17, 171–183. https://doi.org/10.1017/S0305000900013167

Iverson, J. M., Longobardi, E., & Casselli, M. C. 2003. Relationship between gestures and words in children with Down's syndrome and typically developing children in the early stages of communicative development. *International Journal of Language & Communication Disorders* 38, 179–197. https://doi.org/10.1080/1368282031000062891

Jackson-Maldonado, D. (in process). The effect of hippotherapy on communicative abilities in children with Down Syndrome.

Jackson-Maldonado, D., & Conboy, B. T. 2007. Utterance length measures for Spanish-speaking toddlers: The morpheme vs word issue revisited. In J. G. Centeno, L. K. Obler, & R. Anderson (Eds.), *Studying communication disorders in Spanish speakers: Theoretical, research, & clinical aspects*. Clevedon: Multilingual Matters.

Jackson-Maldonado, D., de Santiago, B., & Sánchez Aguilar, N. 2010. Verbal and non-verbal requests in Spanish-speaking children with Down Syndrome. *Down Syndrome Research and Practice* 12(2), 98–102.

Jackson-Maldonado, D., Thal, D., Fenson, L., Marchman, V. A., Newton, T., & Conboy, B. 2003. *Inventarios MacArthur-Bates del Desarrollo de Habilidades Comunicativas. Technical Manual*. Baltimore, MD: Paul H. Brookes.

Jackson-Maldonado, D., Thal, D., Marchman, V., Bates, E., & Gutierrez-Clellen, V. 1993. Early lexical development in Spanish-speaking infants and toddlers. *Journal of Child Language* 20(3), 523–549. https://doi.org/10.1017/S0305000900008461

Kohnert, K., Kan, P. F., & Conboy, B. T. 2010. Lexical and grammatical associations in sequential bilingual preschoolers. *Journal of Speech, Language, and Hearing Research* 53(3), 684–698. https://doi.org/10.1044/1092-4388(2009/08-0126)

López-Ornat, S., Gallego, C., Gallo, P., Karousou, A., Mariscal, S. & Martínez, M. 2005. *Inventarios de Desarrollo Comunicativo MacArthur: Manual* [The MacArthur Communicative Development Inventories : Manual]. Madrid : TEA.

Marchman, V., & Bates, E. 1994. Continuity in lexical and morphological development: A test of the critical mass hypothesis. *Journal of Child Language* 21, 339–366. https://doi.org/10.1017/S0305000900009302

Marchman, V. A., Martínez-Sussmann, C., & Dale, P. S. 2004. The language-specific nature of grammatical development: Evidence from bilingual language learners. *Developmental Science* 7(2), 212–224. https://doi.org/10.1111/j.1467-7687.2004.00340.x

Miller, J. F. 1988. The developmental asynchrony of language development in children with Down Syndrome. In L. Nadel (Ed.), *The psychobiology of Down Syndrome*, (pp. 167–198). Cambridge, MA: The MIT Press.

Miller, J. F. 1992. Development of speech and language in children with Down Syndrome. In I. T. Lott & E. E. McLoy (eds.), *Clinical care for persons with Down Syndrome*, (pp. 39–50). New York, NY: Academic Press.

Reynolds, C. R., & Kampahus, R. W. 2013. *RIAS Escalas de Inteligencia de Reynolds. RIST Test de Inteligencia Breve de Reynolds* (Spanish adaptation by P. S. Santamaría Fernández & I. Fernández Pinto). Madrid: TEA Ediciones.

Roberts, J. E., Price, J., Barnes, E., Nelson, L., Burchinal, M., Hennon, E. A., Moskowitz, L., Edwards, A., Malkin, C., Anderson, K., Misenheimer, J., & Hooper, S. R. 2007. Receptive vocabulary, expressive vocabulary, and speech production of boys with fragile X syndrome in comparison to boys with Down Syndrome. *American Journal on Mental Retardation* 112, 177–193. https://doi.org/10.1352/0895-8017(2007)112[177:RVEVAS]2.0.CO;2

Rondal, J. A. 1978. Developmental sentence scoring procedure and the delay-difference question in language development of Down's syndrome children. *Mental Retardation* 16, 169–171.

Rondal, J. A. 1993. Down syndrome. In D. Bishop & K. Mogford (Eds.), *Language development in exceptional circumstances*, (pp. 165–176). Hillsdale, NJ: Lawrence Erlbaum Associates.

Serrat, E., Sanz-Torrent, M., & Bel, A. 2004. Aprendizaje léxico y desarrollo de la gramática: vocabulario verbal, aceleración morfológica y complejidad sintáctica. *Anuario de Psicología/ The UB Journal of Psychology* 35(2), 221.

Serrat , E., Sanz-Torrent, M., Badia, I., Aguilar- Mediavilla, E., Olmo, R., Lara, M. F., & Serra-Raventós, M. 2010. La relación entre el aprendizaje léxico y el desarrollo gramatical. *Infancia y Aprendizaje* 33(4), 435–448. https://doi.org/10.1174/021037010793139590

Tomasello, M. 1992. *First verbs: A case study of early grammatical development.* New York, NY: Cambridge University Press. https://doi.org/10.1017/CBO9780511527678

Tomasello, M. 2001. The item-based nature of children's early syntactic development. In M. Tomasello & E. Bates (Eds.), *Language development: The essential readings* (pp. 169–186). Malden, MA: Blackwell.

Vicari, S., Caselli, M. C., & Tonucci, F. 2000. Asynchrony of lexical and morphosyntactic development in children with Down Syndrome. *Neuropsychologia* 38, 634–644. https://doi.org/10.1016/S0028-3932(99)00110-4

Vicari, S., Caselli, M. C., Gagliardi, C., Tonucci, F., & Volterra, V. 2002. Language acquisition in special populations: A comparison between Down and Williams syndromes. *Neuropsychologia* 40, 2461–2470. https://doi.org/10.1016/S0028-3932(02)00083-0

Zampini, L., & D'Odorico, L. 2011. Lexical and syntactic development in Italian children with Down's syndrome. *International Journal of Language & Communication Disorders* 46(4): 386–396. https://doi.org/10.3109/13682822.2010.508764

Profiles of grammatical morphology in Spanish-speaking adolescents with Williams Syndrome and Down Syndrome

Eliseo Díez-Itza,[1] Manuela Miranda,[1] Vanesa Pérez[2] and Verónica Martínez[1]
[1]Universidad de Oviedo / [2]Escuelas Universitarias Gimbernat-Cantabria

This chapter presents a comparative perspective on the morphological profiles of Williams Syndrome (WS) and Down Syndrome (DS). The initial research described these neurodevelopmental disorders as cases of specific preservation and delay of grammar, respectively, whereas later approaches have challenged such assumptions. The present study aimed to contribute to this discussion with data from 18 Spanish-speaking adolescents in three groups (WS, DS and typical development). Spontaneous speech was analysed with the tools of the CHILDES Project, transcribing and coding the parts of speech and morphological errors. While errors are less frequent in WS than in DS, their type and distribution remain atypical in both syndromes which points towards differential trajectories of language development.

Keywords: Williams Syndrome, Down Syndrome, morphology, grammatical profiles, atypical language trajectories

Introduction

Comparative studies have contributed significantly in the past three decades to a substantial revision in the definition of Intellectual Disability, within a new paradigm that is more centred on syndrome-specific neurodevelopmental profiles than on global deficits or delays (Schalock et al., 2010). During this period, a growing body of research has emerged on Williams Syndrome (WS), a rare genetic neurodevelopmental syndrome (hemideletion on chromosome 7q11.23) with a phenotype of distinctive facial features, intellectual disability and hypersociability. The studies comparing Williams Syndrome and Down Syndrome started in

https://doi.org/10.1075/z.223.13die

the Salk Institute, within the research program on the neuropsychological profile of WS (Bellugi, Lichtenberger, Jones, Lai, & St. George, 2000) using Down Syndrome (DS) as the comparison group because it was considered the model of "mental retardation", global and homogenous for all functions. The initial study by Salk Institute researchers (Bellugi, Marks, Bihrle, & Sabo, 1988) presented the results of the cognitive and linguistic functioning of three adolescents with WS and concluded that their language, contrary to what had been described in DS, constituted "an island of sparing" in the face of severe cognitive deficits. Therefore, these authors presented WS as a particular or atypical case of "mental retardation", with intact grammatical competence against impaired visuospatial skills, which was interpreted as a genetically based dissociation between language and nonverbal intelligence. Despite certain morphological errors, Bellugi, Bihrle, Jernigan, Trauner, and Doherty (1990) also concluded that the language of six adolescents with WS was "preserved" in comparison with their DS controls matched for sex and chronological and mental age. At the same time, the WS profile was considered "atypical" due to its specific deficits and preservations within and across domains. From these preliminary data on WS and their comparison with those of children with Specific Language Impairment (SLI), Pinker (1991) suggested that they constituted a case of "double dissociation" that would prove the independence between language and general cognition.

However, studies in Romance languages such as Italian, Spanish and French, found atypical morphosyntactic errors, questioning the hypothesis of preserved language in WS (Diez-Itza, Antón, Fernández-Toral, & García, 1998; Karmiloff-Smith, Grant, Berthoud, Davies, Howlin, & Udwin 1997; Volterra, Capirci, Pezzini, Sabbadini, & Vicari, 1996). The debate over the typical or atypical nature of the morphosyntactic profile of WS has been maintained in a series of studies (Benítez-Burraco, Garayzábal, & Cuetos, 2017; Diez-Itza, Martínez, Fernández-Urquiza, & Antón, 2017; Mervis, 2006).

WS profile is interpreted differently from different approaches. From the preservation approach, WS profile is interpreted regarding a system with a typical functioning but in which some components are impaired (Clahsen & Almazan, 1998, 2001; Clahsen, Ring, & Temple, 2004; Krause & Penke, 2002; Zukowski, 2005). Nevertheless, from the neuroconstructivist approach, WS profile is interpreted as the result of an atypical developmental trajectory, arguing that the preservation approach disregards the complex dynamics of development (Karmiloff-Smith, 1998; Hsu & Karmiloff-Smith, 2008; Oliver, Johnson, Karmiloff-Smith, & Pennington, 2000; Thomas et al., 2001; Thomas & Karmiloff-Smith, 2003).

Research concerning the grammatical profile of individuals with DS is not exempt from controversy. While an important agreement exists about the marked difficulties in grammar observed in the individuals with DS, studies differ about the nature and extent of their grammatical impairment (Chapman, Seung, Schwartz, & Kay-Raining Bird, 1998; Diez-Itza & Miranda, 2007; Eadie, Fey, Douglas, & Parson, 2002; Fabbretti, Pizzuto, Vicari, & Volterra, 1997; Finestack & Abbeduto, 2010; Galeote, Soto, Sebastián, Checa, & Sánchez-Palacios, 2014; Lázaro, Garayzábal, & Moraleda, 2013; Martin, Klusek, Estigarribia, & Roberts, 2009; Rutter & Buckley, 1994; Schaner-Wolles, 2004). The hypothesis of preservation of grammar in WS was based on the comparison with DS, but the view that DS presented a homogeneous profile of cognitive and linguistic delay did not correspond with research results that showed linguistic development as asynchronous related to mental age (Fowler, 1990; Miller, 1988). Similarly, later comparative studies suggested that WS did not demonstrate better linguistic abilities than expected for mental age and that the apparent preservation of language in WS was a resulting artefact from comparing it with DS, whose profile presented specific weaknesses in grammar (Vicari, Caselli, Gagliardi, Tonucci, & Volterra, 2002). In fact, even though the difficulties of morphosyntactic production were more prominent in DS, they also appeared to some extent in WS individuals when compared with TD children matched for mental age (Vicari et al., 2004), for verbal age (Diez-Itza et al., 2017), and for chronological age (Benítez-Burraco et al., 2017). Furthermore, the research of early language development showed that both syndromes presented an initial delay and that the later observed differences in the profiles of adolescents were the result of specific asynchronous trajectories of lexical and morphosyntactic development (Mervis & Robinson, 2000; Singer-Harris, Bellugi, Bates, Jones, & Rossen, 1997; Vicari, Caselli, & Tonucci, 2000).

In sum, although the comparative research has shown that DS presents a higher frequency of morphological errors than WS, it is still debated if the frequency of errors in WS is at the level expected for mental and verbal age. The nature of errors in both syndromes is also debated by those who consider that it reflects delays or selective deficits in a system that is comparable to that of the typical development; and those interpreting the morphological profiles as the result of atypical developmental trajectories.

In order to address some of these issues, the study presented in this chapter aimed to investigate the morphological profiles of WS and DS as part of a wider research program that compares the linguistic profiles of WS, DS and Fragile X Syndrome (FXS) with those of TD individuals (The Syndroling Project: Diez-Itza et al., 2014). The specific objectives are centred in the comparison of two groups of adolescents with WS and DS according to (i) the distribution of the part-of-speech categories (nouns, verbs, determiners, prepositions, conjunctions, pronouns, …) in the samples; (ii) the frequency of morphological errors by parts of speech; and (iii) the frequency of each type of morphological errors. Based on prior research, it was predicted that the distribution of parts of speech would not be syndrome-specific.

It was also predicted that morphological errors would not be equally present in all part-of-speech categories. Finally, it was predicted that participants with DS would present a syndrome-specific profile characterised by a higher frequency of morphological errors affecting function words and by a higher frequency of omission errors, while participants with WS would present fewer errors but would also show atypical errors.

Methodology

Participants

The sample was composed of 18 Spanish-speaking adolescents in three groups (3 males and 3 females in each group): a WS group (Mean age 17.06/SD 2.31/range 14.36–20.64), a DS group (Mean age 16.83/SD 1.89/range 14.05–19.06) and a group of typically developing (TD) children (Mean age 5.42/SD 0.34/range 5.01–5.89). The TD children were paired by sex and verbal age (MLU) with the WS group (WS MLU 5.70/SD 2.07/range 3.56–9.17; TD MLU 5.77/SD 2.00/range 3.71–9.00). Given that the MLU of the adolescents in the DS group was significantly lower (DS MLU 2.52/SD 0.98/range 1.29–4.12), their verbal age-equivalent (VAE) was obtained from the *Peabody Picture Vocabulary Test* (PPVT) (DS VAE 5.53/SD 0.43/range 5.0–6.08) and was used as the paired variable with the other groups.

Procedure

The speech samples were obtained from spontaneous conversations with a researcher in natural settings, and they are part of larger corpora within The Syndroling Project (Diez-Itza et al., 2014). Each session, with an estimated duration of 40 minutes, was videotaped and transcribed using the tools of the CHILDES Project (MacWhinney, 2000). To control for length, one sample of 1,000 consecutive tokens from each participant was selected for analyses in the present study.

Morphological analysis was conducted with the MOR program, one of the CLAN programs for the analysis of transcripts in the CHAT format from CHILDES. MOR provides a complete part-of-speech tagging (POST) for every word indicated on the main line of the transcripts, along with the morphological analysis of inflectional and derivational affixes and clitics. For example, the program gives the following analysis for the utterance "**CHI: en el colegio*" (in the school): %mor: prep|in det:art|el&MASC&SG = the n|school (prep: preposition; det: determiner; n: noun).

The parts of speech selected from the POST output to assess the profiles of grammatical morphology were: Articles, Nouns Adjectives, Personal Pronouns, Demonstratives, Possessives, Relative Pronouns, Quantifiers, Adverbs, Verbs, Prepositions and Conjunctions. Further, manual coding of errors included: (i) Errors by parts of speech; and (ii) Type of errors: Omission (OMI), Substitution (SST), and Addition (ADD). Substitution errors included gender, number and person agreement errors, as well as tense inflexion errors (see examples in Table 1). Measurements included absolute and relative frequencies expressed in means and percentages. According to the first objective, we calculated the distribution of the part-of-speech categories within the 1,000-word samples from each participant, using the FREQ program of CHILDES to count the number of words from each category. Then, we calculated the number and percentage of errors by category, which allowed us to assess whether all the categories were affected by morphological errors in the same proportion (%). Furthermore, with the aim of comparing the error profiles independently of the absolute frequency of error, we determined the percentage distribution of errors by parts of speech in each group. This relative distribution indicates the percentage out of the total number of errors corresponding to each part-of-speech category. Similarly, after calculating the total number of errors by types in each group, we determined the percentage out of the total number of errors corresponding to each type (Omission, Substitution and Addition). The Mann-Whitney U test was used to compare differences between groups in the mean frequency of errors by categories and by types.

Table 1. Examples of the type of errors

Type	Utterances	Part of speech
OMI	no *(***lo***) sabía hacer	Personal pronoun
	I did not know to do *(***it***)	
	me gusta *(***el***) sol	Article
	I like ****the*** sun	
SST	****apaguen*** **(apaga)** la luz tú	Verb
	****turn off*** the light you	
	papi ****con*** (y) mami	Conjunction
	daddy ****with*** **(and)** mommy	
ADD	no ****lo*** quiero decirlo	Personal pronoun
	I do not want ***it*** *to say it*	
	Hay***a** veces que acabo	Preposition
	there are ***to*** *sometimes I end up*	

Results

The analyses of the frequencies of distribution of the part-of-speech categories (out of 1,000-word tokens) revealed some differences. Table 2 presents the percentage of words in the categories in which statistically significant differences between some of the groups existed. In the WS group, the nouns frequency (NOU) was less than in the DS group. Conversely, the adolescents of the DS group showed a lower use of personal pronouns (PPR), relative pronouns (RPR) and verbs (VRB) than the adolescents of the WS and TD groups. Differences did not exist regarding the distribution of parts of speech between the WS group and the TD group, except the case of articles (ART), whose frequency of use was lower in the WS group.

Table 2. Percentage of part-of-speech categories use

	DS	WS	TD	DS vs. WS	DS vs. TD	WS vs. TD
	Mean% (SD)	Mean% (SD)	Mean% (SD)	Mann-Whitney Test (Z) (p)		
ART	6.17%	5.95%	6.90%	−.321	−1.444	−2.173
	(10.206)	(7.791)	(2.529)	(.748)	(.180)	(.030)*
NOU	20.79%	14.88%	18.05%	−2.402	−1.444	−1.604
	(29.224)	(21.235)	(29.303)	(.016)*	(.149)	(.109)
PPR	4.70%	7.88%	7.62%	−2.402	−2.882	−.401
	(17.484)	(17.904)	(16.216)	(.016)*	(.004)**	(.688)
RPR	2.39%	4.53%	4.40%	−2.882	−2.882	−.080
	(5.835)	(13.441)	(13.038)	(.004)**	(.004)**	(.936)
VRB	15.14%	20.32%	20.47%	−2.402	−2.082	−.320
	(31.403)	(15.967)	(36.952)	(.016)*	(.037)*	(.749)

Note: ART Articles, NOU Nouns, PPR Personal Pronouns, RPR Relative Pronouns, VRB Verbs.

As for the absolute incidence of morphological errors, it was much greater in the DS group (Mean = 99.56/*SD* = 39.85) than in the WS group (Mean = 7.67/ *SD* = 5.60) and the TD group (Mean = 2.67/*SD* = 2.25), while between these last two groups there were no statistically significant differences. Morphological errors did not affect in the same proportion (%) all part-of-speech categories. Table 3 shows the percentages of error by categories in each group. The DS group presented a significantly greater percentage of errors than the WS and TD groups in all categories, except in demonstratives (DEM) where none of the groups presented errors. The high percentage of errors in Articles (ART), Personal Pronouns (PPR) and Prepositions (PRE) was salient in the DS group. A similar pattern was observed in the WS group, even though the percentages of errors were much lower in this group. Nevertheless, only the percentage of errors in articles (ART) showed significant differences between WS group and TD children.

Table 3. Percentage of errors by part-of-speech categories

	DS	WS	TD	DS vs. WS	DS vs. TD	WS vs. TD
	Mean% (SD)	Mean% (SD)	Mean% (SD)	Mann-Whitney Test (Z) (p)		
ART	41.30% (32.310)	2.01% (1.672)	.25% (.618)	−2.882 (.004)**	−2.989 (.003)**	−2.308 (.021)*
NOU	2.25% (2.191)	.12% (.309)	.10% (.268)	−2.823 (.005)**	−2.823 (.005)**	−.123 (.902)
ADJ	7.19% (3.878)	1.11% (2.721)	1.04% (2.551)	−2.308 (.021)*	−2.308 (.021)*	−.123 (.902)
PPR	32.38% (18.422)	1.76% (.620)	.78% (.897)	−2.882 (.004)**	−2.903 (.004)**	−1.613 (.107)
DEM	0% –	0% –	0% –	– –	– –	– –
POS	10.79% (16.139)	0% (0)	0% (0)	−2.286 (.022)*	−2.286 (.022)*	0 (1.000)
RPR	4.16% (5.733)	0% (0)	0% (0)	−2.286 (.022)*	−2.286 (.022)*	0 (1.000)
QNT	15.03% (11.456)	0% (0)	0% (0)	−3.077 (.002)**	−3.077 (.002)**	0 (1.000)
ADV	1.68% (.521)	0% (0)	.15% (.388)	−3.077 (.002)**	−2.989 (.003)**	−1.000 (.317)
VRB	11.15% (5.634)	1.18% (.899)	.49% (.637)	−2.882 (.004)**	−2.903 (.004)**	−1.129 (.259)
PRE	28.17% (16.780)	2.63% (3.311)	.35% (.558)	−2.882 (.004)**	−2.934 (.004)**	−1.826 (.068)
CON	7.95% (4.420)	.20% (.504)	0% (0)	−2.989 (.003)**	−3.077 (.002)**	−1.000 (.317)

Note: ART Articles, NOU Nouns, ADJ Adjectives, PPR Personal Pronouns, DEM Demonstratives, POS Possessives, RPR Relative Pronouns, QNT Quantifiers, ADV Adverbs, VRB Verbs, PRE Prepositions, CON Conjunctions.

We also compared the relative percentage of errors in each part-of-speech category over the total number of errors. Figure 1 presents the percentage distribution of errors by category out of the total number of errors. In relative terms, the three groups presented distinct profiles. The WS group and the DS group showed both a higher proportion of errors in articles (ART) and a lower proportion of errors in adjectives (ADJ) than TD group. However, their profiles differed in the proportion of errors in personal pronouns (PPR) and verbs (VRB), which was much higher in the WS group, and in the proportion of errors in conjunctions (CON), which was higher in the DS group. The WS group and the TD group showed both a very high proportion of errors in personal pronouns (PPR) and a very low proportion of errors in conjunctions (CON), but they presented different profiles regarding the proportion of errors in the rest of the categories. The WS group showed a higher proportion of errors in articles (ART), verbs (VRB) and prepositions (PRE), and a lower proportion of errors in adjectives (ADJ). Finally, the DS group and the TD group showed both a similar proportion of errors in prepositions (PRE), but the DS group presented a higher proportion of errors in articles (ART) and conjunctions (CON), and a lower proportion of errors in adjectives (ADJ), personal pronouns (PPR) and verbs (VRB). It is necessary to point out that, in Figure 1, the specified categories account for 98.71% of the errors from the WS group and 95.03% of the errors from the TD group, but they account only for 80.71% of the errors from the DS group. This difference reflects the fact that the DS group presented more morphological errors than the other groups, and, as a result, other categories also presented a high number of errors (OTH: NOU, POS, RPR, QNT, ADV). Therefore, the profile of the DS group also differed in that it presented more errors and in all the part-of-speech categories than those of the WS and TD groups.

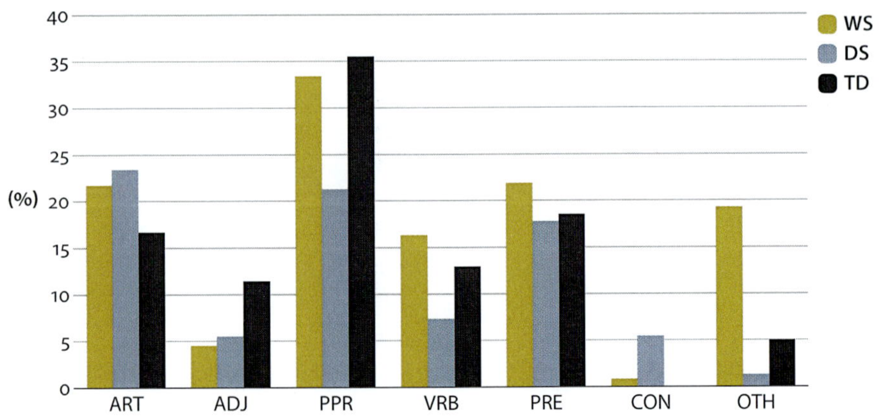

Figure 1. Percentage distribution of errors by part-of-speech categories
Note: *ART* Articles, *ADJ* Adjectives, *PPR* Personal Pronouns, *VRB* Verbs, *PRE* Prepositions, *CON* Conjunctions, *OTH* Other Categories

Concerning the types of error, they were not equally frequent in each group. Table 4 reflects the average number of morphological errors of each type (Omission, Substitution and Addition) that was observed in each group. The DS group showed a significantly higher frequency of all types of error than the WS and TD groups.

Likewise, the WS group showed a significantly higher frequency of Omission and Addition errors than the TD group.

Table 4. Frequency of morphological errors by type of error

	DS	WS	TD	DS vs. WS	DS vs. TD	WS vs. TD
	Mean (SD)	Mean (SD)	Mean (SD)	Mann-Whitney Test (Z) (p)		
OMI	61.36 (34.693)	3.33 (3.932)	.50 (.547)	−2.887 (.004)**	−2.923 (.003)**	−1.996 (.046)*
SST	33.93 (9.108)	3.33 (2.250)	2.16 (2.316)	−2.892 (.004)**	−2.903 (.004)**	−1.083 (.279)
ADD	4.26 (1.990)	1.00 (.632)	0 –	−2.119 (.034)*	−3.077 (.002)**	−2.739 (.006)**

Note: OMI Omission, SST Substitution, ADD Addition

Relative distribution of the types of error represented in Figure 2 also revealed atypical profiles of the DS and WS groups when compared with the TD group. The WS group and the DS group showed both a lower proportion of substitution errors (SST) than the TD group. However, their profiles differed in the proportion of omission errors (OMI), which was much higher in the DS group, and in the proportion of addition errors (ADI), which was much higher in the WS group.

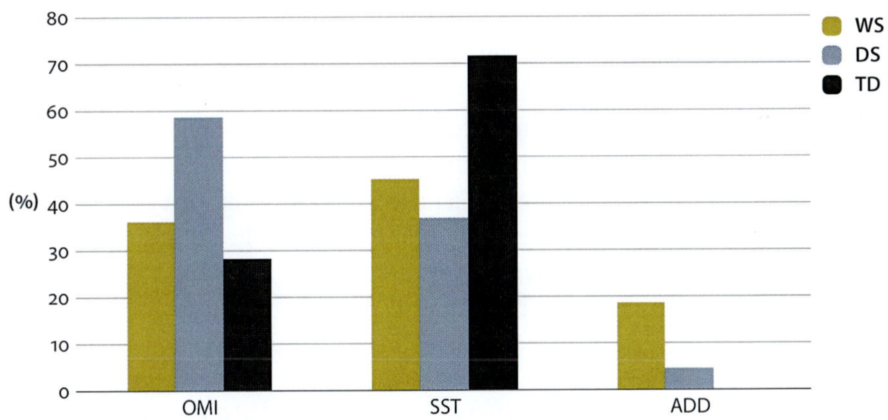

Figure 2. Percentage distribution of errors by types
Note: OMI Omission, SST Substitution, ADD Addition

Discussion

In this chapter, results from a comparative study of the morphological profiles of adolescents with WS and DS were presented. Contrary to our first prediction, the distribution of the part-of-speech categories in the speech samples revealed differences between the groups. The most striking differences concern the DS group, where a lower percentage of verbs, personal pronouns and relative pronouns together with a higher percentage of nouns was observed when compared to the WS and TD groups. Furthermore, the adolescents with WS showed less use of articles than the TD group, a relevant difference that had not been uncovered in the previous study by Diez-Itza et al. (2017). Such results confirm the necessity of taking into account the different proportion of each part-of-speech category in the language samples as a more reliable way of weighting the relative impact of the morphological errors.

The proportion of morphological errors in the DS group, nearly 10% of word tokens, is much higher than in the WS group, where less than 1% of the word tokens are affected by errors. Thus, results of the present study are coincident with previous studies indicating that grammatical morphology constitutes an area of specific weakness in persons with DS, as the observed number of morphological errors lies far beyond that expected for lexical verbal age (Fowler, 1990; Chapman et al., 1998; Miller, 1988; Singer-Harris et al., 1997; Vicari et al., 2000). On the other hand, contrary to our previous findings (Diez-Itza et al., 2017), the rate of morphological errors in the adolescents with WS was not significantly higher than that of the 5-year-old children in the TD group. The disparity between these findings may be attributed to age differences in the samples, as WS participants in the previous study included children, adolescents and adults. Nevertheless, the present study confirmed that grammatical morphology is not intact or preserved in adolescents with WS (Bellugi et al., 1988, 1990; Diez-Itza et al., 1998, 2017; Karmiloff-Smith et al., 1997; Mervis, 2006; Volterra et al., 1996).

When it comes to explaining the nature and the significance of the morphological errors observed in the adolescents with WS, debate arises amongst those who consider that they reflect either a selective impairment of some component (Clahsen & Almazan, 1998, 2001; Clahsen et al., 2004), or they present characteristics that respond to atypical trajectories of development (Thomas et al., 2001; Thomas & Karmiloff-Smith, 2003). Although to a lesser extent, a similar debate exists about whether the apparently deviated grammatical performance observed in the individuals with DS is the result of the asynchronous modular interaction of not deviant developmental patterns (Schaner-Wolles, 2004), or whether differences in the grammatical morphology are not only quantitative but also reveal an atypical trajectory of development (Diez-Itza & Miranda, 2007; Vicari et al., 2002, 2004).

To contribute to these discussions, we analysed the relative proportion of errors, that is to say, their distribution by grammatical categories, as in our previous studies of children and adolescents with DS (Diez-Itza & Miranda, 2007) and with WS (Diez-Itza et al., 2017). Nevertheless, in the present study, in contrast to previous research, we weighted the proportions according to the distribution of the parts of speech in the language samples. As it was already observed in the previous studies, the present findings confirmed our prediction that the percentage of errors would not be equal or homogeneous in all part-of-speech categories, which is against the hypothesis of a generalised grammatical delay in adolescents with DS (Fowler, 1990).

The adolescents with DS in the present study showed a high incidence of error in articles, personal pronouns and connecting words (prepositions and conjunctions), which indicates the same atypical profile observed in the previous study by Diez-Itza & Miranda (2007). Nevertheless, the results of that study should be qualified by considering the relative proportion of the different parts of speech. Relative frequency of errors, both in articles and in connecting words, which was previously estimated at around 30%, in the present study decreases to 25%. Conversely, the estimate of the relative incidence of errors in personal pronouns increases from 10% in the previous study to 20% in the present study. Overall, these three categories continue representing more than two-thirds of the total number of morphological errors. Thus, these results confirm the specific problems that can be observed in DS concerning the production of free morphemes (Fabbretti, Pizzuto, Vicari, & Volterra, 1997). We also found that relative incidence of error in verbs, less than 10%, is even lower than the observed in our previous study, which is consistent with the results in previous studies that observed unexpectedly low error rates in verb inflexion (Eadie et al., 2002; Schaner-Wolles, 2004).

Despite much lower error rates in the WS group, the relative distribution of morphological errors by parts of speech remained atypical in some aspects, which was also observed in the previous study by Diez-Itza et al. (2017). As in the DS group, the great majority of errors of the adolescents with WS were produced in articles, connecting words and personal pronouns. Thus, the advantage of the adolescents with WS in the production of free morphemes was only quantitative but, in relative terms, they presented an atypically high frequency of errors in function words similar to that of individuals with DS (Fabbretti et al., 1997). The main differences between the profiles of both groups lay in the very high relative incidence of errors in personal pronouns, nearly 35%, showed by the individuals with WS, which was also the only salient characteristic shared by the TD group and the WS group.

Finally, the analysis of the types of errors confirmed the prediction of a specific profile of the adolescents with DS characterised by a greater tendency for

Omission errors than for Substitution errors. While the tendency for Omission of free and bound morphemes has been highlighted as a characteristic of the DS profile that is shared with SLI (Eadie et al., 2002), it is important to point out that our results confirm that the tendency for Omission is also significantly greater in the WS group than in the TD group (Diez-Itza et al., 2017). The adolescents with WS also showed a significantly higher frequency of Addition errors than the TD children. Furthermore, the relative proportion of Addition errors in the WS group (18.5%) was much higher than in the DS group (4.5%), which constituted the principal difference between the morphological profiles of WS and DS. Atypical substitutions and additions had been previously described in both syndromes (Vicari et al., 2002; Volterra et al., 1996).

The differences observed in the grammatical profiles of the WS and DS groups could not be explained in terms of preservation of grammatical morphology in WS. Furthermore, differences observed in DS would not only be of grade as suggested by Finestack and Abbeduto (2010) when comparing DS with FXS. On the contrary, the morphological profiles of the WS and DS groups presented differential characteristics compared to those of the 5-year-old TD children, and therefore they may not correspond to a developmental delay (Benítez-Burraco et al., 2017). The results observed in the adolescents with WS and DS seem more consistent with the hypothesis of trajectories or patterns of divergent development from early stages in which the specificities are not yet appreciated (Galeote et al., 2014; Karmiloff-Smith, 1998). In the same vein, the profiles of grammatical morphology observed in adolescence could be interpreted as a developmental outcome of early morphological and phonological processing deficits (Danielsson, Henry, Messer, Carney, & Rönnberg, 2016; Lázaro et al., 2013).

Limitations of the study should be acknowledged. First, this was a preliminary study with a small sample size. Second, individual differences were not analysed even though they have repeatedly been described in DS and WS (Fabbretti et al., 1997; Stojanovik, Perkins, & Howard, 2006). Third, the choice of controls for studies of disordered groups remains controversial as TD controls matched for verbal age necessarily differ in many other aspects (Zukowski, 2005). Forth, while the method based on the analyses of spontaneous speech samples provides an advantage regarding ecological validity, it is not exempt from limitations. In addition to the differences between participants regarding conversational contexts, grammatical production of individuals with intellectual disabilities is less complex in spontaneous speech contexts (Abbeduto, Benson, Short, & Dolish, 1995).

Conclusions

The results of the present study confirmed findings from many previous studies indicating that the linguistic profile of DS shows a specific impairment in grammatical morphology. In contrast to the interpretations suggesting a global and non-specific delay in grammar, it was observed that adolescents with DS presented atypical characteristics in the distribution of the part-of-speech categories and in the frequency of omission of free morphemes. Even though the rate of error was much lower in the WS group than in the DS group, the morphological profile of the WS group also presented certain atypical characteristics that were similar to those observed in the DS group, such as the high relative proportion of errors in free morphemes, while others could be specific, such as the high relative proportion of addition errors. Overall, although it would be necessary to take into account the individual differences, as well as those introduced by the method of elicitation, the results obtained are compatible with dynamic approaches that interpret the distinct morphological profiles of the adolescents with WS and DS as the outcomes of atypical trajectories of development.

References

Abbeduto, L., Benson, G., Short, K., & Dolish, J. 1995. Effects of sampling context in the expressive language of children and adolescents with mental retardation. *Mental Retardation* 33, 279–288.

Bellugi, U., Bihrle, A., Jernigan, T., Trauner, D., & Doherty, S. 1990. Neuropsychological, neurological and neuroanatomical profile of Williams Syndrome. *American Journal of Medical Genetics* 6, 115–125.

Bellugi, U., Lichtenberger, L., Jones, W., Lai, Z., & St. George M. 2000. I. The neurocognitive profile of Williams Syndrome: A complex pattern of strengths and weaknesses. *Journal of Cognitive Neuroscience* 12(supplement 1), 7–29. https://doi.org/10.1162/089892900561959

Bellugi, U., Marks, S., Bihrle, A., & Sabo, H. 1988. Dissociation between language and cognitive functions in Williams Syndrome. In D. Bishop & K. Mogford (Eds.), *Language development in exceptional circumstances* (pp. 177–189). London: Churchill Livingstone.

Benítez-Burraco, A., Garayzábal, E., & Cuetos, F. 2017. Morphology in Spanish-speaking children with Williams syndrome. *Language and Cognition* 9, 728–740. https://doi.org/10.1017/langcog.2017.6

Clahsen, H., & Almazan, M. 1998. Syntax and morphology in Williams syndrome. *Cognition* 68(3), 167–198. https://doi.org/10.1016/S0010-0277(98)00049-3

Clahsen, H., & Almazan, M. 2001. Compounding and inflection in language impairment: Evidence from Williams Syndrome (and SLI). *Lingua* 111(10), 729–757. https://doi.org/10.1016/S0024-3841(00)00047-4

Clahsen, H., Ring, M., & Temple, C. 2004. Lexical and morphological skills in English-speaking children with Williams Syndrome. In S. Bartke & J. Siegmüller (Eds.), *Williams Syndrome across languages* (pp. 221–244). Amsterdam: John Benjamins. https://doi.org/10.1075/lald.36.14cla

Chapman, R. S., Seung, H. K., Schwartz, S. E., & Kay-Raining Bird, E. 1998. Language skills of children and adolescents with Down Syndrome, II: Production deficits. *Journal of Speech, Language, and Hearing Research* 34, 1106–1120. https://doi.org/10.1044/jslhr.4104.861

Danielsson, H., Henry, L., Messer, D., Carney, D. J. P., & Rönnberg, J. 2016. Developmental delays in phonological recoding among children and adolescents with Down Syndrome and Williams Syndrome. *Research in Developmental Disabilities* 55, 64–76. . https://doi.org/10.1016/j.ridd.2016.03.012

Diez-Itza, E., Antón, A., Fernández-Toral, J., & García, M. L. 1998. Language development in Spanish children with Williams Syndrome. In A. Aksu Koç, E. Erguvanli Taylan, A. Sumru Özsoy, & A. Küntay (Eds.), *Perspectives on language acquisition* (pp. 309–324). Istanbul, Turkey: Bogazici University Printhouse.

Diez-Itza, E., Martínez, V., Miranda, M., Antón, A., Ojea, A. I, ... Shiro, M. 2014. The syndroling project: A comparative linguistic analysis of typical development profiles and neurodevelopmental genetic syndromes (Williams, Down, and Fragile X Syndromes). XII *International Congress for the Study of Child Language*, Amsterdam. https://doi.org/10.13140/RG.2.1.3797.7365

Diez-Itza, E., Martínez, V., Fernández-Urquiza, M., & Antón, A. 2017. Morphological profile of Williams Syndrome: Typical or atypical? In A. Auza & R. G. Schwartz (Eds.), *Language development and disorders in Spanish-speaking children* (pp. 311–327). New York, NY: Springer. https://doi.org/10.1007/978-3-319-53646-0_15

Diez-Itza, E., & Miranda, M. 2007. Perfiles gramaticales específicos en el síndrome de Down. *Revista de Logopedia, Foniatría y Audiología* 27(4), 161–172. https://doi.org/10.1016/S0214-4603(07)70085-2

Eadie, P. A., Fey, M. E., Douglas, J. M. & Parsons, C. L. 2002. Profiles of grammatical morphology and sentence imitation in children with specific language impairment and Down Syndrome. *Journal of Speech, Language, and Hearing Research* 45, 720–732. https://doi.org/10.1044/1092-4388(2002/058)

Fabbretti, D., Pizzuto, E., Vicari, S., & Volterra, V. 1997. A story description task in children with Down's Syndrome: lexical and morphosyntactic abilities. *Journal of Intellectual Disability Research* 41(2), 165–179. https://doi.org/10.1111/j.1365-2788.1997.tb00693.x

Finestack, L. H., & Abbeduto, L. 2010. Expressive language profiles of verbally expressive adolescents and young adults with Down Syndrome or Fragile X Syndrome. *Journal of Speech, Language, and Hearing Research* 53(5), 1334–1348. https://doi.org/10.1044/1092-4388(2010/09-0125)

Fowler, A. 1990. Language abilities in children with Down Syndrome: Evidence for a specific syntactic delay. In D. Cicchetti & M. Beeghly (Eds.), *Children with Down Syndrome. A developmental perspective* (pp. 302–328). Cambridge: Cambridge University Press. https://doi.org/10.1017/CBO9780511581786.010

Galeote, M., Soto, P., Sebastián, E., Checa, E., & Sánchez-Palacios, C. 2014. Early grammatical development in Spanish children with Down Syndrome. *Journal of Child Language* 41, 111–131 https://doi.org/10.1017/S0305000912000591

Goldman-Rakic, P. S., 1998. The prefrontal landscape: implications of functional architecture for understanding human mentation and the central executive. In *The Prefrontal Cortex: Executive and Cognitive Functions*, A. C. Roberts, T. W. Robbins, & L. Weiskrantz (eds), 87–102. Oxford: Oxford University Press, Oxford.

Hsu, C. F., & Karmiloff-Smith, A. 2008. Language and Williams Syndrome. *Annual Review of Applied Linguistics* 28, 191–204. https://doi.org/10.1017/S0267190508080070

Karmiloff-Smith, A. 1998. Development itself is the key to understanding developmental disorders. *Trends in Cognitive Sciences* 2(10), 389–398. https://doi.org/10.1016/S1364-6613(98)01230-3

Karmiloff-Smith, A., Grant, J., Berthoud, I., Davies, M., Howlin, P., & Udwin, O. 1997. Language and Williams Syndrome: How intact is "intact"? *Child Development* 68(2), 246–262. https://doi.org/10.1111/j.1467-8624.1997.tb01938.x

Krause, M., & Penke, M. 2002. Inflectional morphology in German Williams Syndrome. *Brain and Cognition* 48, 410–413.

Lázaro, M., Garayzábal, E., & Moraleda, E. 2013. Differences on morphological and phonological processing between typically developing children and children with Down Syndrome. *Research in Developmental Disabilities* 34, 2065–2074. https://doi.org/10.1016/j.ridd.2013.03.027

Levin, H. S., Song, J., Swing-Cobbs, L. & Roberson, G. 2001. Porteus maze performance following traumatic brain injury in children. *Neuropsychology* 15(4), 557-567. https://doi.org/10.1037/0894-4105.15.4.557.

MacWhinney, B. 2000. *The CHILDES project: Tools for analyzing talk* (3rd ed.). Mahwah, NJ: Lawrence Erlbaum Associates.

Martin, G. E., Klusek, J., Estigarribia, B., & Roberts, J. E. 2009. Language characteristics of individuals with Down Syndrome. *Top Language Disorders* 29, 112–132. https://doi.org/10.1097/TLD.0b013e3181a71fe1

Mervis, C. B. 2006. Language abilities in Williams-Beuren Syndrome. In C. A. Morris, H. M. Lenhoff & P. P. Wang (Eds.), *Williams-Beuren Syndrome: Research, evaluation, and treatment*pp. (159–206). Baltimore, MD: Johns Hopkins University Press.

Mervis, C. B., & Robinson, B. F. 2000. Expressive vocabulary ability of toddlers with Williams Syndrome or Down Syndrome: A comparison. *Developmental Neuropsychology* 17, 111–126. https://doi.org/10.1207/S15326942DN1701_07

Miller, J. F. 1988. The developmental asynchrony of language development in children with Down Syndrome. In L. Nadel (Ed.), *The psychobiology of Down Syndrome*pp. (167–198). Cambridge MA: The MIT Press.

Oliver, A., Johnson, M. H., Karmiloff-Smith, A., & Pennington, B. 2000. Deviations in the emergence of representations: A neuroconstructivist framework for analysing developmental disorders. *Developmental Science* 3(1), 1–23. https://doi.org/10.1111/1467-7687.00094

Pinker. S. 1991. Rules of language. *Science* 253, 530–535. https://doi.org/10.1126/science.1857983

Petrides, M. 2000. Dissociable Roles of Mid-Dorsolateral Prefrontal and Anterior Inferotemporal Cortex in Visual Working Memory. *The Journal of Neuroscience* 20(19):7496-7503. https://doi.org/10.1523/jneurosci.20-19-07496.2000.

Rutter, T., & Buckley, S. 1994. The acquisition of grammatical morphemes in children with Down Syndrome. *Down Syndrome Research and Practice* 2, 76 -82. https://doi.org/10.3104/reports.34

Schaner-Wolles, C. 2004. Spared domain-specific cognitive capacities? Syntax and morphology in Williams Syndrome and Down Syndrome. In S. Bartke & J. Siegmüller (Eds.), *Williams Syndrome across languages* (pp. 93–124). Amsterdam: John Benjamins. https://doi.org/10.1075/lald.36.09sch

Schalock, R. L., Borthwick-Duffy, S. A., Bradley, V. J., Buntinx, W. H. E., Coulter, D. L., Craig, E. M., … Yeager, M. H. 2010. *Intellectual disability: Definition, classification, and systems of supports*. Washington, DC: American Association on Intellectual and Developmental Disabilities.

Singer-Harris, N. G., Bellugi, U., Bates, E., Jones, W., & Rossen, M. 1997. Contrasting profiles of language development in children with Williams and Down Syndromes. In D. Thal & J. Reilly (Eds.), *Special issue on Origins of Communication Disorders, Developmental Neuropsychology* 13(3), 345–370. https://doi.org/10.1080/87565649709540683

Stojanovik, V., Perkins, M., & Howard, S. 2006. Linguistic heterogeneity in Williams Syndrome. *Clinical Linguistics & Phonetics* 20(7–8), 547–552, https://doi.org/10.1080/02699200500266422

Thomas, M. S. C., Grant, J., Barham, Z., Gsödl, M., Laing, E., Lakusta, L., … Karmiloff-Smith, A. 2001. Past tense formation in Williams Syndrome. *Language and Cognitive Processes* 16(2–3), 143–176. https://doi.org/10.1080/01690960042000021

Thomas, M. S. C., & Karmiloff-Smith, A. 2003. Modeling language acquisition in atypical phenotypes. *Psychological Review* 110(4), 647–682. https://doi.org/10.1037/0033-295X.110.4.647

Vicari, S., Bates, E., Caselli, M. C., Pasqualetti, P., Gagliardi, C., Tonucci, F., & Volterra, V. 2004. Neuropsychological profile of Italians with Williams Syndrome: An example of a dissociation between language and cognition? *Journal of the International Neuropsychological Society* 10(6), 862–876. https://doi.org/10.1017/S1355617704106073

Vicari, S., Caselli, M. C., Gagliardi, C., Tonucci, F., & Volterra, V. 2002. Language acquisition in special populations: A comparison between Down and Williams Syndromes. *Neuropsychologia* 40(13), 2461–2470. https://doi.org/10.1016/S0028-3932(02)00083-0

Vicari, S., Caselli, M. C., & Tonucci, F. 2000. Asynchrony of lexical and morphosyntactic development in children with Down Syndrome. *Neuropsychologia* 38, 634–644. https://doi.org/10.1016/S0028-3932(99)00110-4

Volterra, V., Capirci, O., Pezzini, G., Sabbadini, L., & Vicari, S. 1996. Linguistic abilities in Italian children with Williams Syndrome. *Cortex* 32(4), 663–677. https://doi.org/10.1016/S0010-9452(96)80037-2

Zukowski, A. 2005. Knowledge of constraints on compounding in children and adolescents with Williams Syndrome. *Journal of Speech, Language, and Hearing Research* 48, 79–92. https://doi.org/10.1044/1092-4388(2005/007)

Evaluative language and component structure of oral narratives in Williams Syndrome

Martha Shiro,[1] Eliseo Díez-Itza[2] and Maite Fernández-Urquiza[2]
[1]Universidad Central de Venezuela / [2]Universidad de Oviedo, España

Williams Syndrome narratives tend to display atypically frequent uses of evaluative language. The aim of the present study is to determine the narrative language profiles of a group of 12 WS participants. We video-recorded their oral recounts of a wordless animated video and compared them to those of typically developing children matched for verbal abilities (matched by MLU). We analyzed narrative structure and evaluative devices referring to internal states and to evidentiality. Our findings suggest that the narrative length and structure of WS and TD groups were similar, but the WS narratives lacked overall coherence and clarity. The use of evaluative language in WS was at the level expected for verbal age, and thus, not significantly excessive.

Keywords: Williams Syndrome, narrative profile, evaluative language

Introduction

Williams Syndrome (WS) is a rare genetic neurodevelopmental disorder caused by the microdeletion on the long arm of chromosome 7 (7q11.23). Individuals with WS have a particular neurocognitive profile which corresponds to a range of intellectual disabilities marked by contrasts between strengths and weaknesses (Bellugi et al., 2000). Initially, some of these contrasts were explained in terms of dissociations between different cognitive domains and, in particular, between preserved language abilities and spatial cognition which is severely affected (Bellugi et al., 1988). Research in languages other than English has found that certain language abilities are also affected, given that asymmetries were detected between the different language components, particularly those related to pragmatic abilities in comparison with grammar skills (Diez-Itza et al., 1998; Karmiloff-Smith et al., 1997; Volterra et al., 1996). Despite a strong tendency of being unusually sociable (Järvinen-Pasley et al., 2008; Jones et al., 2000), individuals with WS were found

https://doi.org/10.1075/z.223.14shi

to be impaired in their pragmatic skills (Fernández-Urquiza et al., 2015; Laws & Bishop, 2004; Stojanovik, 2006), including performance in narrative tasks (Losh et al., 2000; Reilly et al., 1990).

From very early on, children are surrounded by narratives and they start telling stories of their own. As a result, narratives can be easily elicited and are, therefore, a type of extended discourse where developing language skills can be detected in a naturalistic context (Johnstone, 2009). Furthermore, the skills that are required for story telling are developmentally more challenging than the skills involved in day-to-day conversations (Hudson & Shapiro, 1991). Oral narratives require planning for longer turns. As a result, the narrator must use strategies to hold the floor and keep the listener's attention, so that the story would be perceived as interesting and relevant for the interlocutors (Shiro, 2003). Canonical narratives follow a predetermined sequence of components, most of which are present in children's narratives: abstract, orientation, complicating action, high point, resolution and coda (Labov, 1972). Similarly, the narrator is building a story-world, which is displaced from the narrator's world in space and time and which evolves on two planes, the factual and the non-factual (Bruner, 1986). As a result, evaluative devices are required to motivate events and to construct the complex perspective building in story-telling, whereby voices can shift from one character to another and back to the narrator (Shiro 2003, 2008).

There is abundant research on typically developing (TD) children's narratives, focusing not only on narrative discourse and language proficiency, but also on socio-cognitive and emotional development (Astington, 1990; Fivush et al., 2006). Fictional story telling and retelling develop later than personal narratives, as they have a more complex structure, a higher number of characters and episodes, and more evaluative language from a combination of voices, including the speech of characters and onomatopoeia to dramatize the story (Shiro, 2003, 2008).

A series of studies examined the evaluative dimension of the WS pragmatic profile in English-speaking individuals, using the *Frog Story* books (e.g. *Frog where are you?* Mayer, 1969) to elicit narratives (Losh et al., 2000; Reilly et al., 1990, 2004, 2005). The first study addressing this issue provided an original perspective on WS individuals' atypical social cognitive domain (Reilly et al., 1990). Following Labov and Waletzky's (1967) study, they compared the use of evaluative language used by WS and Down Syndrome (DS) IQ-matched adolescents and TD children. The stories produced by WS participants were structurally coherent and grammatically complex as they all included orientation with reference to time, place, characters and their internal states, complicating events and resolution. They also found that the WS group used more evaluative devices than DS or TD controls. In a more recent study, Reilly et al. (2004) reported similar findings when comparing WS children' narratives to those of children with SLI. Evaluative devices such as affective enhancers (reference to emotions, reported speech, onomatopoeia) and audience hookers (dramatization strategies such as affective prosody, use of character voice, emphasis), were used more frequently in the WS narratives, but they showed a lower frequency of cognitive inferences (reference to mental states, character motivation, and causality) when compared to TD and SLI. The high frequency of affective prosody and evaluative devices, even though they enrich WS narratives, attracting the listener's attention and empathy, were considered atypical as only older TD individuals were found to use them in similar ways when their narratives were addressed to preschoolers (Bamberg & Damrad-Frye, 1991).

The use of evaluative devices in narratives, for the purpose of engaging and involving their communicative partner, was also explored by Losh et al. (2000, p. 269), who compared WS and TD children matched for chronological and mental age. Following Reilly et al. (1990), they coded for cognitive inferences (character's motivation, causality and reference to mental states), social engagement devices (sound effects, reported speech and audience hookers) and hedges (levels of un/certainty). The WS children used fewer cognitive inferences than their TD peers but a surprisingly higher frequency of social engagement devices. This feature was considered abnormal and a consequence of their hypersociability, given that they were more engaged in attracting the interlocutor's interest than in focusing on the plot.

Research on WS speakers of Romance languages used a similar methodological framework to determine their narrative profile. Reilly et al. (2005) compared WS speakers of American English, Italian and French. Irrespective of cultural or language differences, the WS individuals displayed an unusual social conduct, and an atypically frequent use of social evaluative expressions. They also report that the frequency of evaluative expressions was highest in Italian WS speakers and lowest in French speakers, concluding thus that these uses may be language dependent. Similarly, Lacroix et al. (2007) found an atypical pragmatic evaluative profile in French speakers, comparing WS children, adolescents, and adults to DS and TD groups matched for chronological and mental age. Evaluative language was also analyzed in two studies exploring the narrative competence of Spanish- and Portuguese-speaking individuals with WS (Garayzábal et al., 2007; Gonçalves et al., 2010). Garayzábal et al. (2007) found that WS participants produced low quality narratives, in terms of narrative structure and coherence as well as in terms of narrative content (topic diversity, events and characters). The only aspect found to be consistent in WS narratives was the reference to affective states and the use of social engagement devices. Gonçalves et al. (2010) also reported a moderate use of emotional and cognitive evaluative devices as well as audience hookers (onomatopoeias, interjections, hesitations, modulation of emotional prosody), indicating that this is the only aspect in which there were no differences between WS and TD chronological age-matched controls. The authors concluded that WS narratives reflect a relative preservation of the social-expressive component of narrative construction, which may compensate for the deficiencies displayed at a global level in narrative production.

In sum, these studies have detected interesting associations between the acquisition of language structures in WS language development, on the one hand, and the uses of language for social purposes, on the other. The findings suggest that the excessive use of evaluative devices seems to be compatible with the ability of WS individuals to express emotions (Lacroix et al., 2007). Particularly, the evaluative dimension of language represents a strength in social expression, which contrasts with important limitations in social perception, explaining thus the paradox observed in the WS population: despite the unusually high motivation to socially interact, WS individuals have difficulties establishing and maintaining social relations (Bellugi et al., 2007).

Furthermore, the pragmatic profile revealed by previous research is not homogeneous in the WS population, showing a relative weakness in narrative organization and a relative strength in evaluation. Thus, as part of a larger project (*The Syndroling Project*, Diez-Itza et al., 2014), in which WS, DS and Fragile X Syndrome (FXS) individuals are compared, our aim in this study is to determine the pragmatic profile in narrative production of WS children, adolescents and adults. Our approach differs slightly from the research reviewed here. First, we compare the WS group with a TD control group matched for language proficiency, rather than chronological or mental age, in order to control for the effects that the differences in language proficiency may have on the narrative skills we intend to examine (Diez-Itza et al., 2017). Second, our elicitation method is more closely related to spontaneous narrative practices as the participants are expected to recount a story based on a short cartoon, a discourse practice that is quite common in natural interactions (Shiro 2003). Finally, our coding scheme is based on pragmatic categories specifically devised for the detailed analysis of oral language corpora, which enable us to better identify and classify the linguistic markers associated with those narrative features (Shiro 2003, 2007).

Thus, the research questions we address in this paper are:

1. How do WS individuals organize their narratives based on a wordless cartoon and how does it compare to TD narratives based on the same cartoon?
2. What evaluative resources do WS participants use in narratives and how do they compare to TD children's evaluative resources in similar narratives?

Method

Participants

Twelve participants with WS took part in the present study. Their mean chronological age was 20;7 (range: 8;10–39;1). All participants had been previously diagnosed with WS using the FISH test (Fluorescence in Situ Hybridization) and presented the typical clinical phenotype. They were matched to a group of 12 five-year-old TD children, on the basis of gender, socio-economic status and mean length of utterance measured in words (MLUw), previously measured in spontaneous conversation, as an indicator of verbal age and language proficiency, particularly grammatical complexity. Previous research indicated that MLUw matched WS and TD groups show similar morphology (Diez-Itza et al., 2017). On this basis, the present study intends to control for the effect of grammatical competence on narrative abilities, specifically those related to narrative structure and evaluation. The WS group had a mean MLUw of 7 (range: 4,4–13,4). The TD group had a mean age of 5;8 (range: 5;4–6;5), and a mean MLUw of 6;6 (range: 4,7–10,3).

Procedure and coding

The participants' narratives were elicited using the six-minute silent film *The Puppy Tale* from the *Tom & Jerry* cartoon series. We chose to use a video to elicit the narratives, rather than the *Frog Stories*, as used by previous research, because we intended to eliminate the visual or memory aid that the presence of the book could have provided, prompting the participant to produce a narrative rather than describe the pictures. Research on narrative development highlights the important effect elicitation methods and prompts can have on narrative production (Castilla-Earls & Eriks-Brophy, 2012; Gazella & Stockman, 2003; Shiro, 2003). We chose a *Tom & Jerry* cartoon because we consider that it is an appropriate prompt for the children in the TD group as well as for the older participants in the WS group. In a comparative study on TD children and adults, Shiro (2001–2002) found that adults not only do well but they also enjoy narrating children's cartoons. Thus, we can compare more reliably the performance of children and adults, using the same video as a prompt.

Immediately after viewing the film, the participants were prompted to tell the story to an experienced researcher whilst being video-recorded. Our aim was to collect narratives which were as ecologically valid as possible.

The narratives were transcribed and coded using the CHAT transcription format provided by the CHILDES Project (MacWhinney, 2000). Total number of utterances, total number of word types and tokens, and mean length of utterance in words (MLUw) were computed by means of the CLAN software. The utterances produced by the child in the interview were further divided into clauses and marked in the transcripts by the researchers. Each transcript was coded for narrative structure and evaluative language. All three authors coded the narrative utterances according to the coding scheme. The coded narrative by one of the authors was revised by the other two and all discrepancies were discussed until agreement was reached.

Our coding scheme, which attempts to give a detailed and integrated view of narrative abilities, was adopted from previous studies on Spanish speaking TD children's narrative profile (Shiro 2003, 2007). We coded for narrative structure only within the child's spontaneous recount of the video, as we identified abstract, orientation, complicating action, resolution and coda. Subsequently, the interviewer asked follow up questions, and we coded the child's responses as additions, if they were related to the story line, or asides if they were unrelated.

The coding scheme for evaluative language has two dimensions: evaluative expressions, understood as the speaker's references to internal states, and evidential markers, understood as the speaker's attitude towards knowledge (Shiro, 2003, 2007; Mushin, 2001). Thus, the evaluative categories included expressions of attributes, emotion, intention, cognition, physical internal states and reported speech (Table 1). The evidential dimension included expressions referring to the speaker's source of knowledge (perception), modes of knowing (causality –cause and purpose-, epistemic and deontic stance, ability), and enhancers (intensifiers-mitigators, comparatives and emphasizers) (Table 2).

Table 1. Examples of evaluative expressions (in bold)

Attribute	he dreamt about **terrible** things.
Cognition	I **don't know** what happened next.
Emotion	and the cat was very **angry** with them.
Intention	all the dogs came **to drink the milk**.
Physical	the cat **was sleeping**.
Reported speech	and he said **you can't come in**.

Table 2. Examples of evidential expressions

Mode of knowing	
Causality	**because** he's having nightmares.
Ability	the little puppy **couldn't come in**.
Deontic	he **had to** go and save them.
Epistemic	it **seemed to be** a cat.

Table 2. (*continued*)

Source of knowledge	
Perception	I saw a mouse saving a dog.
Enhancers	
Intensify	and they made **a lot of** noise.
Compare	the dog was licking **the other** dog.
Emphasize	**oh, yeah, yeah, yeah, it's true!**

Results

The average number of clauses produced in the interview was quite similar for the two groups as shown in Table 3. Even though the average number of clauses produced by the TD group is slightly higher than that of the WS group, the mean number of word tokens is slightly lower. Thus, there is no difference in the amount of speech produced by the two groups. Similarly, there is no difference in the lexical diversity as measured by number of word types, and in the grammatical complexity of their utterances as measured by MLUw.

Table 3. Descriptive measures of narratives

Group	Nr. clauses	Nr. Word Tokens	Nr. Word Types	MLUw
Williams Syndrome	42.83	215.67	88.33	7.01
Range	16–77	93–430	50–152	4.39–13.43
Standard Deviation	17.72	105.33	28.91	2.56
Typical Development	45.42	209.75	86.50	6.4
Range	31–101	132–447	65-163	4.71–10.34
Standard Deviation	19.84	92.34	27.41	1.73

The structure of the interview, i.e. utterances that belonged to the narrative spontaneously produced by the child vs. additions and asides, did not show statistically significant differences (Table 4). The WS group's spontaneous narratives were very similar in length to those of TD children. The TD children produced a higher proportion of additions, directly related to the story, when prompted by the interviewer, whereas the WS individuals produced more talk unrelated to the story.

Table 4. The structure of the interview

Group	Narrative utterances	Additions	Asides
Williams Syndrome	15.0 (53.7%)	8.9 (30.6%)	5.1 (15.7%)
Typical Development	14.2 (51.4%)	11.0 (38.3%)	3.1 (10.3%)

Narrative structure

In Figure 1 we present the average number of clauses devoted to the components that formed the narrative structure. It is worth mentioning that our analysis of the TD group`s narrative structure is based on 11 children's data. One TD child was excluded from this analysis, because he did not recount spontaneously the *Tom & Jerry* video, but was included in the other analyses, given that he did respond adequately to the interviewer's follow up questions, with relevant information on the story plot.

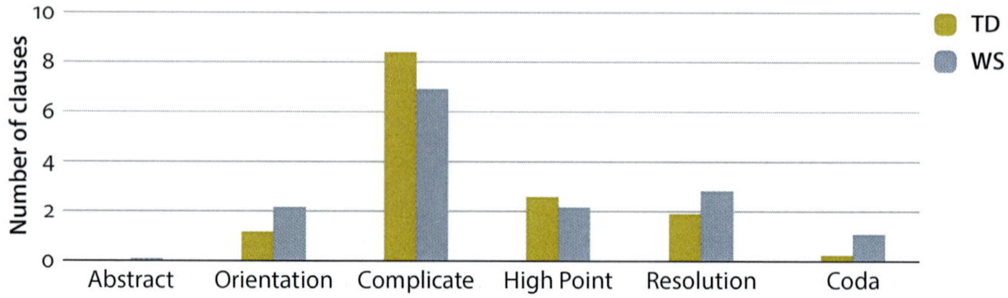

Figure 1. Narrative components

As expected, abstracts were scarcely present. Only one WS child (age 18, MLUw 8.34) began the story with an abstract (*Pues, vi a un ratón que rescataba a un perro* 'I saw a mouse rescuing a dog'). Most participants in both groups (11 WS and 9 TD) produced stories with orientation. However, despite the fact that WS participants devoted a larger proportion of their stories to orientation than their TD peers, the information did not contribute to the clarity of the story. As shown in Example 1, a WS participant's orientation seemingly includes a great number of details, but, actually, it is irrelevant to the future development of the story, as it does not help the interlocutor understand the opening scene of the narrative.

Example 1. Pilar (Age 22;2.19, MLUw 7.86)

> *un cachorrín y un perro estaban en el río, y entonces pues uno iba detrás de otro y cada poco le lamía el chiquitín al grande, como si fuera un lobo, el malo, y entonces llamaba al otro perro con el ladrido*
> ('a puppy and a dog were in the river, one behind the other, and the puppy was licking the big dog, as if he were a wolf, a bad one, and then, he was barking as he was calling the other dog').

All participants, in both groups, included complicating actions in their narratives. In fact, a narrative should have, by definition, at least a sequence of two events that forms a complicating action (Labov, 1972). As expected, the largest part of the narratives in both groups was devoted to complicating action (Figure 1), but the TD group produced, on average, more clauses with complicating actions than the WS group. The complicating action may be detailed in the WS group, but still hard to follow.

Example 2. Valeria (Age 24;3.1 MLUw 13.43)

El ratón salió a la calle a echar un papelito; y un coche que pasó por el puente tiró unos perros por el río; cogió una caña y los cogió; uno quedó, los otros marcharon corriendo; y luego le cogió cariño y se fue con él a su casa; y luego llegó a la casa del ratón y no entraban en la casa del ratón; luego quedó afuera y le indicó por dónde tenía que entrar; luego vio algo de beber, como leche o algo; el gato oyó que estaba alguien bebiendo y apartó al ratón para que no le hiciera daño al perro; luego el ratón fue detrás del perro para ver dónde estaba; luego le echó fuera el gato al perro y cogió una caña el ratón para subirlo arriba con él; luego, al llegar un momentito a casa, cogió el perro y le quitó el manto al gato; el gato se enfadó y lo volvió a echar afuera; luego, volvió otra vez el perro; entonces el gato fue detrás del ratón y del perro y les echó fuera a los dos de la casa.

('The mouse went out and threw a piece of paper in the street; and a car that was crossing the bridge threw some dogs into the river; [he] took a stick and caught them; one stayed, the others ran away; and then [he] got to like him and took him home; and then [he] showed him how to get into the house; then [he] arrived at the mouse's house and [they] couldn't get into the mouse's house; then, [he] saw some drink, like milk or something; the cat heard that somebody was drinking and pushed the mouse to take him up with him; then, as [he] arrived home for a moment, [he] took the dog and took away the blanket from the cat; the cat got angry and threw him out again; then, the dog returned; then the cat followed the mouse and the dog and threw both of them out').

In Example 2, one of the most elaborate in the WS group, Valeria follows quite closely the events reflected in the images on the screen, but the story turns out to be repetitive, there is too much information and the characters are not clearly identified.

Compare this to the complicating action of a 5-year-old TD child's narrative (Example 3), where the same sequence of events is summarized and the characters are identified more clearly (using resources like mentioning their names).

Example 3. José (Age 5;8.3 MLUw 5.55)

[Jerry] encontró un saco, lo sacó del agua y vio que era un perro; entonces empezaron a jugar; entonces los demás perros entraron a la casa y vieron a Tom que estaba dormido; entonces se pusieron a pelear; entonces el gato que era muy fuerte también salió y vio que cayeron al agua.

('[Jerry] found a bag, took it out from the water and saw that there was a dog; then [they] started to play; then the other dogs came into the house and saw

Tom who was asleep; then [they] started fighting; then the cat who was strong came out and saw that [they] fell into the water').

José relies on shared knowledge with the interlocutor and expects that the co-reference of the cat and Tom would be understood as well as the distinction between Jerry, the mouse, and the dog who is introduced in the following clause.

The complicating events lead to a high point in the narratives of 10 (out of 12) WS participants and all 11 TD children. Both groups devoted a similar portion of their stories to the high point (Figure 1). In Example 4, Jaime reaches a high point in his story with a rapid sequence of highly evaluated utterances.

Example 4. Jaime (Age 19;9.12 MLUw 4.94)

Se estaba ahogando, tuvo pesadillas, el gato y tuvo que ir a rescatarles; y el gato silbaba con el paraguas.

('[he] was drowning, had nightmares, the cat, and [he] had to rescue them; and the cat was whistling with the umbrella').

Similarly, most participants (10 out of 12 WS and 9 out of 11 TD) included resolutions in their stories, following the structure of the images on the screen. The WS participants' stories resolution was, on average, slightly longer than that of their TD peers (Figure 1). Thus, Jaime's narrative continues with the resolution:

Example 5. (Jaime Age 19;9.12 MLUw 4.94)

De pronto rescataron al gato ellos dos; el perro y el ratón fueron en busca de él y lo llevaron para la casa, para darle la cosa para curarse bien; y el gato le dio leche y cama; y luego, los perritos, entraron muchos.

('All of a sudden they both rescued the cat; the dog and the mouse were looking for him and took him home, gave him the thing to get well; and the cat gave him milk and bed; and then, the puppies came in, many').

Surprisingly, the majority of WS participants ended their stories with a coda (with the exception of 2 out of 12), whereas only 2 (out of 11) TD children had codas. The presence of codas was significantly higher in the WS group ($t = 4.105$; $p < .001$). The codas consisted of formulaic expressions (e.g. *nada más* 'nothing more', *(y ya) se acabó* 'and it's over').

In sum, the narrative structure is similar in both groups and sometimes it appears to be more elaborate in the WS group (e.g. significantly more WS participants use codas, their orientations are considerably longer). However, a qualitative analysis implies that the more elaborate and extended structure of the components does not contribute to the clarity of the story. TD children tend to be more precise in the introduction of the story characters and less repetitive in the sequence of events.

Narrative evaluation: Evaluative expressions

To determine the uses of narrative evaluation, we coded for markers of subjectivity on two dimensions: the evaluative dimension and the evidential dimension.

As shown in Figure 2, the evaluative categories are very similar in both groups. Almost all participants used all the evaluative categories, references to physical states, cognition and emotion being the most frequent. The average frequencies devoted to each category were quite similar for both groups, with the exception of reference to emotions and internal physical states: on the one hand, WS narratives include more references to emotions than TD narratives, and, on the other, TD narratives include more references to physical states than WS narratives.

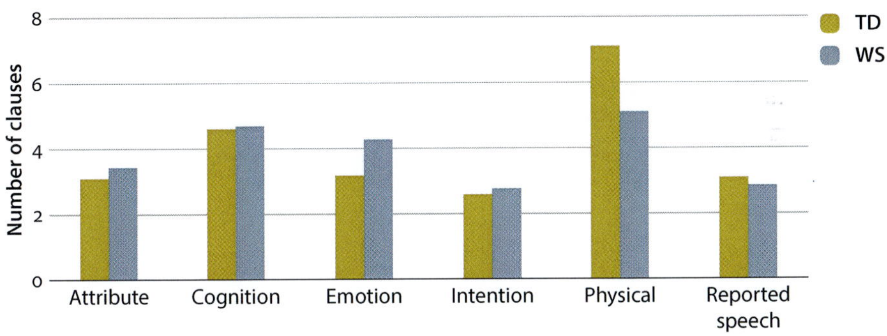

Figure 2. Evaluative expressions

Reported speech has been found to be a characteristic feature of WS narratives. We have not detected major differences between WS and TD narratives in this respect (Figure 2). As studies on WS narratives have found that an important distinction between their stories and those of TD narratives was the presence of markers of social engagement and attention hookers (Losh et al., 2000; Reilly et al., 1990, 2004), we examined the types of reported speech found in our corpus (Figure 3), including here onomatopoeic sounds produced by the participants in the context of narrative production. These expressions help dramatize the story, because the narrator has to mark the different voices in the narrative by changing pitch and intonation.

TD children tend to use more Direct Speech, usually preceded by a reporting clause (underlined in Example 6), whereas WS participants use more free and indirect reporting as well as onomatopoeia (in bold in Example 6). Surprisingly, very few participants used onomatopoeia as a narrative resource, even though studies report frequent use of these expressions, particularly in fictional narratives (Shiro, 2003, 2012, 2014) and more specifically in WS narratives (Reilly et al.,1990).

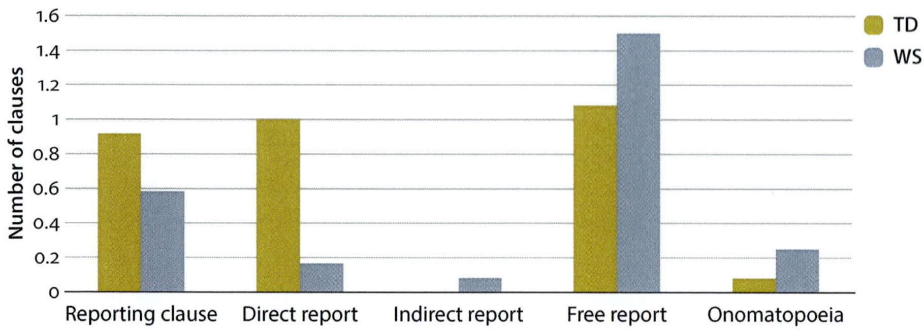

Figure 3. Types of reported speech

Example 6. (Jaime Age 19;9.12 MLUw 4.94)

y el perrito dijo ***guau, guau, guau, guau*** *y dijo el gato* ***[silba]*** *y entró en casa que estaba ahí un gato y dijo el gato* ***miau.***

('and the puppy said **woof woof woof woof** and the cat said (**whistle**) and [he] came into the house where the cat was and the cat said **meow**').

Narrative evaluation: Evidential markers

There are no significant differences between the WS and the TD groups with respect to evidential markers (Figure 4). A closer look at the data shows that some of the evidential markers, such as deontic modality, were barely present in either the WS or in the TD narratives, while others were scarcely used by WS participants when compared to TD children (reference to ability was used by 7 TD children, but only by 1 WS child). Other frequencies were also low, such as causality, but was used more in TD children's stories.

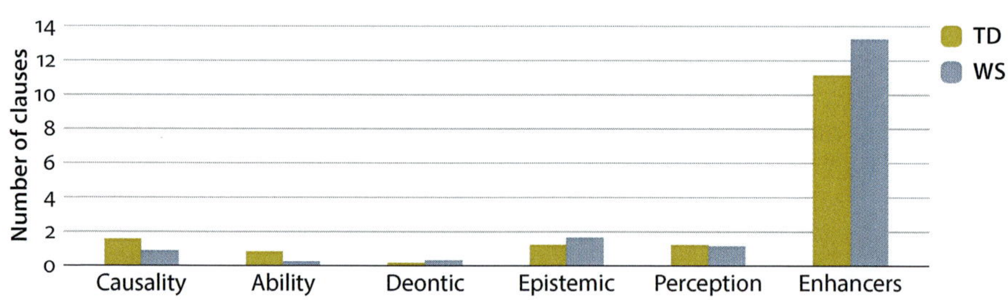

Figure 4. Evidential markers

The major difference in evidential markers was the use of enhancers (intensifiers-mitigators, comparatives and emphasis). All participants used enhancers in their narratives, but WS participants used it more frequently than TD children. This difference implies that WS stories tend to be more emphatic or tentative than TD narratives, as pointed out by other researchers (Garayzábal et al., 2007; Gonçalves et al., 2010).

Discussion and conclusions

In this chapter, we have presented the characteristics of the pragmatic evaluative profile of Spanish-speaking WS individuals in narrative production. We explored the evaluative and evidential devices used in fictional narratives as the participants were prompted to recount a wordless video, an episode of the *Tom & Jerry* television cartoon series. Unlike previous research (Losh et al., 2000; Reilly et al., 1990, 2004, 2005), our control group consisted of TD children matched for MLU with the WS group, controlling thus for language proficiency measured in terms of grammatical complexity. As both groups were capable of producing similar narratives, in terms of extension and structure, we can conclude that the criterion to compare the WS group with a TD control group on the basis of verbal age (MLU) may be adequate. Furthermore, studies have found that verbal age, measured with the Peabody Test, is quite similar to mental age (Diez-Itza et al., 2016; Garayzábal et al., 2007) or to "a posteriori" measures of MLU (Marini et al., 2010). Based on this, it is possible to assume then that our control TD group and the WS group, matched for MLU in the current study, may be also similar in mental age.

As in Reilly et al. (1990), seminal study, we also found that the WS group's stories contain all the components found in canonical narratives, including high points and resolutions, in a similar proportion to the TD group. Thus, both groups showed incipient skills in creating high points in their stories, despite the fact that most studies on children's narratives report that only at a later age do children produce narratives with high points (McCabe & Peterson, 1991; McCabe & Rollins, 1994; Hemphill et al., 1994; Shiro, 2003).

However, the WS group's narratives contained irrelevant details and repetitions, which did not contribute to the overall coherence of the story, as was pointed out by other studies, particularly on WS speakers of Romance languages (Lacroix et al., 2007; Garayzábal et al., 2007; Gonçalves et al., 2010; Reilly et al., 2005). Furthermore, the WS group produced more unrelated responses (asides) to follow-up questions, whereas the TD group elaborated more on the plot (additions). This may indicate that TD children were more focused on the task at hand, as they were able to elaborate and enrich their stories by responding to the interviewer's questions. These findings suggest that there is a dissociation between the micro and the macro-structural narrative skills in the WS population, which may account for the lack of clarity in their narratives, as pointed out previously (Diez-Itza et al., 2016; Garayzábal et al., 2007; Marini et al., 2010).

Unlike other studies (Lacroix et al., 2007; Losh et al., 2000; Reilly et al., 1990, 2004, 2005), our analysis did not find that WS stories had excessive, and therefore atypical, use of evaluative devices when compared to their TD peers. The WS group showed a tendency to an increased use only when referring to emotional states. With respect to the social engagement devices that other studies found as an outstanding feature of WS narratives (Jones et al., 2000; Losh et al., 2000, Reilly et al., 1990), in our study there were no significant differences, in line with the findings of Garayzábal et al. (2007) and Gonçalves et al. (2010). However, the WS group tended to use slightly more expressions of emotion, onomatopoeia and enhancers than the TD group.

There can be several reasons for these different results. On the one hand, as we controlled for language proficiency and as the use of evaluative resources relies heavily on linguistic abilities, the WS individuals may have looked quite similar to TD children in this respect, even though there was a considerable difference in their chronological ages. On the other hand, our findings may differ due to our elicitation method (Castilla-Earls & Eriks-Brophy, 2012; Gazella & Stockman, 2003; Shiro, 2003). Most studies on WS narratives used *Frog Stories* as prompts, which implied that the participants were looking at the illustrations in the book, together with the interviewer, while they were telling the story. We used the *Tom & Jerry* video and, therefore, there was no visual prompt during the story-telling activity. The interviewer's attention was focused solely on the child and, as a result, there was less need for attention hookers in this context, unlike in the multimodal book reading context of the *Frog Stories*, where the child's attention was divided between the book and the interviewer. This fact may explain the finding that WS individuals' excessive use of social engagement devices in narratives is parallel to their atypical use of expressive utterances in collaborative conversation (Lacroix et al., 2007). We found that WS narratives included significantly more codas than the TD group, frequently using closure discourse markers (Diez-Itza et al., 2016).

Similar to previous research, our findings suggest that WS narratives are no less expressive than those of their TD peers, but they lack integrative qualities and are more tentative (due to the frequent use of hedges) and unfocused (with respect to plot clarity) (Garayzábal et al., 2007; Gonçalves et al., 2010; Reilly et al., 2004). It is possible to conclude then, as Bellugi et al. (2007) have done, that WS social engagement, as displayed in their atypically friendly behavior, and their narrative profile present convergent as well as divergent aspects.

The WS participants in this study had similar language proficiency, as measured in grammatical complexity, as the TD control group, but they differed greatly in chronological age, which might constitute a limitation of this study. However, it is safe to assume that comparing WS and TD individuals of the same chronological age would lead to very different results in narrative skills, as the use of evaluative resources in narratives increases greatly with age in TD population (Shiro, 2003, 2007; Bamberg & Damrad-Frye, 1991; Berman, 2004). Therefore, the differences found in groups matched for chronological age would result precisely from the language or intellectual limitations of the WS population.

In sum, the findings of our study imply that WS' narrative profile (including the pragmatic aspects of narrative abilities) is heterogeneous, a feature shared with their language and neuropsychological profiles. Even though pragmatic skills tend to be considered as weak in the WS population, our data suggest that WS individuals were able to construct a story where the principal narrative components were present, the main characters were introduced and the evaluative resources were similar to those of their TD peers, matched for linguistic proficiency. Thus, the conclusion that can be drawn is that the use of evaluative devices in narratives constitutes a relative strength in WS individuals, implying that therapeutic language intervention would be beneficial if it included narratives, taking advantage of this strength in the WS population (Diez-Itza et al., 2018; Semel & Rosner, 2003).

References

Astington, J. 1990. Narrative and the child's theory of mind. In B. Britton & A. Pellegrini (Eds.), *Narrative thought and narrative language* (pp. 151–172). Hillsdale, NJ: Lawrence Erlbaum Associates.

Bamberg, M., & Damrad-Frye, R. 1991. On the ability to provide evaluative comments: Further explorations of children's narrative competencies. *Journal of Child Language* 18(3), 689–710. https://doi.org/10.1017/S0305000900011314

Bellugi, U., Jarvinen-Pasley, A., Doyle, T. F., Reilly, J., Reiss, L., & Korenberg, J. R. 2007. Affect, social behavior, and the brain in Williams Syndrome. *Current Directions in Psychological Science* 16(2), 99–104. https://doi.org/10.1111/j.1467-8721.2007.00484.x

Bellugi, U., Lichtenberger, L., Jones, W., Lai, Z., & St. George, M. 2000. The neurocognitive profile of Williams Syndrome: A complex pattern of strengths and weaknesses. *Journal of Cognitive Neuroscience* 12(supplement 1), 7–29. https://doi.org/10.1162/089892900561959

Bellugi, U., Marks, S., Bihrle, A., & Sabo, H. 1988. Dissociation between language and cognitive functions in Williams Syndrome. In D. Bishop & K. Mogford (Eds.), *Language development in exceptional circumstances* (pp. 177–189). London: Churchill Livingstone.

Berman, R. 2004. Between emergence and mastery: The long developmental route of language acquisition. In R. Berman (Ed.), *Language development across childhood and adolescence* (pp. 9–34). Amsterdam: John Benjamins. https://doi.org/10.1075/tilar.3.05ber

Bruner, J. 1986. *Actual minds, possible worlds*. Cambridge, MA: Harvard University Press.

Castilla-Earls, A. P., & Eriks-Brophy, A. 2012. Spontaneous language measures in monolingual preschool Spanish-speaking children. *Revista de Logopedia, Foniatría y Audiología* 32, 97–108. https://doi.org/10.1016/j.rlfa.2014.06.001

Diez-Itza, E., Antón, A., Fernández, J., & García, M. L. 1998. Language development in Spanish children with Williams Syndrome. In A. Aksu Koç, E. Erguvanli Taylan, A. Sumru, & A. Küntay (Eds.), *Perspectives on language acquisition* (pp. 309–324). Istanbul: Bogazici University Printhouse.

Diez-Itza, E., Martínez, V., & Antón, A. 2016. Narrative competence in Spanish-speaking adults with Williams Syndrome. *Psicothema* 28(3), 291–297. https://doi.org/10.7334/psicothema2015.190

Diez-Itza, E., Martínez, V., Fernández-Urquiza, M., & Antón, A. 2017. Morphological profile of Williams Syndrome: Typical or atypical? In A. Auza & R. G. Schwartz (Eds.), *Language disorders in Spanish-speaking children: Language processing and cognitive functions* (pp. 311–328). New York, NY: Springer. https://doi.org/10.1007/978-3-319-53646-0_15

Diez-Itza, E., Martínez, V., Miranda, M. Antón, A., Ojea, A. I., Fernández-Urquiza, M., Pérez, V., Fernández Toral, J., García, I., & Medina, B. 2014. The Syndroling Project: A comparative linguistic analysis of typical development profiles and neurodevelopmental genetic disorders (Down, Williams and Fragile X Syndromes). *13th International Conference for the Study of Child Language*. Amsterdam.

Diez-Itza, E., Martínez, V., Pérez, V., & Fernández-Urquiza, M. 2018. Explicit oral narrative intervention for students with Williams syndrome. *Frontiers in Psychology 8* <https://www.frontiersin.org/articles/10.3389/fpsyg.2017.02337/full> (15 January 2018). < https://doi.org/10.3389/fpsyg.2017.02337>

Fernández-Urquiza, M., Viejo, A., Cortiñas, S., Huelmo, J., Medina, B., García I., & Diez-Itza, E. 2015. Perfiles pragmáticos comparados de síndromes genéticos neuroevolutivos (S. Williams, S. Down y S. X Frágil). In F. Diéguez-Vide (Ed.), *Temas de lingüística clínica* (pp. 89–90). Barcelona: Horsori Editorial.

Fivush, R., Haden, C. A., & Reese, E. 2006. Elaborating on elaborations. Role of maternal reminiscing style in cognitive and socioemotional development. *Child Development* 77(6), 1568–1588. https://doi.org/10.1111/j.1467-8624.2006.00960.x

Garayzábal, E., Prieto, M. F., Sampaio, A., & Gonçalves, O. 2007. Valoración interlingüística de la producción verbal a partir de una tarea narrativa en el síndrome de Williams. *Psicothema* 19(3), 428–434.

Gazella, J., & Stockman, I. J. 2003. Children's story retelling under different modality and task conditions: Implications for standardizing language sampling procedures. *American Journal of Speech-Language Pathology* 12, 61–72. https://doi.org/10.1044/1058-0360(2003/053)

Gonçalves, Ó., Pinheiro, A., & Sampaio, A. 2010. The narrative profile in Williams Syndrome: There is more to storytelling than just telling a story. *The British Journal of Developmental Disabilities* 56(111), 89–109. https://doi.org/10.1179/096979510799102943

Hemphill, L., Feldman, H. M., Camp, L., Griffin, T. M., Miranda, A. B. & Wolf, D. P. 1994. Developmental changes in narrative and non-narrative discourse in children with and without brain injury. *Journal of Communication Disorders* 27, 107–133. https://doi.org/10.1016/0021-9924(94)90037-X

Hudson, J., & Shapiro, L. 1991. From knowing to telling: The development of children's scripts, stories and personal narratives. In A. McCabe & C. Peterson (Eds.), *Developing narrative structure* (pp. 89–136). Hillsdale, NJ: Lawrence Erlbaum Associates.

Järvinen-Pasley, A., Bellugi, U., Reilly, J., Mills, D. L., Galaburda, A., Reiss, A. L., & Korenberg, J. R. 2008. Defining the social phenotype in Williams Syndrome: A model for linking gene, the brain, and behavior. *Developmental Psychopathology* 20(1), 1–35. https://doi.org/10.1017/S0954579408000011

Johnstone, B. 2009. Stance, style, and the linguistic individual. In A. Jaffe (Ed.), *Sociolinguistic perspectives on stance.* (pp. 29–52). Oxford: Oxford University Press. https://doi.org/10.1093/acprof:oso/9780195331646.003.0002

Jones, W., Bellugi, U., Lai, Z., Chiles, M., Reilly, J., Lincoln, A., & Adolphs, R. 2000. Hypersociability in Williams Syndrome. *Journal of Cognitive Neuroscience* 12(supplement 1), 30–46. https://doi.org/10.1162/089892900561968

Karmiloff-Smith, A., Grant, J., Berthoud, I., Davies, M., Howlin, P., & Udwin, O. 1997. Language and Williams Syndrome: How intact is "intact"? *Child Development* 68(2), 246–262. https://doi.org/10.2307/1131848

Labov, W. 1972. The transformation of experience in narrative syntax. In W. Labov (Ed.), *Language in the inner city* (pp. 354–396). Philadelphia, PA: University of Pennsylvania Press.

Labov, W., & Waletzky, J. 1967. Narrative analysis: Oral versions of personal experience. In J. Helm (ed.), *Essays on the verbal and visual arts* (pp. 12–44). Seattle, WA: University of Washington Press.

Lacroix, A., Bernicot, J., & Reilly, J. 2007. Narration and collaborative conversation in French-speaking children with Williams Syndrome. *Journal of Neurolinguistics* 20(6), 445–461. https://doi.org/10.1016/j.jneuroling.2007.03.004

Laws, G., & Bishop, D. V. M. 2004. Pragmatic language impairment and social deficits in Williams syndrome: A comparison with Down's Syndrome and specific language impairment. *International Journal of Language & Communication Disorders* 39(1), 45–64. https://doi.org/10.1080/13682820310001615797

Losh, M., Bellugi, U., Reilly, J. & Anderson, D. 2000. Narrative as a social engagement tool: The excessive use of evaluation in narratives from children with Williams Syndrome. *Narrative Inquiry* 10(2), 265–290. https://doi.org/10.1075/ni.10.2.01los

MacWhinney, B. 2000. *The CHILDES project: Tools for analyzing talk, Vol. I: Transcription format and programs.* Mahwah, NJ: Lawrence Erlbaum Associates.

Marini, A., Martelli, S., Gagliardi, C., Fabbro, F., & Borgatti, R. 2010. Narrative language in Williams Syndrome and its neuropsychological correlates. *Journal of Neurolinguistics* 23(2), 97–111. https://doi.org/10.1016/j.jneuroling.2009.10.002

Mayer, M. 1969. *Frog, where are you?* New York, NY: Dial Books for Young Readers.

McCabe, A., & Peterson, C. E. (Eds.). 1991. *Developing narrative structure.* Hillsdale, NJ: Lawrence Erlbaum Associates.

McCabe, A., & Rollins, P. 1994. Assessment of preschool narrative skills. *American Journal of Speech and Language Pathology* 3, 367–391. https://doi.org/10.1044/1058-0360.0301.45

Mushin, I. 2001. *Evidentiality and epistemological stance. Narrative retelling.* Amsterdam: John Benjamins. https://doi.org/10.1075/pbns.87

Reilly, J. S., Bernicot, J., Vicari, S., Lacroix, A., & Bellugi, U. 2005. Narratives in children with Williams Syndrome: A cross linguistic perspective. In D. Ravid & H. Bat-Zeev Shyldkrot (Eds.), *Perspectives on language and language development: Essays in honor of Ruth A. Berman* (pp. 303–312). Dordrecht: Kluwer. https://doi.org/10.1007/1-4020-7911-7-22

Reilly, J., Klima, E. S., & Bellugi, U. 1990. Once more with feeling: Affect and language in atypical populations. *Development and Psychopathology* 2, 367–391. https://doi.org/10.1017/S0954579400005782

Reilly, J., Losh, M., Bellugi, U., & Wulfeck, B. 2004. "Frog, where are you?" Narratives in children with specific language impairment, early focal brain injury, and Williams Syndrome. *Brain and Language* 88(2), 229–247. https://doi.org/10.1016/S0093-934X(03)00101-9

Semel, E. M., & Rosner, S. R. 2003. *Understanding Williams Syndrome: Behavioral patterns and interventions*. Mahwah, NJ: Lawrence Erlbaum Associates. https://doi.org/10.4324/9781410607416

Shiro, M. 2001–2002. La construcción de la perspectiva narrativa: El yo y el otro en narraciones de adultos y niños caraqueños. *Cuadernos de Lengua y Habla* 3, 533–549.

Shiro, M. 2003. Genre and evaluation in narrative development. *Journal of Child Language* 30(1), 165–194. https://doi.org/10.1017/S0305000902005500

Shiro M. 2007. *La construcción del punto de vista en los relatos orales de niños en edad escolar: Un análisis discursivo de la modalidad*. Caracas: Universidad Central de Venezuela.

Shiro, M. 2008. Narrative stance in Venezuelan children's stories. In A. McCabe, A. Imbaley, & G. Melzi (Eds.), *Spanish language narration and literacy: Culture, cognition and emotion* (pp. 213–237). Cambridge: Cambridge University Press. https://doi.org/10.1017/CBO9780511815669.012

Shiro, M. 2012. "Y entonces le dijo…" Representación del habla en las narraciones orales de niños venezolanos. *Boletín de Lingüística* 37–38, 119–143.

Shiro Martha. 2014. ¿Quién lo dijo? Las voces en las narraciones de niños venezolanos. In R. Barriga Villanueva (Ed.), *Las narrativas y su impacto en el desarrollo lingüístico infantil* (pp. 173–200). Mexico, DF: Colegio de México.

Stojanovik, V. 2006. Social interaction deficits and conversational inadequacy in Williams Syndrome. *Journal of Neurolinguistics* 19(2), 157–173. https://doi.org/10.1016/j.jneuroling.2005.11.005

Volterra, V., Capirci, O., Pezzini, G., Sabbadini, L., & Vicari, S. 1996. Linguistic abilities in Italian children with Williams Syndrome. *Cortex* 32, 663–677. https://doi.org/10.1016/S0010-9452(96)80037-2

Index